Sleep Disorders and Mental Health

Editors

ANDREW WINOKUR
JAYESH KAMATH

PSYCHIATRIC CLINICS OF NORTH AMERICA

www.psych.theclinics.com

December 2015 • Volume 38 • Number 4

ELSEVIER

1600 John F. Kennedy Boulevard • Suite 1800 • Philadelphia, Pennsylvania, 19103-2899

http://www.theclinics.com

PSYCHIATRIC CLINICS OF NORTH AMERICA Volume 38, Number 4
December 2015 ISSN 0193-953X, ISBN-13: 978-0-323-40268-2

Editor: Lauren Boyle
Developmental Editor: Kristen Helm

Psychiatric Clinics of North America (ISSN 0193-953X) is published quarterly by Elsevier Inc., 360 Park Avenue South, New York, NY 10010-1710. Months of issue are March, June, September, and December. Business and Editorial Offices: 1600 John F. Kennedy Blvd., Suite 1800, Philadelphia, PA 19103-2899. Periodicals postage paid at New York, NY and additional mailing offices. Subscription prices are $300.00 per year (US individuals), $546.00 per year (US institutions), $150.00 per year (US students/residents), $365.00 per year (Canadian individuals), $455.00 per year (international individuals), $687.00 per year (Canadian & international institutions), and $220.00 per year (Canadian & international students/residents). Foreign air speed delivery is included in all Clinics' subscription prices. All prices are subject to change without notice. POSTMASTER: Send address changes to Psychiatric Clinics of North America, Elsevier Health Sciences Division, Subscription Customer Service, 3251 Riverport Lane, Maryland Heights, MO 63043. Customer Service: 1-800-654-2452 (US). From outside the United States, call 1-314-447-8871. Fax: 1-314-447-8029. E-mail: journalscustomerservice-usa@elsevier.com (for print support) and journalsonline support-usa@elsevier.com (for online support).

Reprints. For copies of 100 or more, of articles in this publication, please contact the Commercial Reprints Department, Elsevier Inc., 360 Park Avenue South, New York, New York 10010-1710. Tel.: 212-633-3874, Fax: 212-633-3820, E-mail: reprints@elsevier.com.

Psychiatric Clinics of North America is covered in MEDLINE/PubMed (Index Medicus), Current Contents/Social and Behavioral Sciences, Social Science Citation Index, Embase/Excerpta Medica, and PsycINFO.

Contributors

EDITORS

ANDREW WINOKUR, MD, PhD
Professor, Department of Psychiatry, University of Connecticut School of Medicine, Farmington, Connecticut

JAYESH KAMATH, MD, PhD
Associate Professor of Psychiatry and Immunology; Director, Mood and Anxiety Disorders Program, Department of Psychiatry, University of Connecticut School of Medicine, Farmington, Connecticut

AUTHORS

SABRA M. ABBOTT, MD, PhD
Assistant Professor, Department of Neurology, Northwestern University Feinberg School of Medicine, Chicago, Illinois

ALOK BANGA, MD, MPH, MS
Medical Director, Sierra Vista Hospital, Sacramento, California

RUTH M. BENCA, MD, PhD
Jan and Kathryn Ver Hagen Professor of Translational Medicine; Director, Center for Sleep Medicine and Sleep Research; Professor, Department of Psychiatry, University of Wisconsin, Madison, Wisconsin

ELAINE M. BOLAND, PhD
Postdoctoral Fellow, Behavioral Health, Mental Illness Research Education and Clinical Center, Corporal Michael J. Crescenz Veterans Affairs Medical Center; Department of Psychiatry, Perelman School of Medicine, University of Pennsylvania, Philadelphia, Pennsylvania

ENDA M. BYRNE, PhD
Visiting Scholar, Center for Sleep and Circadian Neurobiology, Perelman School of Medicine, University of Pennsylvania, Philadelphia, Pennsylvania; Research Fellow, Queensland Brain Institute, Brisbane, Australia

KARL DOGHRAMJI, MD
Sleep Medicine Fellowship Director; Professor of Psychiatry, Neurology, and Medicine; Medical Director, Jefferson Sleep Disorders Center, Thomas Jefferson University, Philadelphia, Pennsylvania

PHILIP R. GEHRMAN, PhD
Assistant Professor of Psychiatry, Perelman School of Medicine, University of Pennsylvania, Philadelphia, Pennsylvania

RONAK JHAVERI, MD
Resident in Adult Psychiatry, Department of Psychiatry, University of Connecticut School of Medicine, Farmington, Connecticut

SARAH JILLANI, MBBS
Department of Psychiatry, University of Connecticut School of Medicine, Farmington, Connecticut

JAYESH KAMATH, MD, PhD
Associate Professor of Psychiatry and Immunology; Director, Mood and Anxiety Disorders Program, Department of Psychiatry, University of Connecticut School of Medicine, Farmington, Connecticut

BRENDAN T. KEENAN, MS
Biostatistician, Center for Sleep and Circadian Neurobiology, Perelman School of Medicine, University of Pennsylvania, Philadelphia, Pennsylvania

JOHN KHOURY, MD
Associate Director, Sleep Disorders Center, Abington Neurological Associates, Abington Memorial Hospital (Jefferson Health), Willow Grove, Pennsylvania

THOMAS S. KILDUFF, PhD
Center Director, Biosciences Division, Center for Neuroscience, SRI International, Menlo Park, California

ANDREW D. KRYSTAL, MD, MS
Director of Neurosciences Medicine, Duke Clinical Research Institute; Professor of Psychiatry and Behavioral Sciences, Duke University School of Medicine, Durham, North Carolina

ALLAN I. PACK, MBChB, PhD, FRCP
Chief, Division of Sleep Medicine, Department of Medicine; John Miclot Professor of Medicine; Director, Center for Sleep and Circadian Neurobiology, Perelman School of Medicine, University of Pennsylvania, Philadelphia, Pennsylvania

GARY E. PICKARD, PhD
Professor of Neuroscience, School of Veterinary Medicine and Biomedical Sciences, University of Nebraska, Lincoln, Nebraska; Department of Ophthalmology and Visual Sciences, University of Nebraska Medical Center, Omaha, Nebraska

GALINA PRPICH, MS
Department of Psychiatry, University of Connecticut School of Medicine, Farmington, Connecticut

KATHRYN J. REID, PhD
Research Associate Professor, Department of Neurology, Northwestern University Feinberg School of Medicine, Chicago, Illinois

TIMOTHY A. ROEHRS, PhD
Professor, Department of Psychiatry and Behavioral Neuroscience; Senior Bioscientist, Sleep Disorders and Research Center, Henry Ford Health System, School of Medicine, Wayne State University, Detroit, Michigan

RICHARD J. ROSS, MD, PhD
Professor of Psychiatry, Corporal Michael J. Crescenz Veterans Affairs Medical Center, Perelman School of Medicine, University of Pennsylvania, Philadelphia, Pennsylvania

THOMAS ROTH, PhD
Professor, Department of Psychiatry and Behavioral Neuroscience; Senior Bioscientist, Sleep Disorders and Research Center, Henry Ford Health System, School of Medicine, Wayne State University, Detroit, Michigan

MEREDITH E. RUMBLE, PhD
Assistant Professor, Department of Psychiatry, University of Wisconsin, Madison, Wisconsin

MICHAEL D. SCHWARTZ, PhD
Research Scientist, Biosciences Division, Center for Neuroscience, SRI International, Menlo Park, California

SHIRSHENDU SINHA, MBBS
Addiction Psychiatry Fellow, Department of Psychiatry and Psychology, Mayo School of Graduate Medical Education, Mayo Clinic College of Medicine, Rochester, Minnesota

PATRICIA J. SOLLARS, PhD
Associate Professor of Neuroscience, School of Veterinary Medicine and Biomedical Sciences, University of Nebraska, Lincoln, Nebraska

DAVID C. STEFFENS, MD, MHS
Professor and Chair, Department of Psychiatry, University of Connecticut Health Center, Farmington, Connecticut

SUNDEEP VIRDI, MD, JD
Department of Psychiatry, University of Connecticut School of Medicine, Farmington, Connecticut

KAITLIN HANLEY WHITE, PhD
Research Associate, Department of Psychiatry, University of Wisconsin, Madison, Wisconsin

ANDREW WINOKUR, MD, PhD
Professor, Department of Psychiatry, University of Connecticut School of Medicine, Farmington, Connecticut

KRISTINA F. ZDANYS, MD
Assistant Professor, Department of Psychiatry, University of Connecticut Health Center, Farmington, Connecticut

PHYLLIS C. ZEE, MD, PhD
Benjamin and Virginia T. Boshes Professor, Department of Neurology, Northwestern University Feinberg School of Medicine, Chicago, Illinois

Contents

> Changes in the psychiatric diagnostic guidelines with the transition from Diagnostic and Statistical Manual of Mental Disorders (DSM)-IV to DSM-V include acknowledgment that primary sleep disorders such as insomnia can occur in conjunction with medical and psychiatric disorders. This change in viewpoint regarding the definition of primary sleep disorders opens the way to the recognition that patients with psychiatric disorders demonstrate a high prevalence of sleep disturbances, with complaints of insomnia and excessive daytime sleepiness being especially commonly reported. Recent investigations have pointed to a bidirectional relationship between sleep disturbances and psychiatric disorders.

> Cortical electroencephalographic activity arises from corticothalamocortical interactions, modulated by wake-promoting monoaminergic and cholinergic input. These wake-promoting systems are regulated by hypothalamic hypocretin/orexins, while GABAergic sleep-promoting nuclei are found in the preoptic area, brainstem and lateral hypothalamus. Although pontine acetylcholine is critical for REM sleep, hypothalamic melanin-concentrating hormone/GABAergic cells may "gate" REM sleep. Daily sleep-wake rhythms arise from interactions between a hypothalamic circadian pacemaker and a sleep homeostat whose anatomical locus has yet to be conclusively defined. Control of sleep and wakefulness involves multiple systems, each of which presents vulnerability to sleep/wake dysfunction that may predispose to physical and/or neuropsychiatric disorders.

> There is a growing recognition that the coordinated timing of behavioral, physiologic, and metabolic circadian rhythms is a requirement for a healthy body and mind. In mammals, the primary circadian oscillator is the hypothalamic suprachiasmatic nucleus (SCN), which is responsible for circadian coordination throughout the organism. Temporal homeostasis is recognized as a complex interplay between rhythmic clock gene expression in brain regions outside the SCN and in peripheral organs. Abnormalities in this intricate circadian orchestration may alter sleep patterns and contribute to the pathophysiology of affective disorders.

Sleep disorders are, in part, attributable to genetic variability across individuals. There has been considerable progress in understanding the role of genes for some sleep disorders, such as the identification of a human leukocyte antigen gene for narcolepsy. For other sleep disorders, such as insomnia, little work has been done. Optimizing phenotyping strategies is critical, as is the case for sleep apnea, for which intermediate traits such as obesity and craniofacial features may prove to be more tractable for genetic studies. Rapid advances in genotyping and statistical genetics are likely to lead to greater discoveries in the near future.

Primary sleep disorders include those not attributable to another medical or psychiatric condition: insomnia disorder, hypersomnolence disorder, narcolepsy, obstructive sleep apnea hypopnea syndrome, central sleep apnea syndrome, and the parasomnias. They are commonly encountered and are comorbid with many psychiatric disorders. It is important to recognize these disorders and be comfortable treating them or to know when to refer to a sleep disorders center and sleep specialist. Treatment of a comorbid sleep disorder can improve the overall quality of life, symptoms in mood disorders, and symptoms of excessive daytime sleepiness, and decrease cardiovascular morbidity and mortality.

Sleep deprivation and sleep disorders are commonly seen in children and adolescents. They are often undiagnosed and undertreated. A balance of circadian rhythm and homeostatic drive determine sleep quality, quantity, and timing, which changes across the developmental years. Environmental and lifestyle factors can affect sleep quality and quantity and lead to sleep deprivation. A comprehensive assessment of sleep disorders includes parental report, children's self-report, and school functioning. Diagnostic tools are used in diagnosing and treating sleep disorders.

Sleep disturbances are a common presenting symptom of older-age adults to their physicians. This article explores normal changes in sleep pattern with aging and primary sleep disorders in the elderly. Behavioral factors and primary psychiatric disorders affecting sleep in this population are reviewed. Further discussion examines sleep changes associated with 2 common forms of neurocognitive disorder: Alzheimer disease and Lewy Body Dementia. Common medical illnesses in the elderly are discussed in relation to sleep symptoms. Nonpharmacological and pharmacologic treatment strategies are summarized, with emphasis placed on risk of side effects in older adults. Future targets are considered.

The article provides an overview of common and differentiating self-reported and objective sleep disturbances seen in mood-disordered populations. The importance of considering sleep disturbances in the context of mood disorders is emphasized, because a large body of evidence supports the notion that sleep disturbances are a risk factor for onset, exacerbation, and relapse of mood disorders. In addition, potential mechanisms for sleep disturbance in depression, other primary sleep disorders that often occur with mood disorders, effects of antidepressant and mood-stabilizing drugs on sleep, and the adjunctive effect of treating sleep in patients with mood disorders are discussed.

Sleep disturbance is frequently associated with generalized anxiety disorder, panic disorder, obsessive-compulsive disorder, and posttraumatic stress disorder. This article reviews recent advances in understanding the mechanisms of the sleep disturbances in these disorders and discusses the implications for developing improved treatments.

Sleep disturbances are prevalent in patients with schizophrenia and play a critical role in the morbidity and mortality associated with the illness. Subjective and objective assessments of sleep in patients with schizophrenia have identified certain consistent findings. Findings related to the sleep structure abnormalities have shown correlations with important clinical aspects of the illness. Disruption of specific neurotransmitter systems and dysregulation of clock genes may play a role in the pathophysiology of schizophrenia-related sleep disturbances. Antipsychotic medications play an important role in the treatment of sleep disturbances in these patients and have an impact on their sleep structure.

This article discusses the role sleep and alertness disturbance plays in the initiation, maintenance and relapse of substance use disorders.

The circadian system regulates the timing and expression of nearly all biological processes, most notably, the sleep-wake cycle, and disruption of this system can result in adverse effects on both physical and mental health. The circadian rhythm sleep-wake disorders (CRSWDs) consist of 5 disorders that are due primarily to pathology of the circadian clock or to a misalignment of the timing of the endogenous circadian rhythm with the environment. This article outlines the nature of these disorders, the association of many of these disorders with psychiatric illness, and available treatment options.

Sleep–wake cycle disturbances are prevalent in patients with medical conditions and frequently present as part of a symptom cluster. Sleep disturbances impair functioning and quality of life, decrease adherence to treatments of the primary medical condition, and increase morbidity and mortality. The pathophysiology of sleep disturbances in these patients involves alterations in immune and neuroendocrine function and shares common pathophysiologic pathways with comorbidities such as fatigue and depression. Emphasis is placed on the evaluation and management of medical and psychiatric comorbidities and other factors contributing to sleep problems. Primary treatments include cognitive–behavioral therapy and pharmacotherapy.

Many insomnia medications with high specificity have become available recently. They provide a window into the clinical effects of modulating specific brain systems and establish a new guiding principal for conceptualizing insomnia medications: "mechanism matters." A new paradigm for insomnia therapy in which specific drugs are selected to target the specific type of sleep difficulty for each patient includes administering specific treatments for patients with insomnia comorbid with particular psychiatric disorders. This article reviews insomnia medications and discusses the implications for optimizing the treatment of insomnia occurring comorbid with psychiatric conditions.

PSYCHIATRIC CLINICS OF NORTH AMERICA

RELATED INTEREST

Sleep Medicine Clinics
June 2015 (Vol. 10, No. 2)
Sleep and Psychiatry in Children
John H. Herman and Max Hirshkowitz, *Editors*

THE CLINICS ARE AVAILABLE ONLINE!
Access your subscription at:
www.theclinics.com

PSYCHIATRIC CLINICS OF
NORTH AMERICA

FORTHCOMING ISSUES

March 2016
Bipolar Depression
John L. Beyer, Editor

June 2016
Schizophrenia: Advances and Current Management
Peter F. Buckley, Editor

September 2016
Psychopharmacotherapeutic Side Effects
Rajnish Mago, Editor

RECENT ISSUES

September 2015
Clinical Psychiatry: Recent Advances and Future Directions
David A. Baron and Lawrence S. Gross, editors

June 2015
Young Onset Dementias
Chiadi U. Onyike, Editor

March 2015
Mental Health in the Medical Setting: Delivery, Workforce Needs, and Emerging Best Practices
Peter F. Buckley, Editor

RELATED INTEREST

Sleep Medicine Clinics
June 2015 (Vol. 10, No. 2)
Sleep and Psychiatry in Children
John H. Herman and Max Hirshkowitz, Editors

Preface
Sleep Disorders and Mental Health

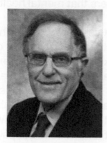 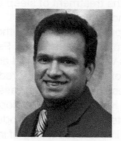

Andrew Winokur, MD, PhD   Jayesh Kamath, MD, PhD
Editors

Mental health care providers are reminded on a daily basis of the prevalence of sleep disorders in the patients to whom they provide care. The first article of this special issue provides an introduction to and overview of the topic of Sleep Disorders and Mental Health, including a summary of the prevalence of sleep disorders in psychiatric populations and a review of studies documenting the functional impact of these sleep abnormalities. The next three articles provide succinct and up-to-date summaries of the neurobiologic mechanisms involved in the regulation of sleep and wakefulness, the control of circadian rhythms, and the genetic factors that are being established as relevant to the control of sleep and circadian rhythms and also representing potential risk factors for a variety of sleep disorders. The remaining articles in this issue address topics of clinical relevance to practicing psychiatrists and psychiatric residents and provide information of interest to medical students and other mental health providers. The fifth article encompasses a comprehensive overview of Primary Sleep Disorders, emphasizing approaches to the recognition, diagnosis, and management (whether directly by the psychiatrist or via referral to a sleep disorders specialist) of this group of disorders. Sleep disturbances are common and have unique importance in the young (children and adolescents) and the elderly, and the interface of sleep disorders with behavior and psychiatric disorders is reviewed extensively in the sixth and seventh articles, including pragmatic guidance on the management of sleep disturbance in these important populations. The next four articles provide reviews of recent research as well as recommendations for practical clinical management of comorbid sleep disturbances with major mental health disorders, including mood disorders, anxiety disorders, including obsessive-compulsive disorder and posttraumatic stress disorder, schizophrenia, and the prevalent and important category of substance use disorders. The twelfth article provides a clinical complement to the coverage of the neurobiology of circadian rhythms described in the third article by presenting an overview of the recognition of and treatment options for circadian rhythm sleep disorders.

Psychiatr Clin N Am 38 (2015) xiii–xiv
http://dx.doi.org/10.1016/j.psc.2015.08.003
0193-953X/15/$ – see front matter © 2015 Published by Elsevier Inc.

psych.theclinics.com

In the next article, commentary is provided on the important and emerging topic of the relevance of sleep disturbances to medical conditions, with a particular focus on cardiovascular and oncologic disorders. Recent literature has emphasized important interrelationships between these major medical conditions and both sleep disorders and psychiatric disorders. The final article presents an update on new developments in insomnia medications and provides what the author aptly describes as a new paradigm in the use of medications for the treatment of sleep disorders that mental health providers should find interesting and useful.

We wish to express our sincere appreciation to the authors of this special issue. The contributors include colleagues from the Department of Psychiatry at the University of Connecticut School of Medicine as well as many noted and acknowledged sleep experts from across the country, all of whom have labored diligently to provide clear, concise, and highly informative presentations of their assigned topic areas. We also appreciate the skilled assistance of Kristen Helm, Developmental Editor, and the publication staff at Elsevier for their outstanding help in producing this special issue. We hope that the information compiled in this issue will be of interest and value to our psychiatric colleagues, to residents and medical students, and to other mental health care providers.

Andrew Winokur, MD, PhD
Department of Psychiatry
University of Connecticut School of Medicine
263 Farmington Avenue
Farmington, CT 06030-6415, USA

Jayesh Kamath, MD, PhD
Department of Psychiatry
University of Connecticut School of Medicine
263 Farmington Avenue
Farmington, CT 06030-6415, USA

E-mail addresses:
awinokur@uchc.edu (A. Winokur)
jkamath@uchc.edu (J. Kamath)

The Relationship Between Sleep Disturbances and Psychiatric Disorders
Introduction and Overview

Andrew Winokur, MD, PhD

KEYWORDS

- Sleep disorders • Insomnia • Polysomnography • Bidirectional

KEY POINTS

- Changes in the diagnostic approach to sleep disorders with Diagnostic and Statistical Manual, Fifth Edition (DSM-V), recognize the importance of coexisting psychiatric disorders.
- Epidemiologic studies confirm the prevalence of sleep disturbances across a broad range of psychiatric disorders.
- Emphasis has been placed on the bidirectional relationship between sleep disturbances and psychiatric disorders.
- Numerous examples have been reported of the relevance of sleep disturbances to the treatment of psychiatric disorders.

This article provides an overview of the relationship between sleep disorders and mental health, starting with a discussion of changes in the approach to the diagnosis of sleep disorders that have accompanied the transition from the Diagnostic and Statistical Manual of Mental Disorders, Fourth Edition (DSM-IV) to the DSM-V, which represents that current diagnostic standard for the field.[1,2] A brief review of data regarding the epidemiology of sleep disorders is followed by a more extensive discussion of the prevalence and impact of sleep abnormalities in patients with various mental health disorders. In recent years, data have been reported that underscore the bidirectional nature of the relationship between sleep abnormalities and psychiatric illness, as is discussed in some detail. Finally, reports from several studies have suggested specific types of relationships between sleep changes and psychiatric disorders, as summarized in **Box 1**.

Disclosures: None to report.
Department of Psychiatry, University of Connecticut School of Medicine, 10 Talcott Notch Road, Third Floor, East Wing, Farmington, CT 06030-6415, USA
E-mail address: awinokur@uchc.edu

Psychiatr Clin N Am 38 (2015) 603–614
http://dx.doi.org/10.1016/j.psc.2015.07.001
0193-953X/15/$ – see front matter © 2015 Elsevier Inc. All rights reserved.

Abbreviations

AD	Alzheimer disease
ADHD	Attention-deficit hyperactivity disorder
CD	Conduct disorder
DSM-IV	Diagnostic and Statistical Manual of Mental Disorders, Fourth Edition
DSM-V	Diagnostic and Statistical Manual, Fifth Edition
EDS	Excessive daytime sleepiness
GAD	Generalized anxiety disorder
HAM-D	Hamilton Depression Rating Scale
MDD	Major depressive disorder
ODD	Oppositional defiant disorder
OSA	Obstructive sleep apnea syndrome
PSG	Polysomnography
REM	Rapid eye movement
REM-L	Rapid eye movement sleep latency

CHANGES IN THE APPROACH TO THE DIAGNOSIS OF SLEEP DISORDERS WITH DIAGNOSTIC AND STATISTICAL MANUAL OF MENTAL DISORDERS, FIFTH EDITION

In DSM-IV, the approach to the diagnosis of sleep disorders included the term primary sleep disorders, which required demonstration that the sleep abnormality occurred in the absence of a psychiatric disorder. An implication of this diagnostic splitting of primary insomnia from psychiatric disorders is the fact that studies examining the efficacy of medications that have recently been evaluated and approved by the US Food and Drug Administration for the treatment of insomnia symptoms, such as zolpidem, zaleplon, or eszopiclone, have been carried out in patients who were shown to meet DSM-IV diagnostic criteria for primary insomnia, including the requirement for the lack of a current primary psychiatric disorder diagnosis. Although the studies that were carried out using this approach provided data that were valuable for the field and also supported regulatory approval of these investigational products for insomnia symptom relief, they excluded from participation patients with psychiatric disorders who were suffering with prominent symptoms of insomnia. As a consequence, Psychiatry faces a translational problem related to a lack of data in patient populations seen in psychiatric practice with regard to the efficacy of approved drugs for insomnia symptoms.

The DSM-V classification of sleep-wake disorders identifies 10 distinct disorders or disorder groups. The authors of the DSM-V chapter on sleep-wake disorders acknowledge interrelationships between sleep disorders and psychiatric disorders in the introduction to this section as follows: "Sleep disorders are often accompanied by depression, anxiety and cognitive changes that must be addressed in treatment planning and management."[2(p361)] They also acknowledge that persistent sleep

---

Box 1
Proposed relevance of sleep parameters to clinical psychiatry

- Prediction of risk for developing a new-onset psychiatric disorder
- Prediction of risk of relapse in stabilized remitted patients
- Prediction of response to pharmacologic treatment
- Biomarker of genetic vulnerability in nonaffected first-degree relatives
- Clues to underlying neurobiological mechanisms linking a sleep disturbance to an associated psychiatric disorder

problems have been reported to represent a significant risk factor for the development of subsequent psychiatric disorders, a point of emphasis for many studies in recent years. The diagnosis of insomnia disorder according to DSM-V criteria includes specifiers to indicate whether the insomnia symptoms occur in the context of a non–sleep disorder mental comorbidity, including substance use disorders, in the context of another medical comorbidity, or with another sleep disorder. Acknowledgment of interrelationships between sleep disorders and psychiatric disorders in DSM-V offers the potential for new avenues of research to investigate the impact of these interactions with respect to diagnosis and treatment issues.

THE PREVALENCE OF SLEEP DISTURBANCES IN PSYCHIATRIC DISORDERS

Epidemiologic studies of the prevalence and impact of sleep disorders are of recent origin, but numerous studies have provided considerable information related to this issue. Several comprehensive review articles have summarized work in this area.[3–6] Insomnia is the most common sleep-wake complaint in the general population, with insomnia symptoms being reported in approximately one-third of subjects surveyed.[7] When specific sleep complaints associated with manifestations of functional impairment are taken into consideration, between 5% and 10% of the general population have been reported to satisfy diagnostic criteria for insomnia.[8] Insomnia has been reported to be more prevalent in older individuals and in women.[9]

Complaints of excessive daytime sleepiness (EDS) represent the second most prevalent clinical manifestation of sleep disturbances. Reports of EDS have ranged from 5% to 15% in the general population in numerous studies.[6,10] Several medical and sleep disorder causes can underlie complaints of EDS, such as obstructive sleep apnea syndrome (OSA), narcolepsy, periodic limb movements syndrome, narcolepsy, and chronic fatigue syndrome. Apart from these medical causes, EDS is often found to be present in the context of a variety of psychiatric disorders.

Although sleep disturbances are prevalent and exert significant negative impact for individuals in the general population, the prevalence and impact of sleep disorders on psychiatric illnesses represent a particularly pressing issue. A summary of selected findings characterizing the intersection of sleep disturbances and psychiatric disorders is presented in later discussion. In a landmark study, Ford and Kamerow[11] reported on a community-based sample of 10,534 respondents who provided data regarding their sleep patterns, among a much more extensive array of information on health behaviors. About 10.2% of the respondents reported experiencing problems with insomnia, whereas 3.2% of the respondents reported manifestations of hypersomnia. About 40.4% of subjects with insomnia and 46.5% of respondents with hypersomnia had a psychiatric disorder as a comorbid entity along with their sleep disorder, whereas only 16.4% of respondents with no sleep complaints had a psychiatric disorder. In patients with a sleep disorder, the most frequently reported comorbid psychiatric disorders were anxiety disorders, depression, and alcohol and substance use disorders. Taylor and colleagues[12] reported on a community-based sample that provided data on sleep complaints and psychiatric disorders. Data obtained from 772 participants revealed that subjects with insomnia were 9.82 times more likely to have a clinically significant depressive disorder than was the case for subjects who did not suffer with insomnia. Moreover, subjects with insomnia were found to have a 17.35 times greater likelihood of having a clinically significant anxiety disorder than subjects with no insomnia symptoms. Buysse and colleagues[13] carried out comprehensive diagnostic assessments on a group of 257 patients who were seen for evaluation at 1 of 5 participating sleep disorders centers, including 216 patients with a presenting complaint of insomnia and 41 patients selected from psychiatric and medical settings without regard to associated sleep complaints. Overall, more than 75% of these patients had a diagnosis of insomnia related to a psychiatric disorder when primary and secondary diagnoses were combined together. Berlin and colleagues[14] assessed 100 consecutive patients on a psychiatric consultation service for evidence of a sleep disorder. Of the 100 psychiatric patients assessed, 80 demonstrated manifestations of a sleep disorder, including 72 patients with insomnia. The investigators noted that 54% of the 80 patients with a sleep disorder did not have the sleep disturbance mentioned in their hospital record. The investigators suggested that this finding indicated the need for more physician education on the identification and diagnosis of sleep disorders.

Sleep problems have been noted to be present in patients with depression from the days of antiquity. Circa 400 BC, the Hippocratic writers stated that melancholia was associated with "aversion to food, despondency, sleeplessness, irritability, restlessness."[15] In contemporary times, numerous studies using clinical assessments, validated rating scales, and laboratory-based polysomnographic (PSG) studies have demonstrated that sleep abnormalities are seen in a high percentage of patients with clinical depression. In studies using PSG techniques to document objectively defined alterations in sleep architecture, 90% of inpatients with major depressive disorder (MDD) demonstrated some form of electroencephalography-verified sleep disturbance.[16] McCall and colleagues[17] conducted evaluations on 88 patients on an inpatient psychiatric unit by means of a structured diagnostic interview and with the use of validated rating scales. Depending on the rating scale used, between 93% and 97% of hospitalized patients reported some form of sleep disturbance.

In patients with bipolar disorder, sleep disturbances are highly prevalent, but the manifestation of the specific sleep disturbance is strongly influenced by the type of mood episode that the patient is experiencing, for example, depressive, manic, or mixed. In the context of a manic or hypomanic episode, reduced total sleep time associated with a reduced sense of need for sleep, as well as normal or frequently increased daytime energy levels, has been reported in 69% to 99% of patients.[18] With respect to bipolar depression, complaints of sleep disturbance are common but the nature of specific sleep disturbance is variable. Some studies have reported that a high percentage of patients with bipolar depression experience insomnia, but this finding has not be replicated in selected other studies.[18] A subset of patients with bipolar depression report symptoms of hypersomnia, frequently associated with complaints of daytime apathy, lethargy, and fatigue.[19,20] In various studies, the rates of hypersomnia in patients with bipolar depression range from 23% to 78%.[18] Symptoms of hypersomnia have also been reported in patients with atypical and seasonal affective disorder.[21–23]

Reports of sleep alterations in patients with schizophrenia are less abundant in comparison with the extensive literature regarding evidence for sleep abnormalities in patients with depression and bipolar disorder. In addition, studies examining sleep disturbances in schizophrenic patients are complicated by several potentially confounding factors, in particular related to the sleep-modulating effects of antipsychotic medications when used in the treatment of schizophrenia. Despite such complicating factors, a substantial body of literature has documented manifestations of sleep disturbance in schizophrenic patients. In a comprehensive review of studies documenting sleep alterations in schizophrenic patients, Monti and Monti[24] included an analysis of reports in never-treated schizophrenic patients and in schizophrenic patients who had been previously treated but were drug-free at the time of evaluation of sleep physiology by PSG. Never-treated schizophrenic patients demonstrated several alterations in sleep physiology, including an increase in the latency to stage 2 sleep, increased wake time after sleep onset, an increase in the number of awakenings after falling asleep, reduced total sleep time and sleep efficiency, and, in 2 studies, reduced latency to rapid eye movement (REM) sleep. In general, sleep findings in previously treated schizophrenic patients who had not been treated with an antipsychotic drug for a period of 2 to 8 weeks demonstrated alterations in sleep that were comparable with the findings described earlier for never-medicated schizophrenic patients. In summary, sleep studies conducted in schizophrenic patients that are designed to minimize the potentially confounding effects of antipsychotic drugs provide strong support for the prominence of sleep disturbances in schizophrenic patients, with the sleep alterations particularly characterized by prolongation of sleep onset and disturbances in sleep continuity.

Several studies have documented sleep disturbances in patients with anxiety disorders. DSM-IV includes 5 primary anxiety disorders, including generalized anxiety disorder (GAD), panic disorder, social anxiety disorder, obsessive-compulsive disorder, and posttraumatic stress disorder, whereas DSM-V approaches anxiety disorder groups in a different manner. Using the traditional DSM-IV approach to the categorization of primary anxiety disorders, all 5 of the major anxiety disorders listed earlier have been linked to prominent sleep disturbances. A review of studies examining sleep alterations in patients with anxiety disorders documented a high prevalence of sleep disturbances in patients with anxiety disorders across all 5 diagnostic categories.[25] Studies in patients with GAD and in patients with panic disorder have reported prominent sleep alterations in 60% to 70% of patients with these disorders.[26,27]

Problems with sleep disorders have long been understood to be prevalent and significant in patients with alcohol and substance use disorders. It has been recognized clinically that patients with sleep disorders, in particular insomnia, frequently self-medicate with alcohol or other substances to induce sleep, as well as potentially use stimulant compounds to promote daytime wakefulness and alertness. Insomnia has been reported to be present in 36% to 72% of patients participating in alcoholism treatment.[28,29]

The early (infancy, childhood, and adolescence) and later (old age and senescence) stages of life are times of dynamic alterations in sleep physiology that are also marked by frequent and significant perturbations in sleep. Prominent behavioral abnormalities can also be encountered in these early and late life stages, establishing a context in which interactions between sleep disturbances and mental health problems can create formidable clinical challenges.

In children with sleep-related breathing disorders, especially OSA or upper airway resistance syndrome, attentional and hyperactivity symptoms are frequently encountered, and some children may be diagnosed with attention-deficit hyperactivity disorder (ADHD) before the recognition and diagnosis of OSA.[30] Children with periodic limb movements of sleep demonstrate an increased liability for inattention and hyperactivity symptoms, and treatment of this sleep disorder sometimes results in improvement in the associated ADHD symptoms. In a study of children with a variety of anxiety disorders, 88% were found to exhibit sleep disturbances.[31] Numerous studies have reported a high overlap between depression and sleep abnormalities.[32]

In elderly individuals, complaints of insomnia or hypersomnia are common, often related to physical symptoms that disturb sleep, a medical condition, or the effects of a prescribed medication.[33] PSG-based studies conducted in elderly individuals have documented decreased total sleep time, reduced sleep efficiency, increased awakenings, decreased slow wave sleep, and laboratory-verified evidence of increased daytime sleepiness. Elderly individuals tend to show advanced sleep phase, a common manifestation of a circadian rhythm sleep alteration with advanced age. The prevalence of insomnia complaints in elderly individuals has been reported to be high in numerous studies, including a report that more than 50% of individuals older than 65 years described sleep problems.[34] In the National Institute of Aging study of 9000 individuals aged 65 years and older, only 12% of respondents reported no sleep complaints.[35] The intersection of sleep disturbances with Alzheimer disease (AD) represents a growing public health problem in light of the pronounced increase in the prevalence of AD and the recognition of the challenging aspects of sleep alterations on the management of patients with AD, particularly the immense burden that falls on caregivers of patients with AD in dealing with the behavioral consequences of this interaction.[36] Alterations of sleep in patients with AD include fragmentation of nocturnal sleep, with frequent and often prolonged awakenings during sleep, daytime sleepiness with frequent napping, REM sleep abnormalities, pronounced alterations in circadian rhythms, and the behavioral agitation syndrome referred to as sundowning in the late afternoon and evening.

Benca and colleagues[25] reported on findings derived from a total of 177 studies involving PSG analyses in patients across a wide range of psychiatric and sleep disorder categories and control subjects. Data available from 7151 patients with psychiatric and sleep disorders and control subjects were analyzed by means of meta-analysis. Patterns of sleep disturbances were identified across the broad range of psychiatric and sleep disorder categories evaluated, which included mood disorders, anxiety disorders, schizophrenia, eating disorders, borderline personality disorder, dementia, insomnia, and narcolepsy. To illustrate findings described in this comprehensive analysis, patients in all the diagnostic categories examined, with the exception of patients with narcolepsy, demonstrated significant disturbances in sleep duration (ie, total sleep time) as compared with the values for control subjects. In addition, patients in all the groups examined, with the exception of patients with narcolepsy and with eating disorders, demonstrated significant prolongation of sleep latency. The meta-analysis also identified other PSG-based manifestations of sleep disturbances that were identified in selected diagnostic groups of psychiatric patients. Complementary to the findings summarized earlier in this section, the comprehensive meta-analysis conducted by Benca and colleagues strongly underscores the rich database confirming the prevalence of sleep abnormalities in a wide range of psychiatric disorders.

The Bidirectional Nature of the Interrelationship Between Sleep Disturbances and Psychiatric Disorders

As noted earlier, sleep disturbances have been recognized to be associated with behavioral disorders since the time of antiquity. In the opinion of the author, a traditional view in Psychiatry has been to attribute the cause of sleep disturbances in psychiatric patients to the underlying primary psychiatric disorder. A potential clinical implication of this belief, although not supported by empirical evidence, is that treatment of the primary psychiatric disorder would automatically lead to the resolution of the associated sleep disturbance.

In a comment entitled "Insomnia and Depression: If it Looks and Walks Like a Duck," Turek[37] observed that much of the literature describing sleep alterations in patients with depression has emphasized the association of MDD to sleep disturbances, but he noted that "psychiatric sleep specialists have been reluctant to use the 'C' word (ie, the 'cause' word)." Turek goes on to assert "Insomnia *causes* depression- and possibly other mood disorders." The commentary by Turek emphasizes the concept that the interrelationships between sleep disturbances and mood disorders (and potentially other psychiatric disorders as well) are complex and nuanced. In recent years, the nature of this interrelationship has most typically been characterized as bidirectional in nature. Data supporting this concept are summarized in the following.

In the report by Ford and Kamerow[11] cited earlier, a subset of the originally enrolled 10,534 community respondents were interviewed and provided information regarding symptoms of sleep disorders and psychiatric disorders both at baseline and at a follow-up evaluation 1 year later.[11] Among a total of 7954 respondents providing data at both baseline and 1-year follow-up, the rate of new psychiatric disorders (primarily depression and anxiety disorders) was significantly higher at 1-year follow-up in subjects with sleep complaints at baseline than was the case for respondents who reported no symptoms of sleep disturbance at baseline. For individuals reporting problems with insomnia at baseline, 57% reported a new-onset psychiatric diagnosis, whereas 64% of respondents with symptoms of hypersomnia at baseline reported a new-onset psychiatric diagnosis at the 1-year follow-up assessment, in contrast to a 24.9% rate of new psychiatric diagnosis at 1-year follow-up in individuals with no sleep disorder symptoms at the baseline or follow-up assessments.

Breslau and colleagues[38] conducted a longitudinal epidemiologic study involving assessment of sleep symptoms and psychiatric disorder diagnoses in young adults recruited from a large health maintenance organization in Michigan. A total of 1007 respondents were interviewed at the baseline assessment, and 979 subjects provided data at a follow-up evaluation 3.5 years after the baseline assessment. Individuals who reported insomnia at baseline demonstrated a 4-fold greater risk for a new-onset depressive episode at the follow-up evaluation 3.5 years later than that seen in subjects with no insomnia symptoms at baseline, whereas subjects who reported symptoms of hypersomnia at the baseline evaluation demonstrated a 2.9-fold increase in risk for a new-onset psychiatric disorder at the 3.5-year follow-up evaluation. A history of insomnia at baseline was also associated with an increased risk for the presentation of an anxiety disorder, illicit drug use disorder, and nicotine dependence at the 3.5-year follow-up visit.

Johnson and colleagues[39] conducted a study to examine the interrelationships as well as the direction of risk between insomnia and both depression and anxiety in a sample of 1676 adolescents aged 13 to 15 years who were recruited from a health maintenance organization in Michigan, along with a participating parent to provide collateral information. A total of 1014 youth-parent pairs provided meaningful data for this study. In this analysis, prior insomnia did not demonstrate a significantly increased risk for the development of a subsequent anxiety disorder, whereas a prior history of an anxiety disorder did demonstrate a significant increase in the risk for developing insomnia. In contrast, youths with prior insomnia demonstrated a 3.8-fold increased risk for developing depression as compared with peers with no history of insomnia, a finding that is comparable with the previous report by Breslau and colleagues,[38] based on their study in young adults.

Steinsbekk and colleagues[31] reported on results from a study identifying symptoms of primary insomnia in children aged 4 years and then conducting assessments for the presence of psychiatric/behavioral disorders that emerged during the next 2 years, based on follow-up assessments and interviews with an informative parent. A total of 795 child-parent pairs provided information for this analysis. The presence of primary insomnia at age 4 years was associated with an increased risk for the development of several psychiatric/behavioral disorders by age 6 years, including MDD, ADHD, conduct disorder (CD), oppositional defiant disorder (ODD), GAD, separation anxiety, and social phobia. The investigators note that when the initial levels of psychiatric symptoms were adjusted for, insomnia positively predicted symptoms of MDD, GAD, social phobia, CD, and ODD.

To extend the discussion of the assessment of bidirectionality in the interrelationships between sleep disturbances and psychiatric disorders, 2 reports that provide systematic reviews of pertinent studies are discussed. Riemann and Vodenholzer[40] conducted a review of the literature to identify "longitudinal epidemiological studies with at least two measurement points 1 year apart measuring insomnia and depression" The researchers identified 8 studies meeting their criteria. Their assessment of findings reported in these 8 studies was "Almost unambiguously insomnia at baseline significantly predicted an increased depression risk at follow-up 1–3 years later."

Alvaro and colleagues[41] conducted a systematic literature review to identify studies that "assessed bidirectionality between a sleep disturbance, and anxiety or depression." The researchers identified a total of 9 informative studies, 8 of which used a longitudinal prospective design. Their literature review indicated a more variable mix of findings with respect to the evidence supporting a bidirectional relationship between sleep disturbances and depression and anxiety. Nevertheless, the conclusion offered by the researchers stated: "Best available evidence suggests that insomnia is bidirectionally related to anxiety and depression."

THE RELEVANCE OF SLEEP DISTURBANCE TO THE CLINICAL PRACTICE OF PSYCHIATRY

During the past 4 decades, several proposals have been suggested for the use of sleep disturbances, whether based on clinical assessment or on PSG analysis, to be applied on a practical basis in clinical treatment of psychiatric disorders. In many cases, more data are needed to establish an adequate evidence base to justify the translation of research investigations into standard clinical practice. Some selected examples of the potential application of research findings regarding sleep disturbances to clinical practice in psychiatry are discussed. Many of these topics are elaborated on in other articles.

Much of the research in the area of sleep disturbances related to psychiatric disorders that has been conducted in recent years has focused on depression. Several alterations in sleep continuity and sleep architecture have been reported in patients with MDD, including numerous studies documenting a finding of short REM latency (REM-L) in a significant percentage of patients with MDD. Studies evaluating REM-L in patients with MDD have pointed to a marked increase in the finding of short REM-L in first-degree relatives of patients with MDD.[42,43] Moreover, first-degree relatives of patients with MDD with short REM-L have an increased risk for developing depression. In other studies, short REM-L was reported to indicate increased risk for developing depression, as well as increased risk for relapse following response to antidepressant medication.[16,44] In other studies, patients with MDD were evaluated with respect to their REM-L profiles as a potential correlate of treatment response. In some studies involving treatment with tricyclic antidepressant drugs, REM-L was significantly correlated with positive antidepressant response.[45,46] In studies examining a different sleep PSG parameter, Kupfer and colleagues[47] reported that an index of slow wave sleep referred to as the delta sleep ratio was significantly linked to the time to develop a recurrence of an episode of depression in patients with MDD who had been successfully treated and were in remission. A final example of a sleep-related variable that has potential clinical relevance relates to the clinical assessment of residual symptoms in patients with MDD who have been treated and are in remission. Studies by Judd and colleagues have emphasized the importance of alleviating all symptoms of depression in conjunction with treatment to reduce the likelihood that patients will suffer relapses or recurrences.[48] Nierenberg and colleagues[49] examined 215 outpatients with MDD who were treated with fluoxetine, with a total of 108 patients being considered full responders, based on a final Hamilton Depression Rating Scale (HAM-D) score of 7 or less. Only 17.6% of recovered patients were free of all symptoms of depression. The most prevalent residual symptoms observed in this group of recovered patients with MDD were sleep-related complaints, including insomnia (reported in 44%) and fatigue (38%).

Sleep disturbances have also been suggested to be clinically relevant to other psychiatric disorders in addition to depression. Herz and Melville[50] identified insomnia as one of the most frequent symptoms reported in advance of exacerbation of psychotic symptoms in schizophrenic patients. Chemerinski and colleagues[51] reported on observations made in a large group of patients with schizophrenia and schizophrenic-spectrum disorders who were evaluated in an inpatient clinical research unit during a planned 3-week washout of antipsychotic medications. Severity of insomnia before antipsychotic discontinuation demonstrated a significant relationship with worsening of psychotic and disorganized symptoms. In addition, Dencker and colleagues[52] reported on findings from a group of patients with schizophrenia who had been stable for at least 2 years. In this report, the development of middle insomnia following discontinuation of antipsychotic medication was associated with an increased risk of relapse of psychotic symptoms.

Sleep disturbances have long been thought to be of clinical relevance to alcohol and substance use disorders. Gillin and colleagues[53] carried out PSG assessments on patients with primary alcoholism who were participating in an inpatient treatment program. They reported that indices that indicate increased REM pressure, including short REM-L, increased REM percentage, and increased REM density, predicted relapse to heavy alcohol use within 3 months of discharge from the inpatient program. Brower and colleagues[54] examined both subjective measures of sleep disturbance and PSG-based assessments and reported that both subjective sleep complaints, including reports of prolonged sleep latency and abnormal sleep in general, and objective PSG parameters, including long sleep latency and short REM-L, were correlated with an increased risk for relapsing to excessive alcohol use.

SUMMARY

Sleep disturbances have been documented to occur with high prevalence in patients with a variety of psychiatric disorders. In recent years, studies using longitudinal epidemiologic assessment methodologies have generated compelling evidence to support a bidirectional relationship between sleep disturbances and psychiatric disorders. Moreover, numerous examples have been cited to support the potential relevance of alterations in sleep parameters to the risk of developing a psychiatric disorder, to the risk of relapsing after having been treated to the point of remission, to potential biomarkers of familial vulnerability to the development of a psychiatric disorder, and to potential correlates and predictors of treatment response. Many of these themes are further elaborated in other articles in this issue.

REFERENCES

1. Diagnostic and statistical manual of mental disorders. 4th edition. Washington, DC: American Psychiatric Association; 1994.
2. Diagnostic and statistical manual of mental disorders. 5th edition. Washington, DC: American Psychiatric Association; 2013.

3. Bixler EO, Kales A, Soldatos CR. Prevalence of sleep disorders in the Los Angeles Metropolitan area. Am J Psychiatry 1979;136(10):1257–62.
4. Ohayon MM. Prevalence of DSM-IV diagnostic criteria of insomnia: distinguishing insomnia related to mental disorders from sleep disorders. J Psychiatr Res 1997; 31(3):333–46.
5. Leger D, Guilleminault C, Dreyfus JP, et al. Prevalence of insomnia in a survey of 12,778 adults in France. J Sleep Res 2000;9(1):35–42.
6. Ohayon MM. Epidemiology of insomnia: what we know and what we still need to learn. Sleep Med Rev 2002;6(2):97–111.
7. National Institutes of Health State of the Science Conferences Statement: manifestations and management of chronic insomnia: pathophysiology and implications for treatment. Sleep 2005;28(9):1049–57.
8. Roth T, Roehrs T, Pies R. Insomnia: pathophysiology and implications for treatment. Sleep Med Rev 2007;11(1):71–9.
9. Buysse DA, Angst J, Gamma A, et al. Prevalence, course and comorbidities of insomnia and depression in young adults. Sleep 2008;31(4):473–80.
10. Karacan I, Thornby JI, Anch M, et al. Prevalence of sleep disturbance in a primary urban Florida county. Soc Sci Med 1976;10:239–44.
11. Ford D, Kamerow D. Epidemiologic study of sleep disturbances and psychiatric disorders. JAMA 1989;262(11):1470–84.
12. Taylor DJ, Lichstein KL, Durrence H, et al. Epidemiology of insomnia, depression and anxiety. Sleep 2005;28(11):1457–64.
13. Buysse DA, Reynolds CF III, Kupfer DJ, et al. Clinical diagnoses in 216 insomnia patients using the International Classification of Sleep Disorders (ICSD), DSM-IV and ICD-10 categories: a report from the APA/NIMH DSM-IV Field Trial. Sleep 1994;17(7):630–7.
14. Berlin RM, Litovitz GL, Diaz MA, et al. Sleep disorders on a psychiatric consultation service. Am J Psychiatry 1984;141(4):582–4.
15. Jackson SW. Melancholia and depression: from Hippocratic times to modern times. New Haven (CT): Yale University Press; 1986. p. 30.
16. Reynolds CF III, Kupfer DJ. Sleep research in affective illness: state of the art circa 1987. Sleep 1987;10(3):199–215.
17. McCall WV, Reboussin BA, Cohen W. Subjective measurement of insomnia and quality of life in depressed inpatients. J Sleep Res 2000;9(1):43–8.
18. Harvey AG. Sleep and circadian rhythms in bipolar disorder: seeking synchrony, harmony and regulation. Am J Psychiatry 2008;165(7):820–9.
19. Goodwin GM, Anderson I, Arango C, et al. ECNP consensus meeting. Bipolar depression. Nice, March 2007. Eur Neuropsychopharmacol 2008;18(7): 535–49.
20. Frye MA. Bipolar depression - a focus on depression. N Engl J Med 2011;364(1): 51–9.
21. Wanders RB, Wardenaar KJ, Penninx BW, et al. Data-driven atypical profiles of depressive symptoms: identification and validation in a large cohort. J Affect Disord 2015;180(1):36–43.
22. Thompson C, Isaacs G. Seasonal affective disorder - a British sample symptomatology in relation to mode of referral and diagnostic subtype. J Affect Disord 1988;14(1):1–12.
23. Tam EM, Lam RW, Robertson HA, et al. Atypical depressive symptoms in seasonal and non-seasonal mood disorders. J Affect Disord 1997;44(1):39–44.
24. Monti JM, Monti D. Sleep disturbance in schizophrenia. Int Rev Psychiatry 2005; 17(4):247–53.

25. Benca RM, Obermeyer WH, Thisted RA, et al. Sleep and psychiatric disorders: a meta-analysis. Arch Gen Psychiatry 1992;49(8):651–68.
26. Fuller KH, Waters WF, Binks PG, et al. Generalized anxiety and sleep architecture: a polysomnographic investigation. Sleep 1997;20(5):370–6.
27. Arriaga F, Paiva T, Matos-Pires PG, et al. The sleep of non-depressed patients with panic disorder: a comparison with normal controls. Acta Psychiatr Scand 1996;93(3):191–4.
28. Roehrs T, Roth T. Medication and substance abuse. In: Kryger MH, Roth T, Dement WC, editors. Principles and practice of sleep medicine. 5th edition. Philadelphia: Elsevier Saunders; 2011. p. 1512–23.
29. Mahfoud Y, Talih F, Streem D, et al. Sleep disorders in substance abusers: how common are they? Psychiatry 2009;6(9):38–42.
30. Chervin RD, Dillon JE, Bassetti C, et al. Symptoms of sleep disorders, inattention, and hyperactivity in children. Sleep 1997;20(12):1185–92.
31. Steinsbekk S, Berg-Nielsen TS, Wichstrøm L. Sleep disorders in preschoolers: comorbidity with psychiatric symptoms. J Dev Behav Pediatr 2013;34(9):633–41.
32. Steinsbekk S, Wichstrøm L. Stability of sleep disorders from preschool to first grade and their bidirectional relationship with psychiatric symptoms. J Dev Behav Pediatr 2015;36(3):243–51.
33. Ancoli-Israel S. Sleep problems in older adults: putting myths to bed. Geriatrics 1997;52(1):20–30.
34. Ancoli-Israel S, Poceta JS, Stepnowsky C, et al. Identification and treatment of sleep problems in the elderly. Sleep Med Rev 1997;1(1):3–17.
35. Foley DJ, Monjan AA, Brown SL, et al. Sleep complaints among elderly persons: an epidemiological study of three communities. Sleep 1995;18(6):425–32.
36. McCurry SM, Reynolds CF III, Ancoli-Israel S, et al. Treatment of sleep disturbances in Alzheimer's disease. Sleep Med Rev 2000;4(6):603–28.
37. Turek FW. Insomnia and depression: if it looks and walks like a duck. Sleep 2005; 28(11):1362–3.
38. Breslau N, Roth T, Rosenthal L, et al. Sleep disturbance and psychiatric disorders: a longitudinal epidemiological study of young adults. Biol Psychiatry 1996;39(6):411–8.
39. Johnson E, Roth T, Breslau N. The association of insomnia with anxiety disorders and depression: exploration of the direction of risk. J Psychiatr Res 2006;40(8): 700–8.
40. Riemann D, Voderholzer U. Primary insomnia: a risk factor to develop depression? J Affect Disord 2003;76(1–3):255–9.
41. Alvaro PK, Roberts RM, Harris JK. A systematic review assessing bidirectionality between sleep disturbances, anxiety and depression. Sleep 2013;36(7):1059–68.
42. Giles DE, Biggs MM, Rush AJ, et al. Risk factors in families of unipolar depression. 1. Psychiatric illness and reduced REM latency. J Affect Disord 1988; 14(1):51–9.
43. Giles DE, Kupfer DJ, Roffwarg HP, et al. Polysomnographic parameters in first-degree relatives of unipolar probands. Psychiatry Res 1989;27(2):127–36.
44. Emslie GJ, Armitage R, Weinberg WA, et al. Sleep polysomnography as a predictor of recurrence in children and adolescents with major depressive disorder. Int J Neuropsychopharmacol 2001;4(2):159–68.
45. Kupfer DJ, Spiker DG, Coble PA, et al. Sleep treatment prediction in endogenous depression. Am J Psychiatry 1981;138(4):429–34.
46. Rush AJ, Giles DE, Jarrett RB, et al. Reduced REM latency predicts response to tricyclic medication in depressed outpatients. Biol Psychiatry 1989;26(1):61–72.

47. Kupfer DJ, Frank E, McEachran AB, et al. Delta sleep ratio: a biological correlate of early recurrence in unipolar affective disorder. Arch Gen Psychiatry 1990; 47(12):1100–5.

48. Judd LL, Paulus MJ, Schettler PJ, et al. Does incomplete recovery from first life-time major depressive episode herald a chronic course of illness? Am J Psychiatry 2000;157(9):1501–4.

49. Nierenberg AA, Keefe BR, Leslie VC, et al. Residual symptoms in depressed patients. Am J Psychiatry 1989;26(1):61–72.

50. Herz MI, Melville C. Relapse in schizophrenia. Am J Psychiatry 1980;137(7): 801–5.

51. Chemerinski E, Ho BC, Flaum M, et al. Insomnia as a predictor for symptom worsening following antipsychotic withdrawal in schizophrenia. Compr Psychiatry 2002;43(5):393–6.

52. Dencker SJ, Malm U, Lepp M. Schizophrenic relapse after drug withdrawal is predictable. Acta Psychiatr Scand 1986;73(2):181–5.

53. Gillin JC, Smith TL, Irwin M, et al. Increased pressure for rapid eye movement sleep at time of hospital admission predicts relapse in nondepressed patients with primary alcoholism at 3-month follow-up. Arch Gen Psychiatry 1994;51(3): 189–97.

54. Brower KJ, Aldrich MS, Hall JM. Polysomnographic and subjective sleep predictors of alcohol relapse. Alcohol Clin Exp Res 1998;22(8):1864–71.

The Neurobiology of Sleep and Wakefulness

Michael D. Schwartz, PhD, Thomas S. Kilduff, PhD*

KEYWORDS

- EEG • Synchronization • Homeostasis • Slow wave activity • NREM sleep
- REM sleep • Neurotransmitter • Hypocretin

KEY POINTS

- The monoaminergic systems of the brainstem, the cholinergic neuronal groups found in the brainstem and basal forebrain and the hypocretin/orexin cells of the hypothalamus are critical for the maintenance of wakefulness.
- Sleep is regulated by GABAergic populations in both the preoptic area and the brainstem; increasing evidence suggests a role for the melanin-concentrating hormone cells of the lateral hypothalamus and the parafacial zone of the brainstem.
- The pons has historically been viewed as critical for the production of REM sleep; recent research implicates descending projections from the hypothalamus and the periaqueductal gray as important for control of pontine REM generators.
- The hypocretin/orexin cells of the posterior and lateral hypothalamus provide excitatory input to all wake-promoting monoaminergic and cholinergic brain nuclei and both promote wakefulness and suppress REM sleep; loss of these cells results in the sleep disorder narcolepsy.
- The circadian organization of sleep and wakefulness arises from the interaction between a pacemaker located in the hypothalamus and a sleep homeostatic mechanism whose anatomical locus is yet to be conclusively defined, but may involve adenosine and cortical neuronal nitric oxide synthase neurons.

Our understanding of the neural control of sleep in large part parallels the history of neuroscience. As new tools and methodologies have become available to the research community, sleep researchers have been quick to take advantage of such techniques. Thus, the description in the following sections progresses from relatively crude methods, such as brain transections and lesion studies, to the application of

This work was supported by NIH R01 HL059658, R01 NS077408, R21 NS087550, R01 NS082876, R21 NS083639 and R21 NS085757.
Disclosures: Within the last 12 months, Dr T.S. Kilduff has received research support from F. Hoffmann La-Roche and received honoraria from Merck Pharmaceuticals and Pfizer.
Biosciences Division, Center for Neuroscience, SRI International, 333 Ravenswood Avenue, Menlo Park, CA 94025, USA
* Corresponding author.
E-mail address: thomas.kilduff@sri.com

Abbreviations

5-HT	5-Hydroxytrytamine (serotonin)
ACh	Acetylcholine
AD	Adenosine
ARAS	Ascending reticular activating system
BF	Basal forebrain
CCK-8	Cholecystokinin-8
CRF	Corticotrophin-releasing factor
CSF	Cerebrospinal fluid
DA	Dopamine
DREADD	Designer receptors exclusively activated by designer drugs
DRN	Dorsal raphe nuclei
EEG	Electroencephalogram
GABA	Gamma-aminobutyric acid
GAL	Galanin
GH	Growth hormone
Glu	Glutamate
HA	Histaminergic
Hcrt	Hypocretin (orexin)
IGF-1	Insulinlike growth factor-1
i.c.v.	Intracerebroventricular
LC	Locus coeruleus
LDT	Laterodorsal tegmental nucleus
MCH	Melanin-concentrating hormone
MnPO	Median preoptic area
nNOS	Neuronal nitric oxide synthase
NPY	Neuropeptide Y
NRD	NREM delta power
NREM	Non–rapid eye movement
PB	Parabrachial
PGD_2	Prostaglandin D2
PGD_2-SZ	Prostaglandin D2-sensitive zone
PLH	Posterolateral hypothalamus
PPT	Pedunculopontine tegmentum nuclei
PZ	Parafacial zone
REM	Rapid eye movement
SCN	Suprachiasmatic nuclei
SLD	Sublaterodorsal tegmental nucleus
SN	Substantia nigra
SWA	Slow wave activity
SWS	Slow wave sleep
TM	Tuberomammillary nuclei
TRH	Thyrotropin-releasing hormone
vlPAG	Ventrolateral periaqueductal gray
VLPO	Ventrolateral preoptic area
VTA	Ventral tegmental area

molecular biology and genetics to create transgenic models. The approach in this section is largely historical, illustrating the insights and principles that have emerged as research has progressed.

The advent of inducible transgenic mouse strains and viral-mediated transfection has enabled the ability to target cell populations in a phenotype-, location-, and time-specific manner. This added precision eliminates many of the caveats associated with more traditional lesion (impossible to isolate heterogeneous cell populations) and knockout methodologies (developmental confounds, lack of anatomic specificity).

Recently, optogenetic and chemogenetic methods have enabled manipulation of specific cell populations with unprecedented precision using light or synthetic ligands, respectively. In optogenetics, neurons of interest are genetically engineered to express light-sensitive opsins that control specialized ion channels. Subsequent illumination of these cells (usually through surgically implanted optical fibers) by specific wavelengths of light can activate or inhibit the cells expressing that opsin without collateral activation of nearby cell types. For example, the blue light-sensitive channelrhodopsin-2 protein opens a sodium ion channel and, when stimulated, will depolarize a cell. Conversely, the yellow/green light-sensitive halorhodopsin opens a chloride ion channel and will inhibit cells when illuminated. Similarly, the DREADD (Designer Receptors Exclusively Activated by Designer Drugs) system relies on a modified G protein–coupled receptor that responds only to a (otherwise biologically inert) synthetic ligand. Following expression of the DREADD receptor in a cell population of choice, the ligand can be injected systemically to activate only that population. This combination of powerful tools for precisely manipulating neuronal activity with the specificity of genetic targeting is revolutionizing the study of neural circuits and their control of behavior.

CORTICAL ACTIVITY DURING SLEEP AND WAKEFULNESS

The electrical activity of the cerebral cortex has been used to distinguish sleep versus wakefulness since the earliest electroencephalogram (EEG) studies of sleep.[1] The firing rate of cortical neurons generally declines during non–rapid eye movement (NREM) sleep relative to wakefulness and rapid eye movement (REM) sleep,[2,3] although a few studies have reported cortical neurons with the opposite firing pattern.[4,5] EEG activity reflects the aggregate firing of large neuronal ensembles and is conventionally referred to by bandwidths with the following approximate frequencies: alpha (9–12 Hz), beta (12–30 Hz), delta (0.5–4.0 Hz), low (30–60 Hz) and high (60–100 Hz) gamma, and theta (5–9 Hz). Several neural circuits have been implicated in the synchronization and desynchronization of cortical activity that distinguish NREM sleep from wakefulness and REM sleep. For example, input from the basal forebrain (BF), likely from both cholinergic and noncholinergic neurons, is critical for the desynchronized EEG characteristic of wakefulness and REM sleep.[6,7] Synchronization of the EEG during NREM sleep depends on a corticothalamocortical loop[8] as well as intrinsic cortical oscillators,[9] whose activities are modulated by several subcortical systems. In this article, the primary focus is how interactions between these subcortical systems produce sleep and wake and their electrophysiologic correlates at the cortical level.

HISTORICAL OVERVIEW
Classic Brainstem Transection Studies

The first investigations relevant to the neurobiology of sleep and wakefulness were conducted in the 1930s. Bremer[10] transected the cat brainstem, observing that sleep/wake cycles remained intact after a low medullary level transection (*encephale isole*), whereas transection between the pons and midbrain (*cerveau isole*) yielded chronic drowsiness. Conversely, electrical stimulation of the midbrain reticular formation caused alerting of the cortex.[11] From these observations arose the concept that the forebrain was kept alert by tonic activity in the reticular formation. This ascending reticular activating system (ARAS) is composed of cholinergic laterodorsal tegmental nucleus (LDT) and pedunculopontine tegmentum nucleus (PPT), noradrenergic locus coeruleus (LC), serotonergic (5-HT) raphe nuclei and dopaminergic ventral tegmental area (VTA), substantia nigra (SN) and periaqueductal gray projections that stimulate the cortex directly and indirectly via the thalamus, hypothalamus and BF.[6,12–18] These aminergic and catecholaminergic populations have numerous interconnections and parallel projections which likely impart functional redundancy and resilience to the system.[6,13,19]

In contrast, transecting the pons rostral to the trigeminal nerve induced constant wakefulness,[20] suggesting that input from a sleep center in the lower pons or medulla inhibited a wakefulness center in the rostral pons. This result established that sleep is an active state of the brain[21]; however, the identity of this lower brainstem sleep center remained a mystery. Although sleep-active neurons were reported in the nucleus tractus solitarius,[22] their location has proven to be elusive. More recently, the medullary parafacial zone (PZ) adjacent to the facial nerve was identified as a sleep-promoting center from anatomic, electrophysiologic, and chemogenetic and optogenetic studies.[23,24] GABAergic PZ neurons inhibit glutamatergic parabrachial (PB) neurons that project to the BF,[25] thereby promoting NREM sleep at the expense of wakefulness and REM sleep. As we shall see later, these populations exert much of their effects via projections to the BF and hypothalamus.

Encephalitis Lethargica: Insights into Sleep/Wake Control from Neuropathology

After World War I, a worldwide influenza epidemic claimed an estimated 25 to 40 million fatalities. One variant of this disease was *encephalitis lethargica*, in which patients entered a coma that often resulted in death. The neuropathologist Constantin von Economo[26] identified distinct types of brain lesions associated with equally distinct effects on sleep and waking. Lesions in the posterior hypothalamus extending into the mesencephalic reticular formation were associated with persistent coma, whereas lesions in the anterior hypothalamus and the adjacent BF were associated with chronic insomnia. von Economo concluded that the posterior hypothalamus was important for the maintenance of wakefulness and the anterior hypothalamic/BF region important for sleep induction.[26]

Nauta[27] subsequently demonstrated that anterior hypothalamic transections severely disrupted sleep and wakefulness, providing direct experimental evidence for von Economo's clinical observations. McGinty and Sterman[28] and others found that preoptic/BF lesions decreased sleep, whereas stimulation of this region facilitated sleep onset.[29] Sleep-active neurons were later described in the BF, particularly the substantia innominata and the horizontal limb of the diagonal band of Broca.[30] Subsequent electrophysiologic, Fos activation, tract tracing, and lesion studies identified the GABAergic ventrolateral preoptic area (VLPO) and the median preoptic area (MnPO) as being sleep-active neuronal populations that project to and inhibit wake-active cell groups.[31–38] These preoptic sleep-promoting groups are themselves inhibited by wake-active monoaminergic stimulation.[39,40] It should be noted that the BF also contains cortically-projecting cholinergic neurons distributed across the diagonal band of Broca, nucleus basalis, and substantia innominata.[41,42] These neurons have been extensively studied for their role in promoting cortical activation and wakefulness. In addition, much research has examined the role of the BF, including the cholinergic neurons therein, in regulating sleep homeostasis; this work is discussed in detail in a later section.

Also consistent with von Economo's earlier observations, lesions of the posterolateral hypothalamus (PLH) were found to increase sleep in rats, cats, and monkeys.[27,43,44] Histaminergic (HA) cells were subsequently identified in the tuberomammillary nuclei (TM) and found to be wake-promoting.[45] Antihistamines have long been known to be soporific, and knockout mice lacking the enzyme responsible for histamine synthesis are hypersomnolent.[46,47] Inhibitory VLPO neurons project to HA TM neurons[48]; HA neurons project widely throughout the brain, including to wake-promoting populations in the brainstem and to the cortex.[49] Injections of the gamma-aminobutyric acid (GABA)$_A$ agonist muscimol into the posterior hypothalamus increased NREM sleep and suppressed REM sleep, whereas injections in the ventral PLH increased both NREM and REM sleep.[50] Together, these results supported the hypothesis that sleep results from functional blockade of a posterior hypothalamic waking center. Although the neurons inactivated by muscimol were thought to be the HA cells, the PLH contains another wake-active neuronal population, the hypocretin/orexin cells, that were yet to be described.

Rapid Eye Movement Sleep: the Role of the Pons and Acetylcholine

REM sleep was first described by Aserinsky and Kleitman[51,52] and Dement and Kleitman[53] and was described in animals in 1959.[54] As cellular neurophysiology entered the neurobiologist's toolbox in the 1960s and early 1970s,[55–57] sleep physiologists characterized the firing rates of cells in specific brain regions across the arousal state continuum from wakefulness to NREM to REM sleep. These firing rate profiles showed that monoaminergic cell groups decrease their firing from wakefulness to REM and are thus called REM-off cells. In contrast, a smaller set of brainstem regions had maximal firing rates during REM (REM-on cells). Because these cell groups were anatomically localized, Hobson and colleagues[58] and McCarley and Hobson[59] proposed that the NREM/REM cycle arises from a reciprocal interaction between these aminergic REM-off cell groups and cholinergic REM-on cell groups in the medial pons. More recent versions of this model recognize that the REM-on and REM-off cells are distributed in a variety of brain regions[60–62] and include both glutamatergic and GABAergic populations.[63,64]

The pons is both necessary and sufficient to generate REM sleep[65,66]; the dorsolateral pons, in particular, is crucial for the genesis of REM sleep.[67,68] Neurons in this region have a REM-on profile with their highest discharge rate occurring during REM sleep.[69,70] Microinjections of carbachol, a mixed cholinergic agonist, into the dorsolateral pons results in a prolonged REM-like state; pontine acetylcholine (ACh) levels are increased during REM sleep relative to NREM and wakefulness.[71] Cholinergic input for REM sleep generation comes from the more rostral PPT and LDT, which project to the cholinoceptive subcoeruleus or sublaterodorsal tegmental nucleus (SLD) and the subjacent nucleus pontis oralis.[72,73] During REM sleep, activation of the dorsolateral pons regulates the varied physiologic manifestations of REM sleep, for example, EEG desynchronization and theta activity, ponto-geniculo-occipital waves, rapid eye movements, and atonia. More recent studies have implicated the melanin-concentrating hormone (MCH)/GABAergic neurons of the hypothalamus as providing critical input to the pontine generator of REM sleep.[64,74]

Lesions of the dorsolateral pons produce REM sleep without atonia in cats; the cats orient, locomote, and engage in what seems to be prey-catching behavior as if they were acting out their dreams.[75,76] Cholinoceptive dorsolateral pontine neurons project to the ventral medulla, where they form synapses with inhibitory neuronal populations that, in turn, project to and inhibit spinal motorneurons, thereby preventing muscle movement during REM. This descending inhibition is thought to be mediated by glycinergic mechanisms[77]; more recent work has implicated GABA[78,79] as well as local inhibition in the ventral horn.[80] A similar condition, REM behavior disorder, exists in humans[81]; interest in the neurophysiological basis of REM behavior disorder has been potentiated by the finding that REM behavior disorder may be a risk factor or predictor of Parkinson disease and other neurodegenerative synucleinopathies.[82,83]

Narcolepsy/Cataplexy

The other sleep disorder related to the dorsolateral pons is narcolepsy. Narcoleptic patients suffer from excessive daytime sleepiness, abnormalities of REM sleep, and sudden attacks of muscle atonia during wakefulness known as cataplexy. Cataplexy is primarily triggered by positive emotional stimuli (laughter, surprise, sexual arousal) that are processed by the limbic system; these stimuli seem to converge on the REM atonia pathway, likely through the prefrontal cortex and the amygdala.[84,85] In narcoleptic dogs, cataplexy can be exacerbated by anticholinesterases, and the muscarinic cholinergic receptor is upregulated in the pons of these dogs.[86,87] Although this upregulation likely affects the same REM atonia pathway described earlier, narcoleptic dogs have been particularly valuable for the insights that they provided into the role of the hypocretin/orexin system in sleep/wake control and muscle atonia.[88]

THE HYPOCRETIN/OREXIN SYSTEM
Discovery of the Hypocretins and the Orexins

Hypocretins 1 and 2 (Hcrt1 and Hcrt2), also known as orexins A and B, are excitatory hypothalamic neuropeptides that were independently described by 2 groups in 1998.[89,90] Since Sakurai and colleagues[91] confirmed the common identity of the Hcrts and the orexins, the authors use the term *Hcrt* here to refer to this system. Although early studies emphasized the role of the Hcrt system in feeding and energy balance, subsequent research focused on sleep-wake regulation based, in part, on the discovery that Hcrt dysfunction underlies the sleep disorder narcolepsy.

Hcrt neurons are found exclusively in the PLH,[89,90,92] numbering between 4000 and 5000 in rats[92–94] and 50,000 and 80,000 in humans.[95] The two Hcrt peptides are derived from a single precursor molecule by proteolytic processing, and Hcrt1 and Hcrt2 are largely colocalized in the same neurons.[96] Hcrt neurons are coextensive, but not colocalized, with MCH neurons.[92,97,98] The Hcrt neurons project widely throughout the brain and spinal cord,[92,96,99,100] including major projections to wake-promoting cell groups, such as the HA cells of the TM,[101] the 5-HT cells of the dorsal raphe nuclei (DRN),[101] the noradrenergic cells of the LC,[102] and cholinergic cells in the LDT, PPT, and BF.[101,103] Afferent input to Hcrt neurons was mapped using a combination of retrograde and anterograde tract tracers[104]; these studies described major projections from the lateral septal nucleus, bed nucleus of the stria terminalis, preoptic area, dorsomedial, ventromedial and posterior hypothalamic nuclei, SN and VTA, and the DRN. Using transgenic mice expressing transneuronal retrograde tracers linked to the Hcrt promoter,[105] genetic tracing studies revealed a more circumscribed set of afferents to the Hcrt neurons from the amygdala, preoptic GABAergic neurons, and 5-HT neurons in the median/paramedian raphe nuclei. Thus, the anatomy of the Hcrt system strongly suggests involvement in numerous physiologic functions, including sleep-wake, feeding, thermoregulation, blood pressure, and neuroendocrine regulation.

To date, the Hcrt peptides have uniformly been reported as excitatory either by eliciting depolarization and/or increased spike frequency.[89] Hcrt directly excites cellular systems involved in waking and arousal, including the LC,[102,106,107] DRN,[108,109] TM,[110–112] LDT,[113,114] cholinergic BF,[115] and both dopamine (DA) and non-DA neurons in the VTA.[116,117] The excitatory effects of Hcrt are mediated by multiple ionic mechanisms,[110,118–125] which, combined with their capacity for neuromodulation,[109,113,118,126–129] suggest that Hcrt exerts potent direct and indirect effects on a variety of physiologic systems, particularly arousal systems. Some of these effects seem to be mediated by colocalized transmitters and modulators including, but not limited to, dynorphin, galanin (GAL), and glutamate (Glu).[130–135] Cellular electrophysiologic studies revealed that, although Hcrt cells are excited by numerous substances,[136–145] they are inhibited by the aminergic transmitters norepinephrine (NE), DA, and 5-HT,[136,139,146–148] as well as by GABA.[136,139,149]

Hcrt signaling is strongly associated with wakefulness. The region of the PLH containing the Hcrt cells has long been implicated in arousal state control.[27] Hcrt neurons are wake-active as measured by Fos expression,[150] electrophysiology,[151–153] or brain/cerebrospinal fluid (CSF) peptide content.[154–156] Hcrt1 increases arousal when infused into the brain,[106,157–162] and optogenetic stimulation or inhibition of Hcrt signaling increases or decreases wakefulness, respectively.[163–167] Hcrt receptor antagonists promote sleep when administered systemically or directly into the brain.[168–171] Indeed, newly developed dual Hcrt receptor antagonists exhibit promise for the effective pharmacologic promotion of sleep without adverse side effects, such as the cognitive performance deficits and dependence that are common to many sleep medications.[172,173]

The Hypocretin System and the Sleep Disorder Narcolepsy

Narcolepsy has a genetic component in both humans and dogs that has proven instrumental in identifying its unique etiology. In narcoleptic dogs, the *canarc-1* gene that transmits narcolepsy was identified as a mutation in the *hcrtr2* gene that results in a truncated, nonfunctional protein.[88] In a remarkable convergence, *Hcrt* null mutant mice exhibited a narcoleptic phenotype, including cataplectic behavioral arrests, sleep-onset REM, and increased and fragmented NREM and REM sleep.[101] Thus, dysfunction of either the Hcrt ligand or one of its receptors can result in narcolepsy. In humans, the HLA class II antigen HLA DQB1*0602 is present in more than 85% of narcoleptic patients with cataplexy but only 12% to 38% of the general population.[174] Such close association with the HLA system has led to the suggestion that narcolepsy may be an autoimmune disease.[175,176] Narcoleptic humans exhibit undetectable levels of Hcrt1 in CSF.[177] Postmortem studies revealed an absence of *preprohcrt* mRNA[178] and an 85% to 95% reduction in the number of Hcrt-containing cells in human narcoleptic brains[95] without any change in either MCH mRNA or the number of MCH cells. The presence of increased staining for glial fibrillary acid protein in the PLH of narcoleptic brains[95,178] suggests that degeneration of the Hcrt cells may cause human narcolepsy. Consistent with this, animal models in which the Hcrt neurons are ablated by selective neurotoxins[179,180] or engineered to degenerate postnatally[181,182] also present a narcoleptic phenotype.

Models for the Role of the Hypocretin System in Arousal State Regulation

It has been proposed that the balance between sleep and wakefulness is maintained by the relative activation of the wake-active systems found in the BF, LDT/PPT, LC, DRN, and TM and the sleep-active systems found in the VLPO.[13,94] These relationships are summarized in **Fig. 1**. During wakefulness, ascending monoaminergic projections from the ARAS nuclei activate wake-promoting cholinergic BF and histaminergic TM cells en route to the cerebral cortex while inhibiting sleep-promoting VLPO and MnPO neurons. LDT/PPT cholinergic neurons ascend to the thalamus, which in turn stimulates the cortex. During NREM sleep, GABAergic output from the VLPO, MnPO, and PZ inhibit these populations. REM sleep is driven by a combination of increased brainstem cholinergic (REM-on) activity and inhibition of

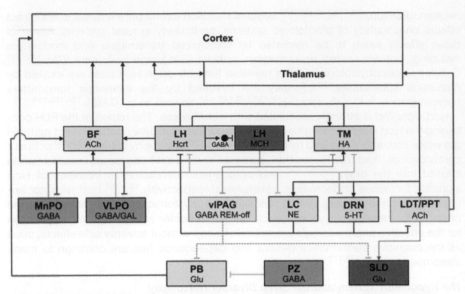

Fig. 1. Major subcortical sleep-wake regulatory populations. Wake-promoting cell groups are green, NREM sleep-promoting cell groups are blue, and REM sleep-related cell groups are red. Green boxes with red outlines indicated wake/REM-active populations. Gray boxes indicate local GABA interneurons. Excitatory connections are marked with arrowheads, and inhibitory connections are indicated by blunted terminals. Dotted lines indicate pathways that are inhibited during REM sleep. LH, lateral hypothalamus.

REM-off populations; MCH neurons in the lateral hypothalamus are proposed to be a part of the REM control mechanism as well. Hcrt signaling promotes waking by activating brainstem and forebrain wake-active populations and is, in turn, inhibited by ascending 5-HT and NE inputs. "In the flip-flop switch model Hcrt has been proposed to consolidate waking and sleep states by stabilizing transitions between sleep and wakefulness.[13] When the Hcrt system is dysfunctional as occurs in human narcolepsy and transgenic mouse models, behavioral state instability results so that the affected individual cannot maintain extended periods of wakefulness of sleep and, instead, shifts rapidly between these states.[183] This flip-flop switch concept was subsequently extended to account for the alternation between NREM and REM sleep.[63]

SLEEP HOMEOSTASIS AND THE TIMING OF SLEEP AND WAKEFULNESS

Common knowledge, as well as scientific observations, suggests that sleep is a homeostatically regulated physiologic response. The longer one is awake, the more likely one is to sleep or, at least, be sleepy. Sleep deprivation impairs cognition; prolonged sleep deprivation results in impaired physiologic function, ultimately resulting in death.[184] This homeostatic property has been incorporated into the 2-process model of sleep regulation,[185,186] which posits that the homeostatic sleep-related process S integrates input from the circadian system (process C) to gate the occurrence of sleep and wakefulness across the day. Process S is proposed to be neurochemical processes that begin to build up at the onset of wakefulness; once a threshold value is reached, sleep will ensue only if process C is in the appropriate circadian phase. This seemingly simplistic model accounts remarkably well for the timing of sleep in humans and rodents.

EEG slow waves in the delta bandwidth (0.5–4.0 Hz) generated by thalamocortical interactions during NREM sleep increase in proportion to prior wake duration. The level of NREM delta power (NRD; also called EEG slow wave activity [EEG SWA]) depends highly on the prior history of sleep and wakefulness: prolonged wakefulness dose-dependently increases NRD while both daytime naps and nighttime sleep decrease NRD, reflecting a diminution of process S. Conversely, NRD itself is highly resistant to circadian modulation.[187,188] Thus, EEG NRD has been suggested to reflect the cortical manifestation of the recovery from prior waking activities[185] and is commonly used as a quantitative measurement of process S.

ANATOMIC SUBSTRATES OF THE 2-PROCESS MODEL
The Suprachiasmatic Nuclei as the Basis for Process C

The hypothalamic suprachiasmatic nuclei (SCN) contain a master circadian pacemaker (or biological clock) in mammals[189–192] and are commonly recognized as the source of process C.[193–195] However, it remains unclear how SCN activity temporally organizes daily sleep-wake rhythms. Early studies relied on SCN lesions to functionally dissect circadian versus homeostatic regulation. The homeostatic response to sleep loss was intact in SCN-lesioned rats with no change in total sleep time per 24 hours,[196,197] whereas similar studies in SCN-lesioned squirrel monkeys and mice and in behaviorally arrhythmic Siberian hamsters reported increased sleep time per 24 hours.[198–200] These results fueled ongoing debate over whether the SCN specifically promotes wakefulness (as in the opponent process model), sleep, or both.[199,201] More recently, Hcrt was proposed as a point of integration between circadian and homeostatic mechanisms based on CSF Hcrt1 levels assayed across the day and in conjunction with sleep deprivation. However, it is unclear to what extent changing Hcrt1 levels in the CSF results from active (eg, circadian or homeostatic) regulation[156,202,203] or is passively driven by increased locomotor activity.[204] Integration of circadian and homeostatic signaling may also occur within the SCN. Indeed, SCN neuronal firing rates are modulated by sleep-wake state and by sleep deprivation,[205,206] and certain sleep-wake states (eg, REM sleep)[207–209] and EEG spectral signatures[188] may be under stronger circadian control than others.

Circadian rhythms arise from interactions between a well-characterized set of dedicated clock genes found throughout the body and central nervous system.[210,211] Genetic disruption of the clock via knockout yields increased waking, increased sleep, or no change of daily sleep-wake amounts depending on the particular gene targeted.[212–216] Sleep deprivation can modulate extra-SCN clock gene expression and binding activity.[217–221] Together, these findings suggest that different clock genes may play distinct roles in regulating or integrating circadian and homeostatic aspects of sleep.

In Search of Substrates for Process S

Although the anatomic substrate for process C had been identified before the development of the 2-process model, a similar substrate for process S has proven more difficult to identify. GABAergic neurons in the MnPO are sleep-active,[34,222] project to wake-active brain regions including the LC, DRN, ventrolateral periaqueductal gray (vlPAG), and the Hcrt neurons[38]; Fos immunohistochemical studies indicate that MnPO activation occurs during sleep deprivation before sleep onset,[223] suggesting that this region is responsive to homeostatic sleep pressure. MnPO neurons also exhibit increased Fos activation during REM sleep deprivation.[224]

A cortical neuronal population that expresses neuronal nitric oxide synthase (nNOS) has recently emerged as a candidate for involvement in process S. Although most cortical neurons express the immediate early gene product Fos during waking, cortical nNOS neurons express Fos during sleep but not during wakefulness.[225] Cortical nNOS neurons, which also coexpress the substance P receptor NK1, represent the rarest subset of GABAergic interneurons and are anatomically and functionally quite distinctive: they are the only nNOS-synthesizing neuronal population reported to be sleep-active[226]; they receive subcortical inputs from sleep-related cholinergic[227] and serotonergic[228] neurons and send long-range rather than local circuit projections.[229–232] Functionally, nNOS cortical neuron activation is positively correlated with NREM bout duration and NRD energy[233] and critically depends on elevated sleep pressure.[234] Furthermore, loss of nNOS signaling in nNOS null mutant mice fragments NREM sleep, attenuates NRD power while increasing delta power in wake, and increases sleepiness while attenuating response to sleep deprivation. Cortical nNOS neurons, thus, seem to be critical integrators in the neuronal network linking state-dependent afferent inputs, homeostatic sleep drive, and EEG SWA.[235]

OTHER NEUROCHEMICALS INVOLVED IN SLEEP/WAKE CONTROL

Although functional neuroanatomical approaches, especially when combined with electrophysiology, have led to many fundamental insights into the control of sleep and waking, there is an equally impressive literature on sleep substances and their contributions to behavioral state. These sparks versus soup approaches are highly complementary, and valuable insights into the control of sleep and wakefulness have arisen from both approaches.

Cytokines and Sleep

Several lymphokines (eg, interleukin-1, tumor necrosis factor alpha), inflammatory molecules, and growth factors promote NREM sleep.[236,237] Interleukin-1 and tumor necrosis factor may regulate physiologic sleep through direct, receptor-mediated modulation of the hypothalamus and serotonergic raphe nuclei. Other immune molecules, such as interleukin-6, promote NREM sleep and are elevated in sleep disorders with excessive daytime sleepiness as a symptom.

Peptides and Sleep

As indicated earlier, Hcrt has wake-promoting activity.[106,160] Several other neuropeptides have also been found to promote wakefulness. Corticotrophin-releasing factor (CRF)[238,239] and adrenocorticotrophic hormone,[240] core components of the hypothalamo-pituitary adrenal axis, promote wakefulness, possibly mediated by CRF activation of CRF receptor-1 on Hcrt cells.[141] Thyrotropin-releasing hormone (TRH) and TRH analogues are wake-promoting in rodents[241,242]; but, in a clinical study, TRH only exerted a weak effect on sleep efficiency.[243] Neuropeptide Y (NPY), a potent inducer of feeding behavior, exerts varied effects on rodent sleep, ranging from sleep suppression to alterations in EEG spectral power.[244–246] In humans, intravenous NPY reduced sleep latency in young men[247] and older men and women.[248] Neuropeptide S[249] and urotensin[250] are also reported to promote wakefulness in rodents.

Among sleep-promoting peptides, growth hormone (GH)–releasing hormone has been extensively studied,[238,251,252] in part because pharmacologic stimulation of slow wave sleep (SWS) results in increased GH release.[253] However, studies of peptides related to the GH system have produced varying results.[246,254–256] Intraperitoneal cholecystokinin-8 (CCK-8) reduced sleep latency and increased NREM sleep in rats and rabbits,[257–259] and centrally administered CCK restored sleep in cats rendered insomniac by serotonin depletion.[259,260] The α-melanocyte–stimulating hormone is sleep-promoting as is corticotropin-like intermediate lobe peptide.[240] Both peripheral[261] and intracerebroventricular (i.c.v.)[262] infusion of insulin increases SWS in rats. These effects could be related to postprandial sleepiness. Insulin also stimulates insulin-like growth factor-1 (IGF-1) receptors, although the molar doses of IGF-1 needed to promote sleep are much lower than that of insulin.[263]

As indicated earlier, the hypothalamic neuropeptide MCH is coextensive, but not colocalized, with Hcrt cells.[92,97,98] MCH has profound effects on both SWS and REM sleep, in particular, when administered i.c.v.[264] Fos is activated in MCH neurons during recovery from REM sleep deprivation.[264,265] MCH neurons are inhibited directly by HA and indirectly by Hcrt via local GABA interneurons.[266,267] Optogenetic studies have implicated MCH neurons in the control of REM sleep[268,269] as well as sleep onset.[270] Other peptides with REM-promoting activity include prolactin,[271,272] vasoactive intestinal polypeptide,[272,273] and pituitary adenylate cyclase-activating polypeptide.[274–277]

Extracellular Adenosine as an Indicator of Sleep Loss

Interest in adenosine (AD) as a potential modulator of sleep and wakefulness arose when the AD receptors were cloned and it was recognized that methylxanthines such as caffeine, a potent wake-promoting substance, were antagonists at AD receptors.[278] AD is the ultimate breakdown product of ATP; therefore, there has also been great interest in a role for AD as a potential link between sleep and restoration of intracellular energy stores.[279,280] Injections of AD or AD analogues typically promote sleep and NREM EEG delta power[281–284]; interestingly, such injections increase delta power even in sleep-satiated animals.[285] AD signaling regulates sleep and waking at targets, including the BF, VLPO, Hcrt neurons, cortex, and brainstem,[280] primarily via inhibitory A_1 receptors and excitatory A_{2A} receptors.[286–289]

Levels of extracellular AD accumulate with time spent awake and decline during recovery sleep in the BF and cortex but weakly, if at all, in other brain regions.[290,291] In the BF, wake-related AD release seems to depend on cholinergic neurons, as cell-specific lesions of these neurons abolish AD increases induced by sleep deprivation.[292,293] Together, these data suggest that AD is an important endogenous regulator of sleep and waking in the brain and that the BF, in particular, is important for adenosinergic influences on sleep homeostasis.[294] Although the source of AD in the BF has proven elusive, expression of inducible nitric oxide synthase (iNOS) in the cholinergic BF neurons seems to be important for the wake-related upregulation of AD.[295–297] Astrocytes may be an important source for AD induced by waking, as abolishing vesicular release specifically in astrocytes attenuated the homeostatic sleep response and blocked the sleep-suppressing effect of an AD A_1 receptor antagonist.[298,299] Given the important role played by astrocytes in regulating neuronal energy stores, it is tempting to speculate that glial-neuronal interactions may be a critical component of regulating sleep need.[300–302]

Melatonin

Melatonin is produced by the pineal gland during the night in both diurnal and nocturnal species. Specific receptors for melatonin are found in the cortex, SCN, and hypothalamic regions involved in thermoregulation. Exogenous melatonin is a popular hypnotic available in both physiologic (0.03 mg) and pharmacologic (1–10 mg) doses. Physiologic doses can help in sleep-onset processes when sleep initiation is attempted at abnormal times, such as occurs following travel across time zones. Melatonin helps to synchronize circadian rhythms in totally blind individuals.[303] Pharmacologic doses may work through nonmelatonin receptors.

Prostaglandin D₂ and Sleep/Wake Regulation

Intracerebral administration of prostaglandin D_2 (PGD_2) induces sleep, especially SWS, in rats and monkeys.[304] Inhibition of the enzyme responsible for PGD_2 synthesis, PGD synthase,[305,306] markedly suppresses sleep; the blockade of PGD_2 receptors inhibits physiologic sleep.[307] CSF levels of PGD_2 undergo significant modulation by the time of day in rats, with a daytime peak and a nighttime trough.[308] CSF levels of PGD_2 in rats increase during sleep deprivation and tend to increase along with an increasing propensity toward sleep under normal conditions.[309] The site of action for PGD_2 has been identified as a sleep-promoting zone (PGD_2-SZ) located on ventral surface of the rostral BF outside the brain parenchyma.[310,311] Administration of a selective AD A_{2a}-R agonist (CGS21680), but not the selective AD A_1-R agonist cyclohexyladenosine, markedly induces sleep when administered to the PGD_2-SZ.[312] The SWS-promoting effect of PGD_2 is inhibited by pretreatment with KF17837, a highly selective A_{2a}-R antagonist,[312] and is blunted in AD A_{2a}-R-deficient mice.[289] It is, therefore, hypothesized that PGD_2 is coupled to A_{2a}-R adenosinergic signaling via the brain parenchyma and that the PGD_2-SZ plays an important role as an interface between these two systems.

Gonadal Steroids and Sleep

Sex and sex hormones have long been reported to modulate sleep and biological timing, but only recently have these phenomena begun to be studied on a more mechanistic level.[313] Women exhibit increased subjective sleep disturbance, particularly insomnia,[314] and increased spindle activity and SWA compared with men.[315–318] Sex differences in SWA are amplified by sleep deprivation, aging, and major depression.[315,319] Sleep spindle activity and REM sleep, but not SWA, also vary across the menstrual cycle.[320–322] Female rodents exhibit increased wakefulness in the dark (active) phase compared with males,[323–328] with the estrus cycle further modulating sleep in female rats[329–331] but not mice.[325] Like humans, female mice exhibit increased spindle frequency activity and NRD compared with males.[324,326] Circulating ovarian steroids, particularly estradiol and progesterone, are important for maintaining many of these effects.[327,330,332–334] Studies exploiting genetic tools to dissociate genetic and gonadal sex, along with use of classic neuroendocrine paradigms, recently showed that sex differences in sleep seem to be developmentally determined by a combination of genetic sex and gonadal hormone exposure.[335,336] Estradiol downregulates the synthetic enzyme for PGD_2,[337] increases Hcrt and Hcrt receptor expression levels,[338,339] and modulates Fos expression in the VLPO and TM.[331]

SUMMARY

Sleep is a regulated physiologic state with clear implications for cognition, performance, and overall well-being. Although beyond the scope of this review, numerous sleep disorders have been described that negatively impact these functions. Sleep disturbances are also common to a number of psychiatric disorders. The neural substrates of sleep and wakefulness form a highly distributed and, to some extent, redundant network, with hypocretin, monoaminergic and cholinergic systems largely promoting wakefulness and GABAergic systems in the preoptic area, hypothalamus and brainstem promoting sleep. The hypocretin/orexin system seems to play a special role in the promotion of wakefulness and suppression of REM sleep by providing excitatory input to the monoaminergic and cholinergic systems. Sleep is not a unitary state but involves a cyclic alternation between NREM and REM sleep; the pons is critical for generating the multiple components (ie, EEG synchronization, eye movements, muscle atonia, and so forth) that characterize REM sleep. The timing of sleep and wakefulness is regulated by an interaction between the circadian pacemaker located in the hypothalamic SCN and a sleep homeostatic system whose anatomic location is yet to be convincingly identified. Among various neurochemicals, extracellular AD accumulates in the BF as wakefulness is extended and inhibits cortically projecting cholinergic neurons, thereby influencing cortical activity. A corticothalamocortical loop plays a major role in generating SWA measured in the EEG; cortical nNOS/NK1 neurons may be important in coordinating and/or propagating SWA within the cortex. Because the control of sleep and wakefulness involves a complex orchestration of the activity of many neural systems, it is readily apparent that many nodes for dysfunction exist that can have implications for both physical and mental health.

ACKNOWLEDGMENTS

The authors thank Drs Sarah Wurts Black, Stephen Morairty, and Gregory Parks for valuable comments on the article.

REFERENCES

1. Loomis AL, Harvey EN, Hobart G. Potential rhythms of the cerebral cortex during sleep. Science 1935;81(2111):597–8.
2. Szymusiak R. Hypothalamic versus neocortical control of sleep. Curr Opin Pulm Med 2010;16(6):530–5.
3. Siegel JM. The neurobiology of sleep. Semin Neurol 2009;29(4):277–96.
4. Rolls ET, Inoue K, Browning A. Activity of primate subgenual cingulate cortex neurons is related to sleep. J Neurophysiol 2003;90(1):134–42.
5. Rudolph M, Pospischil M, Timofeev I, et al. Inhibition determines membrane potential dynamics and controls action potential generation in awake and sleeping cat cortex. J Neurosci 2007;27(20):5280–90.
6. Brown RE, Basheer R, McKenna JT, et al. Control of sleep and wakefulness. Physiol Rev 2012;92(3):1087–187.
7. Saper CB, Fuller PM, Pedersen NP, et al. Sleep state switching. Neuron 2010; 68(6):1023–42.
8. Steriade M, McCormick DA, Sejnowski TJ. Thalamocortical oscillations in the sleeping and aroused brain. Science 1993;262(5134):679–85.
9. Crunelli V, Hughes SW. The slow (<1 Hz) rhythm of non-REM sleep: a dialogue between three cardinal oscillators. Nat Neurosci 2010;13(1):9–17.
10. Bremer F. Cerveau "isole" et physiologie du sommeil. C R Soc Biol (Paris) 1935; 118:1235–41.
11. Moruzzi G, Magoun H. Brainstem reticular formation and activation of the EEG. Electroencephalogr Clin Neurophysiol 1949;1:455–73.
12. Jones BE. From waking to sleeping: neuronal and chemical substrates. Trends Pharmacol Sci 2005;26(11):578–86.
13. Saper CB, Chou TC, Scammell TE. The sleep switch: hypothalamic control of sleep and wakefulness. Trends Neurosci 2001;24(12):726–31.
14. Steriade M, McCarley RW. Brain control of wakefulness and sleep. New York: Kluwer Academic/Plenum Publishers; 2005.
15. Carter ME, Yizhar O, Chikahisa S, et al. Tuning arousal with optogenetic modulation of locus coeruleus neurons. Nat Neurosci 2010;13(12):1526–33.
16. Ito H, Yanase M, Yamashita A, et al. Analysis of sleep disorders under pain using an optogenetic tool: possible involvement of the activation of dorsal raphe nucleus-serotonergic neurons. Mol Brain 2013;6:59.

17. McGinty D, Szymusiak R. Neural control of sleep in mammals. In: Siegel J, editor. Principles and practice of sleep medicine. 5th edition. St Louis (MO): Elsevier; 2011. p. 76–91.
18. Van Dort CJ, Zachs DP, Kenny JD, et al. Optogenetic activation of cholinergic neurons in the PPT or LDT induces REM sleep. Proc Natl Acad Sci U S A 2015;112(2):584–9.
19. Blanco-Centurion C, Gerashchenko D, Shiromani PJ. Effects of saporin-induced lesions of three arousal populations on daily levels of sleep and wake. J Neurosci 2007;27(51):14041–8.
20. Batini C, Moruzzi G, Palestini M, et al. Persistent patterns of wakefulness in the pretrigeminal midpontine preparation. Science 1958;128(3314):30–2.
21. Hess WR. Über die Wechselbeziehungen zwischen psychischen und vegetativen Funktionen. Schweiz Arch Neurol Psychiatr 1925;16:36–55.
22. Eguchi K, Satoh T. Characterization of the neurons in the region of solitary tract nucleus during sleep. Physiol Behav 1980;24(1):99–102.
23. Anaclet C, Ferrari L, Arrigoni E, et al. The GABAergic parafacial zone is a medullary slow wave sleep-promoting center. Nat Neurosci 2014;17(9):1217–24.
24. Anaclet C, Lin JS, Vetrivelan R, et al. Identification and characterization of a sleep-active cell group in the rostral medullary brainstem. J Neurosci 2012; 32(50):17970–6.
25. Fuller PM, Sherman D, Pedersen NP, et al. Reassessment of the structural basis of the ascending arousal system. J Comp Neurol 2011;519(5):933–56.
26. von Economo C. Sleep as a problem of localization. J Nerv Ment Dis 1930;71(3): 249–59.
27. Nauta WJH. Hypothalamic regulation of sleep in rats. An experimental study. J Neurophysiol 1946;9:285–316.
28. McGinty DJ, Sterman MB. Sleep suppression after basal forebrain lesions in the cat. Science 1968;160(833):1253–5.
29. Sterman MB, Clemente CD. Forebrain inhibitory mechanisms: sleep patterns induced by basal forebrain stimulation in the behaving cat. Exp Neurol 1962; 6:103–17.
30. Szymusiak R, McGinty D. Sleep-related neuronal discharge in the basal forebrain of cats. Brain Res 1986;370(1):82–92.
31. Sherin JE, Shiromani PJ, McCarley RW, et al. Activation of ventrolateral preoptic neurons during sleep. Science 1996;271(5246):216–9.
32. Szymusiak R, Alam N, Steininger TL, et al. Sleep-waking discharge patterns of ventrolateral preoptic/anterior hypothalamic neurons in rats. Brain Res 1998; 803(1–2):178–88.
33. Gong H, Szymusiak R, King J, et al. Sleep-related c-Fos protein expression in the preoptic hypothalamus: effects of ambient warming. Am J Physiol Regul Integr Comp Physiol 2000;279(6):R2079–88.
34. Suntsova N, Szymusiak R, Alam MN, et al. Sleep-waking discharge patterns of median preoptic nucleus neurons in rats. J Physiol 2002;543(Pt 2): 665–77.
35. Lu J, Greco MA, Shiromani P, et al. Effect of lesions of the ventrolateral preoptic nucleus on NREM and REM sleep. J Neurosci 2000;20(10):3830–42.
36. Chou TC, Bjorkum AA, Gaus SE, et al. Afferents to the ventrolateral preoptic nucleus. J Neurosci 2002;22(3):977–90.
37. Lu J, Bjorkum AA, Xu M, et al. Selective activation of the extended ventrolateral preoptic nucleus during rapid eye movement sleep. J Neurosci 2002;22(11): 4568–76.

38. Uschakov A, Gong H, McGinty D, et al. Efferent projections from the median preoptic nucleus to sleep- and arousal-regulatory nuclei in the rat brain. Neuroscience 2007;150(1):104–20.
39. Bai D, Renaud LP. Median preoptic nucleus neurons: an in vitro patch-clamp analysis of their intrinsic properties and noradrenergic receptors in the rat. Neuroscience 1998;83(3):905–16.
40. Gallopin T, Fort P, Eggermann E, et al. Identification of sleep-promoting neurons in vitro. Nature 2000;404(6781):992–5.
41. Szymusiak R. Magnocellular nuclei of the basal forebrain: substrates of sleep and arousal regulation. Sleep 1995;18(6):478–500.
42. Rye DB, Wainer BH, Mesulam MM, et al. Cortical projections arising from the basal forebrain: a study of cholinergic and noncholinergic components employing combined retrograde tracing and immunohistochemical localization of choline acetyltransferase. Neuroscience 1984;13(3):627–43.
43. Ranson SW. Somnolence caused by hypothalamic lesions in the monkey. Arch Neurol Psychiatry 1939;41(1):1–23.
44. Swett C, Hobson J. The effects of posterior hypothalamic lesions on behavioral and electrographic manifestations of sleep and waking in cats. Arch Ital Biol 1968;106:270–82.
45. Watanabe T, Taguchi Y, Shiosaka S, et al. Distribution of the histaminergic neuron system in the central nervous system of rats: a fluorescent immunohistochemical analysis with histidine decarboxylase as a marker. Brain Res 1984;295(1):13–25.
46. Parmentier R, Ohtsu H, Djebbara-Hannas Z, et al. Anatomical, physiological, and pharmacological characteristics of histidine decarboxylase knock-out mice: evidence for the role of brain histamine in behavioral and sleep-wake control. J Neurosci 2002;22(17):7695–711.
47. Anaclet C, Parmentier R, Ouk K, et al. Orexin/hypocretin and histamine: distinct roles in the control of wakefulness demonstrated using knock-out mouse models. J Neurosci 2009;29(46):14423–38.
48. Sherin JE, Elmquist JK, Torrealba F, et al. Innervation of histaminergic tuberomammillary neurons by GABAergic and galaninergic neurons in the ventrolateral preoptic nucleus of the rat. J Neurosci 1998;18(12):4705–21.
49. Schwartz JC, Arrang JM, Garbarg M, et al. Histaminergic transmission in the mammalian brain. Physiol Rev 1991;71(1):1–51.
50. Lin JS, Sakai K, Vanni-Mercier G, et al. A critical role of the posterior hypothalamus in the mechanisms of wakefulness determined by microinjection of muscimol in freely moving cats. Brain Res 1989;479(2):225–40.
51. Aserinsky E, Kleitman N. Regularly occurring periods of eye motility, and concomitant phenomena, during sleep. Science 1953;118(3062):273–4.
52. Aserinsky E, Kleitman N. Two types of ocular motility occurring in sleep. J Appl Physiol 1955;8(1):1–10.
53. Dement W, Kleitman N. Cyclic variations in EEG during sleep and their relation to eye movements, body motility, and dreaming. Electroencephalogr Clin Neurophysiol 1957;9(4):673–90.
54. Jouvet M, Michel F, Courjon J. On a stage of rapid cerebral electrical activity in the course of physiological sleep. C R Seances Soc Biol Fil 1959;153:1024–8 [in French].
55. Evarts EV, Bental E, Bihari B, et al. Spontaneous discharge of single neurons during sleep and waking. Science 1962;135:726–8.
56. McCarley RW, Hobson JA. Cortical unit activity in desynchronized sleep. Science 1970;167(919):901–3.

57. Siegel JM, McGinty DJ. Brainstem neurons without spontaneous unit discharge. Science 1976;193(4249):240–2.
58. Hobson JA, McCarley RW, Wyzinski PW. Sleep cycle oscillation: reciprocal discharge by two brainstem neuronal groups. Science 1975;189(4196):55–8.
59. McCarley RW, Hobson JA. Neuronal excitability modulation over the sleep cycle: a structural and mathematical model. Science 1975;189(4196):58–60.
60. McCarley RW. Mechanisms and models of REM sleep control. Arch Ital Biol 2004;142(4):429–67.
61. McCarley RW, Massaquoi SG. Neurobiological structure of the revised limit cycle reciprocal interaction model of REM cycle control. J Sleep Res 1992;1(2):132–7.
62. McCarley RW. Neurobiology of REM and NREM sleep. Sleep Med 2007;8(4): 302–30.
63. Lu J, Sherman D, Devor M, et al. A putative flip-flop switch for control of REM sleep. Nature 2006;441(7093):589–94.
64. Luppi PH, Clement O, Fort P. Paradoxical (REM) sleep genesis by the brainstem is under hypothalamic control. Curr Opin Neurobiol 2013;23(5):786–92.
65. Siegel JM, Nienhuis R, Tomaszewski KS. Rostral brainstem contributes to medullary inhibition of muscle tone. Brain Res 1983;268(2):344–8.
66. Siegel JM, Nienhuis R, Tomaszewski KS. REM sleep signs rostral to chronic transections at the pontomedullary junction. Neurosci Lett 1984;45(3):241–6.
67. Sastre JP, Sakai K, Jouvet M. Are the gigantocellular tegmental field neurons responsible for paradoxical sleep? Brain Res 1981;229(1):147–61.
68. Katayama Y, DeWitt DS, Becker DP, et al. Behavioral evidence for a cholinoceptive pontine inhibitory area: descending control of spinal motor output and sensory input. Brain Res 1984;296(2):241–62.
69. Steriade M, Datta S, Pare D, et al. Neuronal activities in brain-stem cholinergic nuclei related to tonic activation processes in thalamocortical systems. J Neurosci 1990;10(8):2541–59.
70. el Mansari M, Sakai K, Jouvet M. Unitary characteristics of presumptive cholinergic tegmental neurons during the sleep-waking cycle in freely moving cats. Exp Brain Res 1989;76(3):519–29.
71. Kodama T, Takahashi Y, Honda Y. Enhancement of acetylcholine release during paradoxical sleep in the dorsal tegmental field of the cat brain stem. Neurosci Lett 1990;114(3):277–82.
72. Greene RW, Gerber U, McCarley RW. Cholinergic activation of medial pontine reticular formation neurons in vitro. Brain Res 1989;476(1):154–9.
73. Brown RE, Winston S, Basheer R, et al. Electrophysiological characterization of neurons in the dorsolateral pontine rapid-eye-movement sleep induction zone of the rat: intrinsic membrane properties and responses to carbachol and orexins. Neuroscience 2006;143(3):739–55.
74. Clement O, Sapin E, Libourel PA, et al. The lateral hypothalamic area controls paradoxical (REM) sleep by means of descending projections to brainstem GABAergic neurons. J Neurosci 2012;32(47):16763–74.
75. Jouvet M, Delorme F. Locus coeruleus et sommeil paradoxal. C R Seances Soc Biol Fil 1965;159:895–9.
76. Henley K, Morrison AR. A re-evaluation of the effects of lesions of the pontine tegmentum and locus coeruleus on phenomena of paradoxical sleep in the cat. Acta Neurobiol Exp (Wars) 1974;34(2):215–32.
77. Chase MH, Soja PJ, Morales FR. Evidence that glycine mediates the postsynaptic potentials that inhibit lumbar motoneurons during the atonia of active sleep. J Neurosci 1989;9(3):743–51.

78. Brooks PL, Peever JH. Glycinergic and GABA(A)-mediated inhibition of somatic motoneurons does not mediate rapid eye movement sleep motor atonia. J Neurosci 2008;28(14):3535–45.
79. Brooks PL, Peever JH. Identification of the transmitter and receptor mechanisms responsible for REM sleep paralysis. J Neurosci 2012;32(29):9785–95.
80. Krenzer M, Anaclet C, Vetrivelan R, et al. Brainstem and spinal cord circuitry regulating REM sleep and muscle atonia. PLoS One 2011;6(10):e24998.
81. Schenck CH, Bundlie SR, Patterson AL, et al. Rapid eye movement sleep behavior disorder. A treatable parasomnia affecting older adults. JAMA 1987; 257(13):1786–9.
82. Boeve BF, Silber MH, Saper CB, et al. Pathophysiology of REM sleep behaviour disorder and relevance to neurodegenerative disease. Brain 2007;130(Pt 11): 2770–88.
83. McCarter SJ, St Louis EK, Boeve BF. REM sleep behavior disorder and REM sleep without atonia as an early manifestation of degenerative neurological disease. Curr Neurol Neurosci Rep 2012;12(2):182–92.
84. Burgess CR, Oishi Y, Mochizuki T, et al. Amygdala lesions reduce cataplexy in orexin knock-out mice. J Neurosci 2013;33(23):9734–42.
85. Oishi Y, Williams RH, Agostinelli L, et al. Role of the medial prefrontal cortex in cataplexy. J Neurosci 2013;33(23):9743–51.
86. Boehme RE, Baker TL, Mefford IN, et al. Narcolepsy: cholinergic receptor changes in an animal model. Life Sci 1984;34(19):1825–8.
87. Kilduff TS, Bowersox SS, Kaitin KI, et al. Muscarinic cholinergic receptors and the canine model of narcolepsy. Sleep 1986;9(1 Pt 2):102–6.
88. Lin L, Faraco J, Li R, et al. The sleep disorder canine narcolepsy is caused by a mutation in the hypocretin (orexin) receptor 2 gene. Cell 1999;98(3):365–76.
89. de Lecea L, Kilduff TS, Peyron C, et al. The hypocretins: hypothalamus-specific peptides with neuroexcitatory activity. Proc Natl Acad Sci U S A 1998;95(1): 322–7.
90. Sakurai T, Amemiya A, Ishii M, et al. Orexins and orexin receptors: a family of hypothalamic neuropeptides and G protein-coupled receptors that regulate feeding behavior. Cell 1998;92(4):573–85.
91. Sakurai T, Amemiya A, Ishii M, et al. Orexins and orexin receptors: a family of hypothalamic neuropeptides and G protein-coupled receptors that regulate feeding behavior. Cell 1998;92(5):696.
92. Peyron C, Tighe DK, van den Pol AN, et al. Neurons containing hypocretin (orexin) project to multiple neuronal systems. J Neurosci 1998;18(23): 9996–10015.
93. Harrison TA, Chen CT, Dun NJ, et al. Hypothalamic orexin A-immunoreactive neurons project to the rat dorsal medulla. Neurosci Lett 1999;273(1):17–20.
94. Kilduff TS, Peyron C. The hypocretin/orexin ligand-receptor system: implications for sleep and sleep disorders. Trends Neurosci 2000;23(8):359–65.
95. Thannickal T, Moore RY, Nienhuis R, et al. Reduced number of hypocretin neurons in human narcolepsy. Neuron 2000;27(3):469–74.
96. Date Y, Ueta Y, Yamashita H, et al. Orexins, orexigenic hypothalamic peptides, interact with autonomic, neuroendocrine and neuroregulatory systems. Proc Natl Acad Sci U S A 1999;96(2):748–53.
97. Broberger C, De Lecea L, Sutcliffe JG, et al. Hypocretin/orexin- and melanin-concentrating hormone-expressing cells form distinct populations in the rodent lateral hypothalamus: relationship to the neuropeptide Y and agouti gene-related protein systems. J Comp Neurol 1998;402(4):460–74.

98. Elias CF, Saper CB, Maratos-Flier E, et al. Chemically defined projections linking the mediobasal hypothalamus and the lateral hypothalamic area. J Comp Neurol 1998;402(4):442–59.
99. Nambu T, Sakurai T, Mizukami K, et al. Distribution of orexin neurons in the adult rat brain. Brain Res 1999;827(1–2):243–60.
100. van den Pol AN. Hypothalamic hypocretin (orexin): robust innervation of the spinal cord. J Neurosci 1999;19(8):3171–82.
101. Chemelli RM, Willie JT, Sinton CM, et al. Narcolepsy in orexin knockout mice: molecular genetics of sleep regulation. Cell 1999;98(4):437–51.
102. Horvath TL, Peyron C, Diano S, et al. Hypocretin (orexin) activation and synaptic innervation of the locus coeruleus noradrenergic system. J Comp Neurol 1999; 415(2):145–59.
103. Espana RA, Reis KM, Valentino RJ, et al. Organization of hypocretin/orexin efferents to locus coeruleus and basal forebrain arousal-related structures. J Comp Neurol 2005;481(2):160–78.
104. Yoshida K, McCormack S, Espana RA, et al. Afferents to the orexin neurons of the rat brain. J Comp Neurol 2006;494(5):845–61.
105. Sakurai T, Nagata R, Yamanaka A, et al. Input of orexin/hypocretin neurons revealed by a genetically encoded tracer in mice. Neuron 2005;46(2): 297–308.
106. Hagan JJ, Leslie RA, Patel S, et al. Orexin A activates locus coeruleus cell firing and increases arousal in the rat. Proc Natl Acad Sci U S A 1999;96(19):10911–6.
107. Soffin EM, Evans ML, Gill CH, et al. SB-334867-A antagonises orexin mediated excitation in the locus coeruleus. Neuropharmacology 2002;42(1):127–33.
108. Brown RE, Sergeeva O, Eriksson KS, et al. Orexin A excites serotonergic neurons in the dorsal raphe nucleus of the rat. Neuropharmacology 2001;40(3): 457–9.
109. Liu RJ, van den Pol AN, Aghajanian GK. Hypocretins (orexins) regulate serotonin neurons in the dorsal raphe nucleus by excitatory direct and inhibitory indirect actions. J Neurosci 2002;22(21):9453–64.
110. Eriksson KS, Sergeeva O, Brown RS, et al. Orexin/hypocretin excites the histaminergic neurons of the tuberomammillary nucleus. J Neurosci 2001;21(23): 9273–9.
111. Bayer L, Eggermann E, Serafin M, et al. Orexins (hypocretins) directly excite tuberomammillary neurons. Eur J Neurosci 2001;14(9):1571–5.
112. Yamanaka A, Tsujino N, Funahashi H, et al. Orexins activate histaminergic neurons via the orexin 2 receptor. Biochem Biophys Res Commun 2002;290(4): 1237–45.
113. Burlet S, Tyler CJ, Leonard CS. Direct and indirect excitation of laterodorsal tegmental neurons by hypocretin/orexin peptides: implications for wakefulness and narcolepsy. J Neurosci 2002;22(7):2862–72.
114. Takahashi K, Koyama Y, Kayama Y, et al. Effects of orexin on the laterodorsal tegmental neurones. Psychiatry Clin Neurosci 2002;56(3):335–6.
115. Eggermann E, Serafin M, Bayer L, et al. Orexins/hypocretins excite basal forebrain cholinergic neurones. Neuroscience 2001;108(2):177–81.
116. Borgland SL, Taha SA, Sarti F, et al. Orexin A in the VTA is critical for the induction of synaptic plasticity and behavioral sensitization to cocaine. Neuron 2006; 49(4):589–601.
117. Korotkova TM, Sergeeva OA, Eriksson KS, et al. Excitation of ventral tegmental area dopaminergic and nondopaminergic neurons by orexins/hypocretins. J Neurosci 2003;23(1):7–11.

118. van den Pol AN, Gao XB, Obrietan K, et al. Presynaptic and postsynaptic actions and modulation of neuroendocrine neurons by a new hypothalamic peptide, hypocretin/orexin. J Neurosci 1998;18(19):7962–71.
119. Ivanov A, Aston-Jones G. Hypocretin/orexin depolarizes and decreases potassium conductance in locus coeruleus neurons. Neuroreport 2000;11(8):1755–8.
120. Hoang QV, Bajic D, Yanagisawa M, et al. Effects of orexin (hypocretin) on GIRK channels. J Neurophysiol 2003;90(2):693–702.
121. Hoang QV, Zhao P, Nakajima S, et al. Orexin (hypocretin) effects on constitutively active inward rectifier K+ channels in cultured nucleus basalis neurons. J Neurophysiol 2004;92(6):3183–91.
122. Hwang LL, Chen CT, Dun NJ. Mechanisms of orexin-induced depolarizations in rat dorsal motor nucleus of vagus neurones in vitro. J Physiol 2001;537(Pt 2):511–20.
123. Yang B, Ferguson AV. Orexin-A depolarizes dissociated rat area postrema neurons through activation of a nonselective cationic conductance. J Neurosci 2002;22(15):6303–8.
124. Yang B, Ferguson AV. Orexin-A depolarizes nucleus tractus solitarius neurons through effects on nonselective cationic and K+ conductances. J Neurophysiol 2003;89(4):2167–75.
125. Yang B, Samson WK, Ferguson AV. Excitatory effects of orexin-A on nucleus tractus solitarius neurons are mediated by phospholipase C and protein kinase C. J Neurosci 2003;23(15):6215–22.
126. Follwell MJ, Ferguson AV. Cellular mechanisms of orexin actions on paraventricular nucleus neurones in rat hypothalamus. J Physiol 2002;545(Pt 3):855–67.
127. Smith BN, Davis SF, Van Den Pol AN, et al. Selective enhancement of excitatory synaptic activity in the rat nucleus tractus solitarius by hypocretin 2. Neuroscience 2002;115(3):707–14.
128. Xi MC, Fung SJ, Yamuy J, et al. Hypocretinergic facilitation of synaptic activity of neurons in the nucleus pontis oralis of the cat. Brain Res 2003;976(2):253–8.
129. Davis SF, Williams KW, Xu W, et al. Selective enhancement of synaptic inhibition by hypocretin (orexin) in rat vagal motor neurons: implications for autonomic regulation. J Neurosci 2003;23(9):3844–54.
130. Chou TC, Lee CE, Lu J, et al. Orexin (hypocretin) neurons contain dynorphin. J Neurosci 2001;21(19):RC168.
131. Hakansson M, de Lecea L, Sutcliffe JG, et al. Leptin receptor- and STAT3-immunoreactivities in hypocretin/orexin neurones of the lateral hypothalamus. J Neuroendocrinol 1999;11(8):653–63.
132. Risold PY, Griffond B, Kilduff TS, et al. Preprohypocretin (orexin) and prolactin-like immunoreactivity are coexpressed by neurons of the rat lateral hypothalamic area. Neurosci Lett 1999;259(3):153–6.
133. Torrealba F, Yanagisawa M, Saper CB. Colocalization of orexin a and glutamate immunoreactivity in axon terminals in the tuberomammillary nucleus in rats. Neuroscience 2003;119(4):1033–44.
134. Henny P, Brischoux F, Mainville L, et al. Immunohistochemical evidence for synaptic release of glutamate from orexin terminals in the locus coeruleus. Neuroscience 2010;169(3):1150–7.
135. Schone C, Apergis-Schoute J, Sakurai T, et al. Coreleased orexin and glutamate evoke nonredundant spike outputs and computations in histamine neurons. Cell Rep 2014;7(3):697–704.
136. Li Y, Gao XB, Sakurai T, et al. Hypocretin/Orexin excites hypocretin neurons via a local glutamate neuron-A potential mechanism for orchestrating the hypothalamic arousal system. Neuron 2002;36(6):1169–81.

137. Yamanaka A, Beuckmann CT, Willie JT, et al. Hypothalamic orexin neurons regulate arousal according to energy balance in mice. Neuron 2003;38(5):701–13.
138. Hara J, Gerashchenko D, Wisor JP, et al. Thyrotropin-releasing hormone increases behavioral arousal through modulation of hypocretin/orexin neurons. J Neurosci 2009;29(12):3705–14.
139. Yamanaka A, Muraki Y, Tsujino N, et al. Regulation of orexin neurons by the monoaminergic and cholinergic systems. Biochem Biophys Res Commun 2003;303(1):120–9.
140. Wollmann G, Acuna-Goycolea C, van den Pol AN. Direct excitation of hypocretin/orexin cells by extracellular ATP at P2X receptors. J Neurophysiol 2005;94(3): 2195–206.
141. Winsky-Sommerer R, Yamanaka A, Diano S, et al. Interaction between the corticotropin-releasing factor system and hypocretins (orexins): a novel circuit mediating the stress response. J Neurosci 2004;24(50):11439–48.
142. Acuna-Goycolea C, van den Pol A. Glucagon-like peptide 1 excites hypocretin/orexin neurons by direct and indirect mechanisms: implications for viscera-mediated arousal. J Neurosci 2004;24(37):8141–52.
143. Tsujino N, Yamanaka A, Ichiki K, et al. Cholecystokinin activates orexin/hypocretin neurons through the cholecystokinin A receptor. J Neurosci 2005;25(32):7459–69.
144. Burdakov D, Alexopoulos H. Metabolic state signalling through central hypocretin/orexin neurons. J Cell Mol Med 2005;9(4):795–803.
145. Burdakov D, Jensen LT, Alexopoulos H, et al. Tandem-pore K+ channels mediate inhibition of orexin neurons by glucose. Neuron 2006;50(5):711–22.
146. Li Y, van den Pol AN. Direct and indirect inhibition by catecholamines of hypocretin/orexin neurons. J Neurosci 2005;25(1):173–83.
147. Muraki Y, Yamanaka A, Tsujino N, et al. Serotonergic regulation of the orexin/hypocretin neurons through the 5-HT1A receptor. J Neurosci 2004;24(32): 7159–66.
148. Yamanaka A, Muraki Y, Ichiki K, et al. Orexin neurons are directly and indirectly regulated by catecholamines in a complex manner. J Neurophysiol 2006;96(1): 284–98.
149. Xie X, Crowder TL, Yamanaka A, et al. GABA(B) receptor-mediated modulation of hypocretin/orexin neurones in mouse hypothalamus. J Physiol 2006;574(Pt 2): 399–414.
150. Estabrooke IV, McCarthy MT, Ko E, et al. Fos expression in orexin neurons varies with behavioral state. J Neurosci 2001;21(5):1656–62.
151. Lee MG, Hassani OK, Jones BE. Discharge of identified orexin/hypocretin neurons across the sleep-waking cycle. J Neurosci 2005;25(28):6716–20.
152. Mileykovskiy BY, Kiyashchenko LI, Siegel JM. Behavioral correlates of activity in identified hypocretin/orexin neurons. Neuron 2005;46(5):787–98.
153. Takahashi K, Lin JS, Sakai K. Neuronal activity of orexin and non-orexin waking-active neurons during wake-sleep states in the mouse. Neuroscience 2008; 153(3):860–70.
154. Kiyashchenko LI, Mileykovskiy BY, Maidment N, et al. Release of hypocretin (orexin) during waking and sleep states. J Neurosci 2002;22(13):5282–6.
155. Salomon RM, Ripley B, Kennedy JS, et al. Diurnal variation of cerebrospinal fluid hypocretin-1 (Orexin-A) levels in control and depressed subjects. Biol Psychiatry 2003;54(2):96–104.
156. Zeitzer JM, Buckmaster CL, Parker KJ, et al. Circadian and homeostatic regulation of hypocretin in a primate model: implications for the consolidation of wakefulness. J Neurosci 2003;23(8):3555–60.

157. Bourgin P, Huitron-Resendiz S, Spier AD, et al. Hypocretin-1 modulates REM sleep through activation of locus coeruleus neurons. J Neurosci 2000;20(20): 7760–5.
158. Espana RA, Baldo BA, Kelley AE, et al. Wake-promoting and sleep-suppressing actions of hypocretin (orexin): basal forebrain sites of action. Neuroscience 2001;106(4):699–715.
159. Methippara MM, Alam MN, Szymusiak R, et al. Effects of lateral preoptic area application of orexin-A on sleep-wakefulness. Neuroreport 2000;11(16):3423–6.
160. Piper DC, Upton N, Smith MI, et al. The novel brain neuropeptide, orexin-A, modulates the sleep-wake cycle of rats. Eur J Neurosci 2000;12(2):726–30.
161. Xi M, Morales FR, Chase MH. Effects on sleep and wakefulness of the injection of hypocretin-1 (orexin-A) into the laterodorsal tegmental nucleus of the cat. Brain Res 2001;901(1–2):259–64.
162. Morairty SR, Wisor J, Silveira K, et al. The wake-promoting effects of hypocretin-1 are attenuated in old rats. Neurobiol Aging 2011;32(8):1514–27.
163. Adamantidis AR, Zhang F, Aravanis AM, et al. Neural substrates of awakening probed with optogenetic control of hypocretin neurons. Nature 2007; 450(7168):420–4.
164. Carter ME, Adamantidis A, Ohtsu H, et al. Sleep homeostasis modulates hypocretin-mediated sleep-to-wake transitions. J Neurosci 2009;29(35): 10939–49.
165. Carter ME, Brill J, Bonnavion P, et al. Mechanism for Hypocretin-mediated sleep-to-wake transitions. Proc Natl Acad Sci U S A 2012;109(39):E2635–44.
166. Tsunematsu T, Kilduff TS, Boyden ES, et al. Acute optogenetic silencing of orexin/hypocretin neurons induces slow-wave sleep in mice. J Neurosci 2011; 31(29):10529–39.
167. Tsunematsu T, Tabuchi S, Tanaka KF, et al. Long-lasting silencing of orexin/hypocretin neurons using archaerhodopsin induces slow-wave sleep in mice. Behav Brain Res 2013;255:64–74.
168. Vazquez-DeRose J, Schwartz MD, Nguyen AT, et al. Hypocretin/orexin antagonism enhances sleep-related adenosine and GABA neurotransmission in rat basal forebrain. Brain Struct Funct 2014. [Epub ahead of print].
169. Winrow CJ, Gotter AL, Cox CD, et al. Promotion of sleep by suvorexant-a novel dual orexin receptor antagonist. J Neurogenet 2011;25(1–2):52–61.
170. Brisbare-Roch C, Dingemanse J, Koberstein R, et al. Promotion of sleep by targeting the orexin system in rats, dogs and humans. Nat Med 2007;13(2):150–5.
171. Morairty SR, Revel FG, Malherbe P, et al. Dual hypocretin receptor antagonism is more effective for sleep promotion than antagonism of either receptor alone. PLoS One 2012;7(7):e39131.
172. Morairty S, Wilk AJ, Lincoln WU, et al. The hypocretin/orexin antagonist almorexant promotes sleep without impairment of performance in rats. Front Neurosci 2014;8:3.
173. Uslaner JM, Tye SJ, Eddins DM, et al. Orexin receptor antagonists differ from standard sleep drugs by promoting sleep at doses that do not disrupt cognition. Sci Transl Med 2013;5(179):179ra144.
174. Mignot E. Genetic and familial aspects of narcolepsy. Neurology 1998;50(2 Suppl 1):S16–22.
175. Mignot E, Tafti M, Dement WC, et al. Narcolepsy and immunity. Adv Neuroimmunol 1995;5(1):23–37.
176. Partinen M, Kornum BR, Plazzi G, et al. Narcolepsy as an autoimmune disease: the role of H1N1 infection and vaccination. Lancet Neurol 2014;13(6):600–13.

177. Nishino S, Ripley B, Overeem S, et al. Hypocretin (orexin) deficiency in human narcolepsy. Lancet 2000;355(9197):39–40.
178. Peyron C, Faraco J, Rogers W, et al. A mutation in a case of early onset narcolepsy and a generalized absence of hypocretin peptides in human narcoleptic brains. Nat Med 2000;6(9):991–7.
179. Gerashchenko D, Kohls MD, Greco MA, et al. Hypocretin-2-saporin lesions of the lateral hypothalamus produce narcoleptic-like sleep behavior in the rat. J Neurosci 2001;21(18):7273–83.
180. Gerashchenko D, Blanco-Centurion C, Greco MA, et al. Effects of lateral hypothalamic lesion with the neurotoxin hypocretin-2-saporin on sleep in Long-Evans rats. Neuroscience 2003;116(1):223–35.
181. Hara J, Beuckmann CT, Nambu T, et al. Genetic ablation of orexin neurons in mice results in narcolepsy, hypophagia, and obesity. Neuron 2001;30(2): 345–54.
182. Tabuchi S, Tsunematsu T, Black SW, et al. Conditional ablation of orexin/hypocretin neurons: a new mouse model for the study of narcolepsy and orexin system function. J Neurosci 2014;34(19):6495–509.
183. Mochizuki T, Crocker A, McCormack S, et al. Behavioral state instability in orexin knock-out mice. J Neurosci 2004;24(28):6291–300.
184. Rechtschaffen A, Gilliland MA, Bergmann BM, et al. Physiological correlates of prolonged sleep deprivation in rats. Science 1983;221(4606):182–4.
185. Borbely AA. A two process model of sleep regulation. Hum Neurobiol 1982;1(3): 195–204.
186. Daan S, Beersma DG, Borbely AA. Timing of human sleep: recovery process gated by a circadian pacemaker. Am J Physiol 1984;246(2 Pt 2): R161–83.
187. Yasenkov R, Deboer T. Circadian regulation of sleep and the sleep EEG under constant sleep pressure in the rat. Sleep 2010;33(5):631–41.
188. Yasenkov R, Deboer T. Interrelations and circadian changes of electroencephalogram frequencies under baseline conditions and constant sleep pressure in the rat. Neuroscience 2011;180:212–21.
189. Stephan FK, Zucker I. Circadian rhythms in drinking behavior and locomotor activity are eliminated by suprachiasmatic lesions. Proc Natl Acad Sci U S A 1972; 69(6):1583–6.
190. Moore RY, Eichler VB. Loss of circadian adrenal corticosterone rhythm following suprachiasmatic nucleus lesion in the rat. Brain Res 1972;42:201–6.
191. Ralph MR, Foster RG, Davis FC, et al. Transplanted suprachiasmatic nucleus determines circadian period. Science 1990;247(4945):975–8.
192. Inouye S-IT, Kawamura H. Persistence of circadian rhythmicity in a hypothalamic 'island' containing the suprachiasmatic nucleus. Proc Natl Acad Sci U S A 1979; 76:5962–6.
193. Ibuka N, Inouye SI, Kawamura H. Analysis of sleep-wakefulness rhythms in male rats after suprachiasmatic nucleus lesions and ocular enucleation. Brain Res 1977;122(1):33–47.
194. Ibuka N, Kawamura H. Loss of circadian rhythm in sleep-wakefulness cycle in the rat by suprachiasmatic nucleus lesions. Brain Res 1975;96(1):76–81.
195. Mouret J, Coindet J, Debilly G, et al. Suprachiasmatic nuclei lesions in the rat: alterations in sleep circadian rhythms. Electroencephalogr Clin Neurophysiol 1978;45(3):402–8.
196. Tobler I, Borbely AA, Groos G. The effect of sleep deprivation on sleep in rats with suprachiasmatic lesions. Neurosci Lett 1983;42(1):49–54.

197. Mistlberger RE, Bergmann BM, Waldenar W, et al. Recovery sleep following sleep deprivation in intact and suprachiasmatic nuclei-lesioned rats. Sleep 1983;6(3):217–33.
198. Easton A, Meerlo P, Bergmann B, et al. The suprachiasmatic nucleus regulates sleep timing and amount in mice. Sleep 2004;27(7):1307–18.
199. Edgar DM, Dement WC, Fuller CA. Effect of SCN lesions on sleep in squirrel monkeys: evidence for opponent processes in sleep-wake regulation. J Neurosci 1993;13(3):1065–79.
200. Larkin JE, Yokogawa T, Heller HC, et al. Homeostatic regulation of sleep in arrhythmic Siberian hamsters. Am J Physiol Regul Integr Comp Physiol 2004; 287(1):R104–11.
201. Mistlberger RE. Circadian regulation of sleep in mammals: role of the suprachiasmatic nucleus. Brain Res Brain Res Rev 2005;49(3):429–54.
202. Deboer T, Overeem S, Visser NA, et al. Convergence of circadian and sleep regulatory mechanisms on hypocretin-1. Neuroscience 2004;129(3):727–32.
203. Fujiki N, Yoshida Y, Ripley B, et al. Changes in CSF hypocretin-1 (orexin A) levels in rats across 24 hours and in response to food deprivation. Neuroreport 2001; 12(5):993–7.
204. Wu MF, John J, Maidment N, et al. Hypocretin release in normal and narcoleptic dogs after food and sleep deprivation, eating, and movement. Am J Physiol Regul Integr Comp Physiol 2002;283(5):R1079–86.
205. Deboer T, Detari L, Meijer JH. Long term effects of sleep deprivation on the mammalian circadian pacemaker. Sleep 2007;30(3):257–62.
206. Deboer T, Vansteensel MJ, Detari L, et al. Sleep states alter activity of suprachiasmatic nucleus neurons. Nat Neurosci 2003;6(10):1086–90.
207. Cambras T, Weller JR, Angles-Pujoras M, et al. Circadian desynchronization of core body temperature and sleep stages in the rat. Proc Natl Acad Sci U S A 2007;104(18):7634–9.
208. Lee ML, Swanson BE, de la Iglesia HO. Circadian timing of REM sleep is coupled to an oscillator within the dorsomedial suprachiasmatic nucleus. Curr Biol 2009;19(10):848–52.
209. Wurts SW, Edgar DM. Circadian and homeostatic control of rapid eye movement (REM) sleep: promotion of REM tendency by the suprachiasmatic nucleus. J Neurosci 2000;20(11):4300–10.
210. Reppert SM, Weaver DR. Coordination of circadian timing in mammals. Nature 2002;418(6901):935–41.
211. Takahashi JS, Hong HK, Ko CH, et al. The genetics of mammalian circadian order and disorder: implications for physiology and disease. Nat Rev Genet 2008; 9(10):764–75.
212. Dudley CA, Erbel-Sieler C, Estill SJ, et al. Altered patterns of sleep and behavioral adaptability in NPAS2-deficient mice. Science 2003;301(5631):379–83.
213. Laposky A, Easton A, Dugovic C, et al. Deletion of the mammalian circadian clock gene BMAL1/Mop3 alters baseline sleep architecture and the response to sleep deprivation. Sleep 2005;28(4):395–409.
214. Naylor E, Bergmann BM, Krauski K, et al. The circadian clock mutation alters sleep homeostasis in the mouse. J Neurosci 2000;20(21):8138–43.
215. Shiromani PJ, Xu M, Winston EM, et al. Sleep rhythmicity and homeostasis in mice with targeted disruption of mPeriod genes. Am J Physiol Regul Integr Comp Physiol 2004;287(1):R47–57.
216. Wisor JP, O'Hara BF, Terao A, et al. A role for cryptochromes in sleep regulation. BMC Neurosci 2002;3:20.

217. Curie T, Maret S, Emmenegger Y, et al. In vivo imaging of the central and peripheral effects of sleep deprivation and suprachiasmatic nuclei lesion on PERIOD-2 protein in mice. Sleep 2015. [Epub ahead of print].
218. Franken P, Thomason R, Heller HC, et al. A non-circadian role for clock-genes in sleep homeostasis: a strain comparison. BMC Neurosci 2007;8:87.
219. Mongrain V, La Spada F, Curie T, et al. Sleep loss reduces the DNA-binding of BMAL1, CLOCK, and NPAS2 to specific clock genes in the mouse cerebral cortex. PLoS One 2011;6(10):e26622.
220. Thompson CL, Wisor JP, Lee CK, et al. Molecular and anatomical signatures of sleep deprivation in the mouse brain. Front Neurosci 2010;4:165.
221. Wisor JP, Pasumarthi RK, Gerashchenko D, et al. Sleep deprivation effects on circadian clock gene expression in the cerebral cortex parallel electroencephalographic differences among mouse strains. J Neurosci 2008;28(28):7193–201.
222. Suntsova N, Guzman-Marin R, Kumar S, et al. The median preoptic nucleus reciprocally modulates activity of arousal-related and sleep-related neurons in the perifornical lateral hypothalamus. J Neurosci 2007;27(7):1616–30.
223. Gvilia I, Xu F, McGinty D, et al. Homeostatic regulation of sleep: a role for preoptic area neurons. J Neurosci 2006;26(37):9426–33.
224. Gvilia I, Turner A, McGinty D, et al. Preoptic area neurons and the homeostatic regulation of rapid eye movement sleep. J Neurosci 2006;26(11):3037–44.
225. Gerashchenko D, Wisor JP, Burns D, et al. Identification of a population of sleep-active cerebral cortex neurons. Proc Natl Acad Sci U S A 2008;105(29):10227–32.
226. Pasumarthi RK, Gerashchenko D, Kilduff TS. Further characterization of sleep-active neuronal nitric oxide synthase neurons in the mouse brain. Neuroscience 2010;169(1):149–57.
227. Vaucher E, Linville D, Hamel E. Cholinergic basal forebrain projections to nitric oxide synthase-containing neurons in the rat cerebral cortex. Neuroscience 1997;79(3):827–36.
228. Cauli B, Tong XK, Rancillac A, et al. Cortical GABA interneurons in neurovascular coupling: relays for subcortical vasoactive pathways. J Neurosci 2004; 24(41):8940–9.
229. Tomioka R, Okamoto K, Furuta T, et al. Demonstration of long-range GABAergic connections distributed throughout the mouse neocortex. Eur J Neurosci 2005; 21(6):1587–600.
230. Tomioka R, Rockland KS. Long-distance corticocortical GABAergic neurons in the adult monkey white and gray matter. J Comp Neurol 2007;505(5):526–38.
231. Higo S, Akashi K, Sakimura K, et al. Subtypes of GABAergic neurons project axons in the neocortex. Front Neuroanat 2009;3:25.
232. Higo S, Udaka N, Tamamaki N. Long-range GABAergic projection neurons in the cat neocortex. J Comp Neurol 2007;503(3):421–31.
233. Morairty SR, Dittrich L, Pasumarthi RK, et al. A role for cortical nNOS/NK1 neurons in coupling homeostatic sleep drive to EEG slow wave activity. Proc Natl Acad Sci U S A 2013;110(50):20272–7.
234. Dittrich L, Morairty SR, Warrier DR, et al. Homeostatic sleep pressure is the primary factor for activation of cortical nNOS/NK1 neurons. Neuropsychopharmacology 2015;40(3):632–9.
235. Kilduff TS, Cauli B, Gerashchenko D. Activation of cortical interneurons during sleep: an anatomical link to homeostatic sleep regulation? Trends Neurosci 2011;34(1):10–9.
236. Krueger JM, Obal FJ, Fang J, et al. The role of cytokines in physiological sleep regulation. Ann N Y Acad Sci 2001;933:211–21.

237. Majde JA, Krueger JM. Links between the innate immune system and sleep. J Allergy Clin Immunol 2005;116(6):1188–98.
238. Ehlers CL, Reed TK, Henriksen SJ. Effects of corticotropin-releasing factor and growth hormone-releasing factor on sleep and activity in rats. Neuroendocrinology 1986;42(6):467–74.
239. Opp M, Obal F Jr, Krueger JM. Corticotropin-releasing factor attenuates interleukin 1-induced sleep and fever in rabbits. Am J Physiol 1989;257(3 Pt 2): R528–35.
240. Chastrette N, Cespuglio R, Jouvet M. Proopiomelanocortin (POMC)-derived peptides and sleep in the rat. Part 1–hypnogenic properties of ACTH derivatives. Neuropeptides 1990;15(2):61–74.
241. Nishino S, Arrigoni J, Shelton J, et al. Effects of thyrotropin-releasing hormone and its analogs on daytime sleepiness and cataplexy in canine narcolepsy. J Neurosci 1997;17(16):6401–8.
242. Riehl J, Honda K, Kwan M, et al. Chronic oral administration of CG-3703, a thyrotropin releasing hormone analog, increases wake and decreases cataplexy in canine narcolepsy. Neuropsychopharmacology 2000;23(1):34–45.
243. Hemmeter U, Rothe B, Guldner J, et al. Effects of thyrotropin-releasing hormone on the sleep EEG and nocturnal hormone secretion in male volunteers. Neuropsychobiology 1998;38(1):25–31.
244. Zini I, Merlo Pich E, Fuxe K, et al. Actions of centrally administered neuropeptide Y on EEG activity in different rat strains and in different phases of their circadian cycle. Acta Physiol Scand 1984;122(1):71–7.
245. Ehlers CL, Somes C, Lopez A, et al. Electrophysiological actions of neuropeptide Y and its analogs: new measures for anxiolytic therapy? Neuropsychopharmacology 1997;17(1):34–43.
246. Szentirmai E, Krueger JM. Central administration of neuropeptide Y induces wakefulness in rats. Am J Physiol Regul Integr Comp Physiol 2006;291(2): R473–80.
247. Antonijevic IA, Murck H, Bohlhalter S, et al. Neuropeptide Y promotes sleep and inhibits ACTH and cortisol release in young men. Neuropharmacology 2000; 39(8):1474–81.
248. Held K, Antonijevic I, Murck H, et al. Neuropeptide Y (NPY) shortens sleep latency but does not suppress ACTH and cortisol in depressed patients and normal controls. Psychoneuroendocrinology 2006;31(1):100–7.
249. Xu YL, Reinscheid RK, Huitron-Resendiz S, et al. Neuropeptide S: a neuropeptide promoting arousal and anxiolytic-like effects. Neuron 2004;43(4): 487–97.
250. Huitron-Resendiz S, Kristensen MP, Sanchez-Alavez M, et al. Urotensin II modulates rapid eye movement sleep through activation of brainstem cholinergic neurons. J Neurosci 2005;25(23):5465–74.
251. Obal F Jr, Alfoldi P, Cady AB, et al. Growth hormone-releasing factor enhances sleep in rats and rabbits. Am J Physiol 1988;255(2 Pt 2):R310–6.
252. Steiger A. Neurochemical regulation of sleep. J Psychiatr Res 2007;41(7): 537–52.
253. Van Cauter E, Plat L, Scharf MB, et al. Simultaneous stimulation of slow-wave sleep and growth hormone secretion by gamma-hydroxybutyrate in normal young Men. J Clin Invest 1997;100(3):745–53.
254. Havlicek V, Rezek M, Friesen H. Somatostatin and thyrotropin releasing hormone: central effect on sleep and motor system. Pharmacol Biochem Behav 1976;4(4):455–9.

255. Rezek M, Havlicek V, Hughes KR, et al. Cortical administration of somatostatin (SRIF): effect on sleep and motor behavior. Pharmacol Biochem Behav 1976; 5(1):73–7.

256. Szentirmai E, Kapas L, Krueger JM. Ghrelin microinjection into forebrain sites induces wakefulness and feeding in rats. Am J Physiol Regul Integr Comp Physiol 2007;292(1):R575–85.

257. Rojas-Ramirez JA, Crawley JN, Mendelson WB. Electroencephalographic analysis of the sleep-inducing actions of cholecystokinin. Neuropeptides 1982;3(2):129–38.

258. Kapas L, Obal F Jr, Alfoldi P, et al. Effects of nocturnal intraperitoneal administration of cholecystokinin in rats: simultaneous increase in sleep, increase in EEG slow-wave activity, reduction of motor activity, suppression of eating, and decrease in brain temperature. Brain Res 1988;438(1–2):155–64.

259. Kapas L, Obal F Jr, Opp MR, et al. Intraperitoneal injection of cholecystokinin elicits sleep in rabbits. Physiol Behav 1991;50(6):1241–4.

260. Prospero-Garcia O, Ott T, Drucker-Colin R. Cerebroventricular infusion of cholecystokinin (CCK-8) restores REM sleep in parachlorophenylalanine (PCPA)-pretreated cats. Neurosci Lett 1987;78(2):205–10.

261. Sangiah S, Caldwell DF, Villeneuve MJ, et al. Sleep: sequential reduction of paradoxical (REM) and elevation of slow-wave (NREM) sleep by a non-convulsive dose of insulin in rats. Life Sci 1982;31(8):763–9.

262. Danguir J, Nicolaidis S. Chronic intracerebroventricular infusion of insulin causes selective increase of slow wave sleep in rats. Brain Res 1984; 306(1–2):97–103.

263. Obal F Jr, Kapas L, Bodosi B, et al. Changes in sleep in response to intracerebral injection of insulin-like growth factor-1 (IFG-1) in the rat. Sleep Res Online 1998;1(2):87–91.

264. Verret L, Goutagny R, Fort P, et al. A role of melanin-concentrating hormone producing neurons in the central regulation of paradoxical sleep. BMC Neurosci 2003;4:19.

265. Hanriot L, Camargo N, Courau AC, et al. Characterization of the melanin-concentrating hormone neurons activated during paradoxical sleep hypersomnia in rats. J Comp Neurol 2007;505(2):147–57.

266. Apergis-Schoute J, Iordanidou P, Faure C, et al. Optogenetic evidence for inhibitory signaling from orexin to MCH neurons via local microcircuits. J Neurosci 2015;35(14):5435–41.

267. Parks GS, Olivas ND, Ikrar T, et al. Histamine inhibits the melanin-concentrating hormone system: implications for sleep and arousal. J Physiol 2014;592(Pt 10): 2183–96.

268. Jego S, Glasgow SD, Herrera CG, et al. Optogenetic identification of a rapid eye movement sleep modulatory circuit in the hypothalamus. Nat Neurosci 2013; 16(11):1637–43.

269. Tsunematsu T, Ueno T, Tabuchi S, et al. Optogenetic manipulation of activity and temporally controlled cell-specific ablation reveal a role for MCH neurons in sleep/wake regulation. J Neurosci 2014;34(20):6896–909.

270. Konadhode RR, Pelluru D, Blanco-Centurion C, et al. Optogenetic stimulation of MCH neurons increases sleep. J Neurosci 2013;33(25):10257–63.

271. Roky R, Valatx JL, Jouvet M. Effect of prolactin on the sleep-wake cycle in the rat. Neurosci Lett 1993;156(1–2):117–20.

272. Obal F Jr, Opp M, Cady AB, et al. Prolactin, vasoactive intestinal peptide, and peptide histidine methionine elicit selective increases in REM sleep in rabbits. Brain Res 1989;490(2):292–300.

273. Riou F, Cespuglio R, Jouvet M. Hypnogenic properties of the vasoactive intestinal polypeptide in rats. C R Seances Acad Sci III 1981;293(12):679–82 [in French].
274. Fang J, Payne L, Krueger JM. Pituitary adenylate cyclase activating polypeptide enhances rapid eye movement sleep in rats. Brain Res 1995;686(1):23–8.
275. Aguilar-Roblero R, Verduzco-Carbajal L, Rodriguez C, et al. Circadian rhythmicity in the GABAergic system in the suprachiasmatic nuclei of the rat. Neurosci Lett 1993;157:199–202.
276. Ahnaou A, Basille M, Gonzalez B, et al. Long-term enhancement of REM sleep by the pituitary adenylyl cyclase-activating polypeptide (PACAP) in the pontine reticular formation of the rat. Eur J Neurosci 1999;11(11):4051–8.
277. Ahnaou A, Laporte AM, Ballet S, et al. Muscarinic and PACAP receptor interactions at pontine level in the rat: significance for REM sleep regulation. Eur J Neurosci 2000;12(12):4496–504.
278. Yanik G, Glaum S, Radulovacki M. The dose-response effects of caffeine on sleep in rats. Brain Res 1987;403(1):177–80.
279. Benington JH, Heller HC. Restoration of brain energy metabolism as the function of sleep. Prog Neurobiol 1995;45(4):347–60.
280. Scharf MT, Naidoo N, Zimmerman JE, et al. The energy hypothesis of sleep revisited. Prog Neurobiol 2008;86(3):264–80.
281. Dunwiddie TV, Worth T. Sedative and anticonvulsant effects of adenosine analogs in mouse and rat. J Pharmacol Exp Ther 1982;220(1):70–6.
282. Feldberg W, Sherwood SL. Injections of drugs into the lateral ventricle of the cat. J Physiol 1954;123(1):148–67.
283. Radulovacki M, Virus RM, Djuricic-Nedelson M, et al. Adenosine analogs and sleep in rats. J Pharmacol Exp Ther 1984;228(2):268–74.
284. Radulovacki M, Virus RM, Rapoza D, et al. A comparison of the dose response effects of pyrimidine ribonucleosides and adenosine on sleep in rats. Psychopharmacology 1985;87(2):136–40.
285. Benington JH, Kodali SK, Heller HC. Stimulation of A1 adenosine receptors mimics the electroencephalographic effects of sleep deprivation. Brain Res 1995;692(1–2):79–85.
286. Bjorness TE, Kelly CL, Gao T, et al. Control and function of the homeostatic sleep response by adenosine A1 receptors. J Neurosci 2009;29(5):1267–76.
287. Dunwiddie TV, Masino SA. The role and regulation of adenosine in the central nervous system. Annu Rev Neurosci 2001;24:31–55.
288. Huang ZL, Qu WM, Eguchi N, et al. Adenosine A2A, but not A1, receptors mediate the arousal effect of caffeine. Nat Neurosci 2005;8(7):858–9.
289. Urade Y, Eguchi N, Qu WM, et al. Sleep regulation in adenosine A2A receptor-deficient mice. Neurology 2003;61(11 Suppl 6):S94–6.
290. Porkka-Heiskanen T, Strecker RE, McCarley RW. Brain site-specificity of extracellular adenosine concentration changes during sleep deprivation and spontaneous sleep: an in vivo microdialysis study. Neuroscience 2000;99(3):507–17.
291. Porkka-Heiskanen T, Strecker RE, Thakkar M, et al. Adenosine: a mediator of the sleep-inducing effects of prolonged wakefulness. Science 1997;276(5316):1265–8.
292. Blanco-Centurion C, Xu M, Murillo-Rodriguez E, et al. Adenosine and sleep homeostasis in the basal forebrain. J Neurosci 2006;26(31):8092–100.
293. Kalinchuk AV, McCarley RW, Stenberg D, et al. The role of cholinergic basal forebrain neurons in adenosine-mediated homeostatic control of sleep: lessons from 192 IgG-saporin lesions. Neuroscience 2008;157(1):238–53.

294. Strecker RE, Morairty S, Thakkar MM, et al. Adenosinergic modulation of basal forebrain and preoptic/anterior hypothalamic neuronal activity in the control of behavioral state. Behav Brain Res 2000;115(2):183–204.

295. Kalinchuk AV, Lu Y, Stenberg D, et al. Nitric oxide production in the basal forebrain is required for recovery sleep. J Neurochem 2006;99(2):483–98.

296. Kalinchuk AV, McCarley RW, Porkka-Heiskanen T, et al. The time course of adenosine, nitric oxide (NO) and inducible NO synthase changes in the brain with sleep loss and their role in the non-rapid eye movement sleep homeostatic cascade. J Neurochem 2011;116(2):260–72.

297. Kalinchuk AV, Porkka-Heiskanen T, McCarley RW, et al. Cholinergic neurons of the basal forebrain mediate biochemical and electrophysiological mechanisms underlying sleep homeostasis. Eur J Neurosci 2015;41(2):182–95.

298. Halassa MM, Florian C, Fellin T, et al. Astrocytic modulation of sleep homeostasis and cognitive consequences of sleep loss. Neuron 2009;61(2):213–9.

299. Schmitt LI, Sims RE, Dale N, et al. Wakefulness affects synaptic and network activity by increasing extracellular astrocyte-derived adenosine. J Neurosci 2012; 32(13):4417–25.

300. Magistretti PJ. Neuron-glia metabolic coupling and plasticity. J Exp Biol 2006; 209(Pt 12):2304–11.

301. Petit JM, Gyger J, Burlet-Godinot S, et al. Genes involved in the astrocyte-neuron lactate shuttle (ANLS) are specifically regulated in cortical astrocytes following sleep deprivation in mice. Sleep 2013;36(10):1445–58.

302. Petit JM, Tobler I, Allaman I, et al. Sleep deprivation modulates brain mRNAs encoding genes of glycogen metabolism. Eur J Neurosci 2002;16(6):1163–7.

303. Lewy AJ. Melatonin and human chronobiology. Cold Spring Harb Symp Quant Biol 2007;72:623–36.

304. Onoe H, Ueno R, Fujita I, et al. Prostaglandin D2, a cerebral sleep-inducing substance in monkeys. Proc Natl Acad Sci U S A 1988;85(11):4082–6.

305. Matsumura H, Takahata R, Hayaishi O. Inhibition of sleep in rats by inorganic selenium compounds, inhibitors of prostaglandin D synthase. Proc Natl Acad Sci U S A 1991;88(20):9046–50.

306. Takahata R, Matsumura H, Kantha SS, et al. Intravenous administration of inorganic selenium compounds, inhibitors of prostaglandin D synthase, inhibits sleep in freely moving rats. Brain Res 1993;623(1):65–71.

307. Qu WM, Huang ZL, Xu XH, et al. Lipocalin-type prostaglandin D synthase produces prostaglandin D2 involved in regulation of physiological sleep. Proc Natl Acad Sci U S A 2006;103(47):17949–54.

308. Pandey HP, Ram A, Matsumura H, et al. Concentration of prostaglandin D2 in cerebrospinal fluid exhibits a circadian alteration in conscious rats. Biochem Mol Biol Int 1995;37(3):431–7.

309. Ram A, Pandey HP, Matsumura H, et al. CSF levels of prostaglandins, especially the level of prostaglandin D2, are correlated with increasing propensity towards sleep in rats. Brain Res 1997;751(1):81–9.

310. Gerashchenko D, Beuckmann CT, Kanaoka Y, et al. Dominant expression of rat prostanoid DP receptor mRNA in leptomeninges, inner segments of photoreceptor cells, iris epithelium, and ciliary processes. J Neurochem 1998;71(3):937–45.

311. Matsumura H, Nakajima T, Osaka T, et al. Prostaglandin D2-sensitive, sleep-promoting zone defined in the ventral surface of the rostral basal forebrain. Proc Natl Acad Sci U S A 1994;91(25):11998–2002.

312. Satoh S, Matsumura H, Suzuki F, et al. Promotion of sleep mediated by the A2a-adenosine receptor and possible involvement of this receptor in the sleep

induced by prostaglandin D2 in rats. Proc Natl Acad Sci U S A 1996;93(12): 5980–4.

313. Mong JA, Baker FC, Mahoney MM, et al. Sleep, rhythms, and the endocrine brain: influence of sex and gonadal hormones. J Neurosci 2011;31(45): 16107–16.

314. Zhang B, Wing YK. Sex differences in insomnia: a meta-analysis. Sleep 2006; 29(1):85–93.

315. Armitage R, Hoffmann R, Trivedi M, et al. Slow-wave activity in NREM sleep: sex and age effects in depressed outpatients and healthy controls. Psychiatry Res 2000;95(3):201–13.

316. Dijk DJ, Beersma DG, Bloem GM. Sex differences in the sleep EEG of young adults: visual scoring and spectral analysis. Sleep 1989;12(6):500–7.

317. Manber R, Armitage R. Sex, steroids, and sleep: a review. Sleep 1999;22(5): 540–55.

318. Mourtazaev MS, Kemp B, Zwinderman AH, et al. Age and gender affect different characteristics of slow waves in the sleep EEG. Sleep 1995;18(7): 557–64.

319. Armitage R, Hoffmann RF. Sleep EEG, depression and gender. Sleep Med Rev 2001;5(3):237–46.

320. Driver HS, Dijk DJ, Werth E, et al. Sleep and the sleep electroencephalogram across the menstrual cycle in young healthy women. J Clin Endocrinol Metab 1996;81(2):728–35.

321. Baker FC, Driver HS, Paiker J, et al. Acetaminophen does not affect 24-h body temperature or sleep in the luteal phase of the menstrual cycle. J Appl Physiol 2002;92(4):1684–91.

322. Shechter A, Varin F, Boivin DB. Circadian variation of sleep during the follicular and luteal phases of the menstrual cycle. Sleep 2010;33(5):647–56.

323. Fang J, Fishbein W. Sex differences in paradoxical sleep: influences of estrus cycle and ovariectomy. Brain Res 1996;734(1–2):275–85.

324. Franken P, Dudley CA, Estill SJ, et al. NPAS2 as a transcriptional regulator of non-rapid eye movement sleep: genotype and sex interactions. Proc Natl Acad Sci U S A 2006;103(18):7118–23.

325. Koehl M, Battle S, Meerlo P. Sex differences in sleep: the response to sleep deprivation and restraint stress in mice. Sleep 2006;29(9):1224–31.

326. Paul KN, Dugovic C, Turek FW, et al. Diurnal sex differences in the sleep-wake cycle of mice are dependent on gonadal function. Sleep 2006;29(9):1211–23.

327. Paul KN, Laposky AD, Turek FW. Reproductive hormone replacement alters sleep in mice. Neurosci Lett 2009;463(3):239–43.

328. Yamaoka S. Modification of circadian sleep rhythms by gonadal steroids and the neural mechanisms involved. Brain Res 1980;185(2):385–98.

329. Colvin GB, Whitmoyer DI, Lisk RD, et al. Changes in sleep-wakefulness in female rats during circadian and estrous cycles. Brain Res 1968;7(2):173–81.

330. Colvin GB, Whitmoyer DI, Sawyer CH. Circadian sleep-wakefulness patterns in rats after ovariectomy and treatment with estrogen. Exp Neurol 1969;25(4): 616–25.

331. Hadjimarkou MM, Benham R, Schwarz JM, et al. Estradiol suppresses rapid eye movement sleep and activation of sleep-active neurons in the ventrolateral preoptic area. Eur J Neurosci 2008;27(7):1780–92.

332. Deurveilher S, Rusak B, Semba K. Estradiol and progesterone modulate spontaneous sleep patterns and recovery from sleep deprivation in ovariectomized rats. Sleep 2009;32(7):865–77.

333. Schwartz MD, Mong JA. Estradiol suppresses recovery of REM sleep following sleep deprivation in ovariectomized female rats. Physiol Behav 2011;104(5): 962–71.
334. Schwartz MD, Mong JA. Estradiol modulates recovery of REM sleep in a time-of-day-dependent manner. Am J Physiol Regul Integr Comp Physiol 2013;305(3): R271–80.
335. Cusmano DM, Hadjimarkou MM, Mong JA. Gonadal steroid modulation of sleep and wakefulness in male and female rats is sexually differentiated and neonatally organized by steroid exposure. Endocrinology 2014;155(1):204–14.
336. Ehlen JC, Hesse S, Pinckney L, et al. Sex chromosomes regulate nighttime sleep propensity during recovery from sleep loss in mice. PLoS One 2013; 8(5):e62205.
337. Mong JA, Devidze N, Frail DE, et al. Estradiol differentially regulates lipocalin-type prostaglandin D synthase transcript levels in the rodent brain: evidence from high-density oligonucleotide arrays and in situ hybridization. Proc Natl Acad Sci U S A 2003;100(1):318–23.
338. Silveyra P, Catalano PN, Lux-Lantos V, et al. Impact of proestrous milieu on expression of orexin receptors and prepro-orexin in rat hypothalamus and hypophysis: actions of Cetrorelix and Nembutal. Am J Physiol Endocrinol Metab 2007;292(3):E820–8.
339. Silveyra P, Cataldi NI, Lux-Lantos V, et al. Gonadal steroids modulated hypocretin/orexin type-1 receptor expression in a brain region, sex and daytime specific manner. Regul Pept 2009;158(1–3):121–6.

The Neurobiology of Circadian Rhythms

 CrossMark

Patricia J. Sollars, PhD[a],*, Gary E. Pickard, PhD[a,b]

KEYWORDS

- Biological rhythms • Suprachiasmatic nucleus
- Intrinsically photosensitive retinal ganglion cells • Circadian oscillator • Clock

KEY POINTS

- The suprachiasmatic nucleus (SCN) is the primary circadian oscillator in the brain responsible for temporal coordination.
- A set of clock genes forms interlocking transcription/translation feedback loops.
- A rhythm in SCN neural activity represents the functional output of the clock.
- The SCN is entrained to the day/night cycle via the retinohypothalamic tract.
- A recently discovered retinal ganglion cell (RGC) photoreceptor innervates the SCN.

INTRODUCTION

Daily rhythms in nature, such as the opening and closing of flowers or patterns of sleep and wakefulness and their association with the perpetual alteration of night and day, were recognized in antiquity, although their origins were not questioned until the eighteenth century. The French Astronomer Jean-Jacques d'Ortous de Mairan conducted an investigation into whether the leaves of the mimosa plant opened in response to light.[1] Although de Mairan's experiments were the first to question the origin of such daily rhythms, Augustin Pyramus de Candolle[2] is credited with the first suggestion that they arose through an internal timekeeping mechanism. In 1832, de Candolle concluded that the rhythm of mimosa leaf folding and unfolding observed under constant light conditions must come "from within the plant,"[2] and because rhythms observed under such conditions express a period of only approximately 24 hours,

This work was supported by NIH R01 NS077003 and R01 AI056346.

Disclosures: Drs P.J. Sollars and G.E. Pickard have no conflicts and nothing to disclose.

[a] School of Veterinary Medicine and Biomedical Sciences, University of Nebraska, Fair Street and East Campus Loop, Lincoln, NE 68583, USA; [b] Department of Ophthalmology and Visual Sciences, University of Nebraska Medical Center, 600 S 42nd Street, Omaha, NE 68198, USA

* Corresponding author.

E-mail address: patricia.sollars@unl.edu

Abbreviations	
BMAL1	Brain and muscle ARNT-like 1 protein
Brn3b	Brain-specific homeobox/POU domain protein 3B
CLOCK	Circadian locomotor output cycles kaput
CRY	Cryptochrome
EPSC	Excitatory postsynaptic current
GABA	γ-Aminobutyric acid
GR	Glucocorticoid receptor
IGL	Intergeniculate leaflet
ipRGC	Intrinsically photosensitive retinal ganglion cell
KO	Knockout
MAPK	p42/p44 mitogen-activated protein kinase
PACAP	Pituitary adenylate cyclase–activating polypeptide
PER	Period
PLR	Pupillary light reflex
PRC	Phase response curve
PVN	Paraventricular nucleus
RGC	Retinal ganglion cell
RHT	Retinohypothalamic tract
SAD	Seasonal affective disorder
SCN	Suprachiasmatic nucleus
SPZ	Subparaventricular zone
Vglut2	Vesicular glutamate transporter 2
VIP	Vasoactive intestinal polypeptide
VP	Vasopressin

they have come to be called *circadian* rhythms, from the Latin *circa* (about) and *dies* (day). Almost a half a century later, Charles and Frank Darwin came to a similar conclusion regarding leaf movements, writing further that "we may conclude that the periodicity of their movements is to a certain extent inherited."[3] As time progressed, investigators became increasingly aware that not only plants but all organisms, including humans, displayed daily rhythms that were generated by an internal timekeeping system or endogenous biological clock.[4–8]

THE SUPRACHIASMATIC NUCLEUS IS A CIRCADIAN OSCILLATOR

The SCN is the primary circadian oscillator in the brain and is located in the ventral periventricular zone of the hypothalamus, dorsal to the optic chiasm and medial to the anterior hypothalamic area. Each of the paired suprachiasmatic nuclei is composed of a heterogeneous group of approximately 10,000 interconnected small neurons that express circadian rhythms in both gene expression and in the rate of action potential firing.[9] Although recognized early on as a distinct hypothalamic nucleus in a variety of species,[10] its function remained unspecified until the demonstration of a retinal projection terminating in the SCN, the retinohypothalamic tract (RHT).[11,12] Such a projection was thought to be a critical component of clock function, because it would enable direct synchronization with the environmental day/night cycle, so identification of the RHT focused attention on this region of the anterior hypothalamus as a potential site of the biological clock.

SCN ablation studies were then conducted, with the observation that complete destruction of the SCN rendered animals arrhythmic. This led to the suggestion that the SCN was the site of at least 1 component of a circadian clock that is normally entrained by retinal signals transmitted via the RHT.[13,14] SCN metabolic activity, electrophysiologic recording of the SCN both in vivo and in vitro, and transplantation of fetal anterior hypothalamic tissue containing the SCN into SCN-lesioned hosts of the same or different species subsequently confirmed that (1) the SCN is the site of a circadian oscillator whose neurons rhythmically alter their metabolism and firing rate and (2) the SCN is required for the expression of behavioral circadian rhythms (**Fig. 1**).[15–22] There was also an indication, however, from some transplantation studies that the circadian timing system may be composed of a distributed multioscillator system[21] and, as discussed later, it is now recognized that almost all cells and tissues in the body are circadian clocks.[23–25]

THE SUPRACHIASMATIC NUCLEUS MOLECULAR CIRCADIAN OSCILLATOR IS LINKED TO THE NEURAL ACTIVITY RHYTHM

Insights into the molecular mechanisms of the mammalian SCN circadian clock emerged from work conducted in the fruit fly. These studies identified 3 mutant alleles of a single gene (*period* [*per*]) that had the properties of either increasing or decreasing the circadian period or of eliminating circadian rhythmicity altogether.[26] After the discovery of the mammalian homologue of *per* in 1997,[27,28] great strides have been made in defining the core molecular components that underlie the generation of circadian oscillations in the SCN.[29]

The cell autonomous circadian oscillations of SCN neurons are generated by 2 interlocking transcription/translation feedback loops that function together to generate high-amplitude circadian rhythms of gene expression. Four integral clock proteins form the core of the SCN molecular clock: 2 activators (circadian locomotor output cycles kaput [CLOCK] and brain and muscle ARNT-like 1 [BMAL1]) and 2 repressors (period [PER] and cryptochrome [CRY]) as well as kinases and phosphatases that regulate the localization and stability of these integral clock proteins. CLOCK and BMAL1 dimerize in the cytoplasm of SCN neurons, and, after translocation to the nucleus, they initiate transcription of target genes, including *per* and *cry*, by binding to E-box elements within the enhancer and promoter sequences of these genes. A feedback loop results from the translocation of PER:CRY heterodimers back to the nucleus where they repress their own transcription by acting on the CLOCK:BMAL1 complex. As PER and CRY proteins are degraded via ubiquitin-dependent pathways, repression on CLOCK:-BMAL1 is eased and the cycle is repeated. Post-translational modifications play an important role in establishing the circadian period of the oscillation. An additional interlocking feedback loop involves the positive regulator, retinoid-related orphan receptor (ROR), and the negative regulator, orphan nuclear receptor (REV-ERBα), that adds robustness to the oscillations and helps maintain accurate circadian timing (**Fig. 2**).[29]

Circadian oscillations in core clock genes must be linked to the functional output of the SCN, the daily fluctuation of spontaneous action potential firing of SCN neurons. Firing is greatest during the day (6–10 Hz) and low at night (<1 Hz) without regard to whether the behavior of the organism is diurnal or nocturnal.[16–18,30–32] Alterations in components of the molecular clock that increase or decrease the period of the cycle alter the frequency of the spontaneous firing rate of SCN neurons, whereas elimination of the molecular oscillation abolishes the firing rate rhythm. These findings support the interpretation that the intracellular molecular clock drives the expression of rhythms in the frequency of action potential firing in SCN neurons.[33,34] *Per1* may play an important role in the link because there is a positive correlation between *Per1* promoter activity and spike frequency in individual SCN neurons, suggesting a fixed-phase relationship between molecular clock and electrical activity.[35,36] The precise causal link between the molecular oscillations of clock genes within SCN neurons and their rhythm of neuronal firing rate, however, remain unclear.

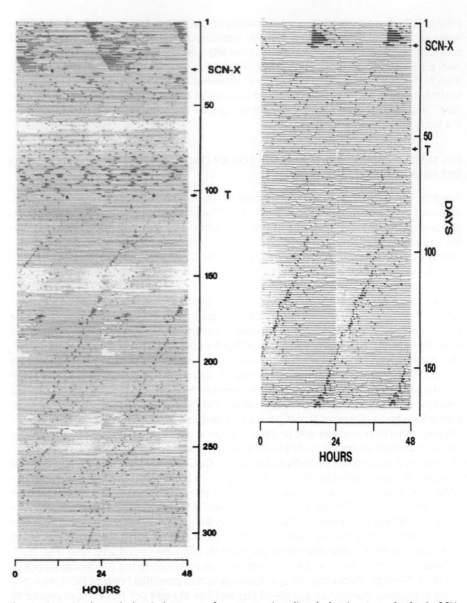

Fig. 1. Anterior hypothalamic heterografts restore circadian behavior to arrhythmic SCN-lesioned hosts. Wheel-running activity record of SCN-lesioned hamsters bearing a fetal mouse anterior hypothalamic heterograft (*left*) or a fetal rat anterior hypothalamic heterograft (*right*). Note that the period of the restored circadian rhythm on the left is typical of that of an intact mouse (ie, <24 h), but the restored rhythm on the right is not typical of that of an intact rat (ie, >24 h). SCN-X, day of complete, bilateral SCN lesion; T, day of fetal anterior hypothalamic implantation. (*Adapted from* Sollars PJ, Kimble DP, Pickard GE. Restoration of circadian behavior by anterior hypothalamic heterografts. J Neurosci 1995;15:2109–22; with permission.)

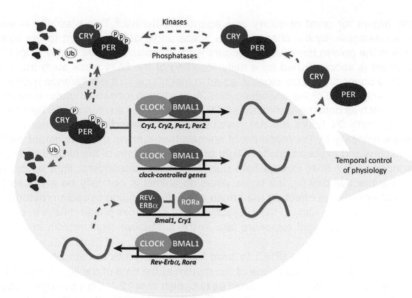

Fig. 2. Molecular architecture of the mammalian circadian clock. (*From* Partch CL, Green CB, Takahashi JS. Molecular architecture of the mammalian circadian clock. Trends Cell Biol 2014;24:91; with permission.)

Ion channels play a major role in neuronal excitability and several ion channels in SCN neurons seem under circadian clock control.[33,37] Ionic mechanisms that seem to contribute to the oscillation in SCN firing include persistent Na^+ currents, L-type Ca^{2+} currents, hyperpolarization-activated currents (I_H), large-conductance Ca^{2+}-activated K^+ (BK) currents, and fast delayed rectifier K^+ currents, although much remains to be learned.[38] There have been suggestions that membrane ion currents may also feed back to regulate the molecular clock, perhaps via voltage-dependent regulation of Ca^{2+} currents and subsequent second-messenger action of intracellular Ca^{2+} on gene transcription.[39–41] Fluxes in intracellular calcium are important for light-induced resetting of the SCN clock (discussed later), but recent work has shown that rhythmic electrical activity does not seem required for molecular oscillations in invertebrate clock neurons.[42] Rhythmic spontaneous firing of the SCN clock is, however, the critical functional output of the SCN and is required for overt behavioral rhythmicity.[43]

THE RETINOHYPOTHALAMIC TRACT ENTRAINS THE SUPRACHIASMATIC NUCLEUS CIRCADIAN CLOCK TO THE DAY/NIGHT CYCLE

The SCN circadian oscillator derives functional utility from its ability to be entrained to the day/night cycle. Simply stated, entrainment of the SCN oscillator to the day/night cycle means that the period of the endogenous SCN circadian oscillation becomes equal to that of the light/dark cycle.[44] Entrainment provides a predictable and appropriate phase relationship to the day/night cycle, in effect enabling recognition of local time; thus, the SCN circadian oscillator is said to function as a biological clock.[45] Entrainment differs from simple synchronization to changes in the light/dark cycle because the rhythm generation is neither passive nor driven and entrainment, therefore, allows for great plasticity and adaptive potential.[9] This plasticity is evidenced, for example, by the change in the phase angle of entrainment to the light/dark cycle in the golden hamster that occurs with seasonal changes in day length.[46]

Entrainment is accomplished by a daily resetting of the SCN clock such that the light-induced phase shift of the clock is equal in magnitude to the difference between the free-running period of the endogenous SCN oscillation (observed under constant conditions, such as constant darkness) and the period of the environmental light/dark cycle (ie, typically 24 hours but not restricted to this period). This mechanism is described empirically by the response of animals free-running under constant darkness conditions and exposed briefly to light at different phases of the circadian cycle. The response of the SCN to brief light pulses is phase dependent: light exposure during the subjective day (ie, the times when an animal is normally be exposed to daylight) has virtually no effect on the phase of the free-running circadian rhythm. In contrast, light exposure early in the subjective night produces phase delays in circadian rhythms, whereas light exposure late in the subjective night results in phase advances.

The phase response curve (PRC) to brief light pulses plots the amplitude of the phase shift as a function of the phase of the rhythm at the time of the light stimulation with the onset of activity arbitrarily defined as circadian time 12.[47] Effective light pulses can be as brief as 1 s and as dim as 0.05 lux.[48,49] Thus, entrainment is critically dependent on phase shifts occurring at dusk and/or dawn because the portion of the circadian day sensitive to light is coincident with the twilight transitions in the day/night cycle. Because light experienced around dusk (or light offset under laboratory conditions) produces phase delays, it is, therefore, the prominent photic cue used for entrainment when the period of the endogenous SCN circadian oscillation is less than 24 hours, as is typical for most strains of laboratory mouse. Light exposure late in the subjective night results in phase advances of the SCN and thus light around dawn (or light onset in the laboratory) is the salient photic cue used to reset the SCN clock of organisms, such as most strains of laboratory rat as well as humans, with a period greater than 24 hours.[50,51]

Although it is clear that signals transmitted from the retina to the SCN via the RHT are necessary for entrainment, the photoreceptors or the type of RGCs that mediated the effects of light on the SCN clock were unresolved until relatively recently. After the pioneering descriptions of the vertebrate retina by Santiago Ramón y Cajal in the late 1800s,[52] it was believed that the retinal rods and cones were the only photoreceptors in mammals. Keeler, in 1927,[53] provided the first suggestion that a nonrod, noncone photoreceptor might exist when he reported that some mice, despite having no photoreceptors in the outer retina,[54] retained their ability to constrict the iris in response to light stimulation (ie, the pupillary light reflex [PLR]).[54] Although it was suggested that RGCs might somehow be light sensitive and, therefore, responsible for the observed behavior of the iris, Keeler's prescient suggestion did not gain traction. Reports of mice lacking rods and cones but retaining their ability to entrain their circadian activity rhythms to a light/dark cycle appeared many decades later.[55,56] Additional studies in the late 1990s using transgenic mice lacking rod and cone photoreceptors reported that these animals also retained several irradiance-dependent responses, including photoentrainment of their circadian locomotor behavior, the PLR, and light-induced suppression of nocturnal pineal melatonin secretion.[57,58] Although these studies and other reports[59–62] provided strong support for the existence of a nonrod, noncone photoreceptor in the mammalian retina, the prospect that a third photoreceptor in the retina had been missed for over a century was met with considerable skepticism.[63]

SUPRACHIASMATIC NUCLEUS–PROJECTING RETINAL GANGLION CELLS EXPRESS MELANOPSIN AND ARE INTRINSICALLY PHOTOSENSITIVE

Using cultured dermal melanophores from *Xenopus laevis*, Provencio and colleagues[64] identified the photopigment responsible for the light-induced dispersion of melansomes. This opsin, now called melanopsin, is a member of the opsin family of G protein–coupled receptors and it shares the greatest sequence homology to octopus (invertebrate) rhodopsin. Melanopsin mRNA was expressed in frog dermal melanophores, in the brain, and in the retina but not in typical retinal photoreceptors.[64] In mammals, melanopsin was found expressed in the ganglion cell layer of the retina, providing the basis for the suggestion that RGCs expressing the novel mammalian opsin were directly photosensitive.[65] These findings were soon extended by the demonstration that melanopsin was expressed in SCN-projecting RGCs.[66]

The prediction that SCN-projecting RGCs were photosensitive was borne out in early 2002 through a set of landmark reports by Berson and colleagues[67] and Hattar and colleagues.[68] Berson and coworkers[67] recorded from SCN-projecting RGCs in the rat retina and showed that when these neurons were isolated pharmacologically and physically from all rod and cone synaptic input, they depolarized and generated action potentials in response to photic stimulation; that is, these ganglion cells were intrinsically photosensitive. It was also shown that these intrinsically photosensitive RCGs (ipRGCs) expressed melanopsin.[68] The discovery of melanopsin by Provencio and colleagues[64,65] and the reports describing ipRGCs in the rodent retina[67,68] laid the foundation for what has become an exciting and rapidly growing new subdivision of retinal biology.[63,69-72]

MULTIPLE INTRINSICALLY PHOTOSENSITIVE RETINAL GANGLION CELL SUBTYPES WITH WIDESPREAD AXONAL PROJECTIONS

Since the initial description of ipRGC projections to the SCN via the RHT, it has become evident that there are multiple morphologic and physiologic ipRGC subtypes that send their axons to many areas of the brain, and their diverse functions are actively being investigated. At least 5 ipRGC subtypes have now been described (M1–M5) and there are preliminary reports of additional subtypes.[70] M1 ipRGCs (initially identified as the SCN-projecting RGCs)[67] have the greatest abundance of melanopsin protein in the plasma membrane and the most robust intrinsic response to light stimulation among all the ipRGC subtypes. In addition to the melanopsin-mediated intrinsic response to light, all ipRGCs receive rod and cone photoreceptor inputs via bipolar cells. In dim light, rods and cones drive ipRGCs whereas the response to bright light is an integration of photoreceptor drive and melanopsin-mediated depolarization. At least 2 ipRGC subtypes (M1 and M2) innervate the mouse SCN and a vast majority of these (approximately 80%) are of the M1 subtype,[73] although the functional significance of these 2 ipRGC subtypes innervating the SCN remains to be determined. M1 ipRGCs can be further parsed based on their expression of the brain-specific homeobox/POU domain protein 3B (Brn3b) transcription factor; Brn3b-negative ipRGCs innervate the SCN.[74] Brn3b-positive M1 ipRGCs send collaterals to the intergeniculate leaflet (IGL), a component of the circadian timing system[75] and to the olivary pretectal nucleus (the midbrain nucleus that regulates the PLR), the medial amygdala, lateral habenula, and superior colliculus.[76,77]

SUPRACHIASMATIC NUCLEUS CIRCADIAN GATING OF RESPONSES TO LIGHT STIMULATION

Illumination of the retina evokes excitatory postsynaptic currents (EPSCs) in a subpopulation of SCN neurons. These responses have long latencies and are sustained,[78] similar to the responses of M1 ipRGCs to light.[79] The light-induced EPSCs are the result of glutamate release from the RHT and are mediated by both ionotropic and metabotropic glutamate receptors. Where examined to date, the location of these indirectly light-responsive neurons in the SCN has been found to correspond to the terminal field of the RHT, primarily within the ventral and lateral aspects of the SCN, although species differences in the RHT terminal field exist and RHT fibers can be found throughout almost all of the SCN in several species.[77,80] The excitatory response to N-methyl-D-aspartate is larger during the night than during the day whereas α-amino-3-hydroxy-5-methyl-4-isoxazoleproprionic acid/kainite–induced currents do not show a day/night difference.[81,82] In addition to glutamate, most (if not all) SCN-projecting ipRGCs also synthesize pituitary adenylate cyclase–activating polypeptide (PACAP)[83] and PACAP may act as a modulator of the glutamatergic input to the SCN.[84] Recent work has reported that when the vesicular glutamate transporter has been selectively knocked out in ipRGCs (vesicular glutamate transporter 2 [Vglut2] conditional knockouts [KOs]), mice retain the ability to entrain to light/dark cycles, albeit not normally,[85] indirectly suggesting that RHT release of PACAP alone may be sufficient to entrain the SCN to the light/dark cycle.[85–87]

Obrietan and colleagues[88] have provided evidence that p42/p44 mitogen-activated protein kinase (MAPK) signal transduction plays an important role in gating the responsiveness of the SCN to light. The MAPK pathway in the SCN is induced by light in a phase-dependent manner, couples light to transcriptional activation, and mediates light-induced phase shifts.[89–91] MAPK activation is also triggered by glutamate and PACAP.[92] The Ras-like G-protein Dexras1 also seems a critical factor in this process. Dexras1 null mice exhibit a restructured PRC to light at night and a loss of gating to photic resetting during the subjective day.[93] The exact mechanisms by which the SCN clock gates its responses to light, shifting its phase during the subjective night but not during the subjective day, remains to be fully elucidated.

The study of light-induced SCN gene activity resulting in pacemaker resetting was initiated by the seminal observation that light induces a rapid and transient expression of the transcription factor c-Fos within the SCN during the same circadian phases that light shifts the SCN oscillation.[94,95] The per genes (per1 and per2) in the SCN are photo-inducible with a phase dependence similar to that of light-induced behavioral phase shifts, suggesting that light-induced induction of per is a pivotal component of phase resetting.[96,97] Daan and colleagues[98] offered an intriguing 2-component molecular model for light-induced phase shifting in the SCN, inspired by earlier work suggesting that per1-mediated phase advances and per2-mediated phase delays. A subsequent analysis, however, of phase shift responses to light in mice lacking functional per (per1 and per2) or cry (cry1 and cry2) genes revealed that all 4 genotypes of mice retain the capacity for both advancing and delaying responses to light.[99] Thus, the molecular mechanism underlying the biphasic response of the SCN to light also remains to be determined.

RHT stimulation increases SCN neuron spike rate and intracellular calcium levels when the spike rate is low at night, and it has been suggested that the light-evoked increase in Ca^{2+} may play a role in shifting the molecular oscillations.[100,101] Although light has little effect on the SCN clock during the subjective day, light stimulation can substantially boost the firing rate of individual SCN neurons that display rhythmic baseline firing (ie, clock cells).[32] This increase in spiking activity during the subjective day does not, however, translate into clock gene (per1 or per2) induction and resetting of the molecular clock. The resistance of the clock to phase shift during the subjective day may be because intracellular calcium levels have plateaued at a high level during this phase of the circadian cycle.[100] Light-evoked increases in action potential firing during the subjective day do little to further increase intracellular calcium levels in SCN clock cells.[101] As in mammals, the pacemaker cells in the marine snail *Bulla gouldiana* respond to light stimulation at all phases of the circadian cycle, whereas light-induced phase shifts of the circadian pacemaker are restricted to the subjective night. An examination of this model system has shown that light shifts the snail pacemaker only during the subjective night because depolarization of clock cells opens calcium channels during the night when these channels are normally closed.[102] Thus, after even very bright light stimulation during the subjective day, the increase in SCN action potential firing rate may have little influence on SCN molecular clock function. Nevertheless, the increased SCN output at this phase may be sufficient to alter the activity of descending autonomic circuits if the light stimulation is of sufficient duration and intensity.[103]

SUPRACHIASMATIC NUCLEUS FUNCTIONAL ORGANIZATION

The SCN oscillator is composed of thousands of autonomous cellular oscillators that are coupled in a complex neural network that is critically important for the generation of coherent circadian rhythms.[104] In addition, the left and right SCNs are coupled to each other, and, under certain conditions, each SCN can function as an independent clock.[105,106] A vast majority of SCN neurons synthesize γ-aminobutyric acid (GABA), and there is an extensive GABAergic plexus throughout the SCN, consistent with intra-SCN communication.[104] In addition, all GABAergic neurons use at least 1 additional peptide neurotransmitter (vasoactive intestinal polypeptide [VIP], vasopressin [VP], gastrin-releasing peptide, substance P, somatostatin, calbindin, calretinin, enkephalin, neurotensin, or cholecystokinin).[80] There are considerable species differences in the clustering of peptide-expressing cells in the SCN,[80] but based on the rat model in which VIP neurons are located primarily ventrolaterally and VP cells are found primarily in the dorsomedial aspect, the SCN has historically been divided into 2 subdivisions.[80] The geniculohypothalamic tract arising from neuropeptide Y neurons in the IGL and the RHT arising from ipRGCs, terminate primarily, although not exclusively, in the ventrolateral VIP subdivision in the rat. Another organizational scheme that has arisen is the core and shell,[107] although it has been suggested that this is an oversimplification of SCN functional organization.[80] The distribution of VIP and VP neurons in the SCN seems dependent both on the circadian phase when the tissue is examined and the species being studied, with considerable overlap in the distribution of these peptide-expressing neurons (see Morin and Allen[80] for a comprehensive review). Interactions among SCN neurons are required for robust and coherent SCN function, with GABA and VIP playing a prominent role, whereas the coupling between regional SCN pacemakers may be dependent on the photoperiodic environment.[108–111]

Although GABA is typically associated with inhibitory postsynaptic responses in the mature brain, GABA-evoked excitation has been reported in the SCN of adult animals. GABA-evoked excitation during the day was originally suggested to contribute to the higher level of firing rate of SCN neurons noted during this phase of the circadian cycle.[112] It is unclear, however, whether GABA-evoked excitation is restricted to particular phases of the circadian cycle and/or to particular cell types or subregions of the nucleus.[113,114] The cellular mechanisms underlying GABA-evoked excitation in the SCN are unknown although it is well documented that the expression and function of cation-chloride cotransporters are responsible for the shift in GABAergic responses during development.[115] There is a heterogeneous distribution of cation-chloride cotransporters within the SCN,[116,117] although it is not known if their expression and/or function, regulated by the lysine-deficient protein kinase 1-Sps1-related proline/alanine-rich kinase/oxidative stress-related kinase 1 complex, is under circadian regulation.[118] It was recently suggested that GABA-evoked excitation in the SCN may be regulated by day length and, therefore, may play a role in seasonal adjustments of SCN activity.[119]

SEROTONERGIC MODULATION OF PHOTIC INPUT TO THE SUPRACHIASMATIC NUCLEUS

The SCN receives a robust serotonergic input arising from ascending projections of serotonin neurons in the median raphe nucleus that modulates RHT input.[120,121] Although SCN neurons express several serotonin receptor subtypes, the best-documented mechanism by which serotonin alters the response of the SCN to light is via presynaptic serotonin$_{1B}$ receptors located on RHT terminals, inhibiting ipRGC glutamate release.[122–126] This inhibitory function might suggest that knocking out serotonin$_{1B}$ receptors would enhance the effect of light on SCN-mediated behavior. Mice lacking serotonin$_{1B}$ receptors have, however, an attenuated response to light,[127] most likely because serotonin$_{1B}$ receptors are also located presynaptically on GABAergic terminals in the SCN.[128] Thus, although serotonin$_{1B}$ receptor KO mice have increased glutamatergic transmission via the RHT, there is apparently a concomitant increase in GABAergic transmission within the SCN that may spill over to attenuate RHT input via GABA$_B$ receptors also located presynaptically on RHT terminals.[129] The attenuated response to light in the serotonin$_{1B}$ receptor KO mouse results in a delayed-phase angle of entrainment compared with wild-type mice under short-day (winter-like) conditions, whereas entrainment to standard 12 hours light:12 hours dark conditions is unaffected.[130] Thus, the circadian response to light in mice lacking serotonin$_{1B}$ receptors phenocopies people suffering from recurring winter depression or seasonal affective disorder (SAD), who typically manifest a phase-delayed circadian system.[131] Various lines of clinical evidence point to a significant role for serotonin in the pathophysiology of SAD, and alterations in the function of serotonin$_{1B}$ receptors have been shown associated with depression-like states.[132,133]

OUTPUTS FROM THE SUPRACHIASMATIC NUCLEUS

SCN temporal signals drive rhythms in behavior, physiology, metabolism, and hormone secretion. This function is accomplished via the 3 major output pathways that exit the SCN: (1) a rostral pathway into the medial preoptic area that continues into the paraventricular nucleus of the thalamus (relaying SCN signals to the medial prefrontal cortex)[134,135]; (2) a pathway that runs caudally along the base of the brain to the retrochiasmatic area and into the capsule of the ventromedial nucleus; and (3) the largest of these pathways that travels in an arc dorsally and caudally giving off terminals along the way to innervate the area immediately dorsal to the SCN, the ventral subparaventricular zone (vSPZ), and a region ventral to the hypothalamic paraventricular nucleus (PVN), the dorsal SPZ.[134,136] Some of these fibers continue caudally to the dorsomedial nucleus of the hypothalamus, which in turn participates in the regulation of the hypocretin/orexin system,[137] helping to consolidate wakefulness.[138] SCN projections into the periventricular portion of the PVN convey circadian signals to descending circuits that synapse in the preganglionic sympathetic neurons of the spinal cord that regulate many autonomic functions, including rhythmic pineal melatonin secretion.[139,140] There are also sparse projections to corticotropin-releasing hormone cells in the PVN that contribute to the circadian rhythm of corticosterone secretion and to the ventrolateral preoptic nucleus, which promotes sleep.[134]

The SPZ is an especially important relay for SCN signals, and lesions in this area reduce the amplitude or disrupt multiple circadian rhythms, including rhythmic sleep, body temperature, locomotor activity, and neural activity in structures outside the SCN. The SPZ may be the region in the hypothalamus that translates SCN signals to determine whether an animal's behavior is nocturnal or diurnal.[141] As an integration site of SCN signals with other homeostatic drives, the SPZ allows for plasticity in the timing of behavior. An example of such behavioral plasticity is seen when food access is restricted to a few hours in daytime. Under these conditions, locomotor activity shifts phase from the night into the day and eventually causes nocturnal torpor (natural hypothermia).[142,143]

Although homogeneous in its cytoarchitecture, the SPZ can be divided into functional quadrants that are interconnected to each other and the SCN. The dorsal subdivision is critical for relaying SCN signals regulating body temperature rhythms whereas the ventral subdivision seems more important for relaying SCN signals that control rhythms of sleep and locomotor activity.[144–146] The medial region of the SPZ receives afferent fibers mainly from the dorsomedial aspect of the SCN. On the other hand, the lateral SPZ receives signals from the ventrolateral SCN and RHT afferents that extend beyond the boundaries of the SCN. These extra-SCN retinal inputs to the lateral SPZ may be part of a functional subdivision of the RHT[147] and may have contact with neuroendocrine cells in the hypothalamus, providing direct input to neuroendocrine and autonomic circuits as a parallel pathway for photic regulation of homeostatic control.[103,148]

THE SUPRACHIASMATIC NUCLEUS REGULATES PERIPHERAL CIRCADIAN OSCILLATORS

Over the past decade it has become clear that the SCN is not the only circadian oscillator in mammalian systems. Several regions of the brain outside the SCN have the capacity to generate circadian oscillations in neural activity and virtually all organs of the body contain autonomous circadian oscillators.[149–153] The oscillators outside the SCN use the same core clock genes that generate circadian oscillations in the SCN, and 5% to 10% of the transcriptome in peripheral tissues display circadian rhythms (ie, up to approximately 10% of the genes are clock-driven genes) although the subset of rhythmic transcripts is distinct among the various tissues, reflecting their specific functions.[154] The most significant difference between the SCN oscillator and the vast majority of peripheral oscillators is that the latter depend on SCN-derived signals to maintain sustained rhythms due to the lack of strong coupling between cells in peripheral tissues compared with the tightly coupled neural network of the SCN.

In addition, although photic cues entrain the SCN and contribute to coupling among SCN neurons, peripheral tissues have no direct access to signals from the retina and thus are dependent on the SCN both for entrainment to the day/night cycle and for maintaining intercellular coupling. The full scope and nature of the SCN-regulated signals that entrain and couple peripheral oscillators are not, however, completely understood. For example, rhythms in body temperature that are regulated by the SCN may play an important role in maintaining synchrony between cells in peripheral organs.[155,156] Yet another example is observed in daily feeding rhythms: restricting the feeding of a nocturnal animal to daytime hours alone shifts the phase of clock gene RNA expression in the liver and other peripheral tissues, whereas the SCN remains normally entrained to the light/dark cycle.[157]

Lastly, a crucially important temporal signal that helps maintain synchrony among peripheral (and central) oscillators is the SCN-regulated daily rhythm in glucocorticoids (cortisol in humans and corticosterone in rodents). Glucocorticoids are potent transcriptional regulators. The robust corticosterone rhythm is critically important in synchronizing subordinate circadian oscillators in the periphery. This is accomplished through the action of glucocorticoid receptors (GRs) on glucocorticoid-responsive elements within the promoter and enhancer sequences of the *per1* and *per2* genes.[158–160] The rhythmic expression of a diverse set of genes in the central nervous system is dependent on rhythmic corticosterone secretion,[150,161–166] although there are no GRs in the SCN. It has been shown that manipulation of corticosterone rhythms alters the speed of re-entrainment to shifted light/dark cycles[167,168] and rhythmic regulation of GRs leads to phase-dependent changes in the sensitivity to glucocorticoids,[169] emphasizing the need for the coordination of central and peripheral oscillators. Serotonin synthesis in the dorsal raphe nucleus is dependent on the high-amplitude corticosterone rhythm,[164,170] and flattening in the cortisol rhythm due to increased basal levels is common for patients suffering from major depression.[171–174] Moreover, there may also be an association between the daily cortisol rhythm and SAD: SAD patients may have both the phase-delayed circadian system (discussed previously) and a reduced daily cortisol rhythm.[175] Recent studies using animal models with entrainment to winter-like (short-day) cycles have observed that when animals exhibit behavioral activity rhythms that are substantially delayed under these conditions, the amplitude of the corticosterone rhythm is reduced by 50%.[176]

Studies, such as those reported in this article and many others currently under way, continue to reinforce the notion that the precise regulation of circadian timing, whether driven or merely coordinated by the central circadian pacemaker in the SCN, is crucial to the sustenance of both physical and mental health. Much work remains to be done to uncover the full range of the mechanisms through which this regulation is effected, but each discovery yields new opportunities to help restore the temporal balance that is required to live in harmony with the ineluctable cyclicity of the earth's rotation.

REFERENCES

1. de Mairan M. Observation botanique. Paris: Historie de l'Academie Royale des Sciences; 1729. p. 1.
2. de Candolle A. Physiologie vegetale, ou Exposition des forces et des fonctions vitals des vegetaux. Paris: Bechet jeune; 1832.
3. Darwin C, Darwin F. The power of movements in plants. London: John Murray; 1880.
4. Johnson MS. Effect of continuous light on periodic spontaneous activity of white-footed mice (Peromyscus). J Exp Zool 1939;82:315–28.
5. Pittendrigh CS. On temperature independence in the clock-system controlling emergence time in Drosophlia. Proc Natl Acad Sci U S A 1954;40:1018–29.
6. Aschoff J. Exogenous and endogenous components in circadian rhythms. Cold Spring Harb Symp Quant Biol 1960;25:11–28.
7. Hamner KC, Finn JC, Sirohi GS, et al. The biological clock at the South Pole. Nature 1962;195:476–80.
8. Richter CP. Biological clocks in medicine and psychiatry. Springfield (IL): Thomas; 1965.
9. Pickard GE, Sollars PJ. The suprachiasmatic nucleus. In: Masland R, Albright TD, editors. The senses: vision, vol. 1. San Diego (CA): Academic Press; 2008. p. 537–55.

10. Crosby EC, Woodburne RT. The comparative anatomy of the preoptic area and the hypothalamus. In: Fulton JF, editor. The hypothalamus. Baltimore (MD): Williams and Wilkins; 1939. p. 52–169.
11. Moore RY, Lenn NJ. A retinohypothalamic projection in the rat. J Comp Neurol 1972;146:1–14.
12. Hendrickson AE, Wagoner N, Cowan WM. An autoradiographic and electron microscopic study of retinohypothalamic connections. Z Zellforsch Mikrosk Anat 1972;135:1–26.
13. Stephan FK, Zucker I. Circadian rhythms in drinking behavior and locomotor activity of rats are eliminated by hypothalamic lesions. Proc Natl Acad Sci U S A 1972;69:1583–6.
14. Moore RY, Eichler VB. Loss of circadian adrenal corticosterone rhythm following suprachiasmatic lesions in the rat. Brain Res 1972;42:201–6.
15. Schwartz WJ, Gainer H. Suprachiasmatic nucleus: use of 14^C-labeled deoxyglucose uptake as a functional marker. Science 1977;197:1089–91.
16. Inouye SIT, Kawamura H. Persistence of circadian rhythmicity in a mammalian hypothalamic "island" containing the suprachiasmatic nucleus. Proc Natl Acad Sci U S A 1979;76:5962–6.
17. Inouye SIT, Kawamura H. Characteristics of a circadian pacemaker in the suprachiasmatic nucleus. J Comp Physiol 1982;146:153–66.
18. Green DJ, Gillette R. Circadian rhythm of firing rate recorded from single cells in the rat suprachiasmatic brain slice. Brain Res 1982;245:198–200.
19. Sawaki Y, Nihonmatsu I, Kawamura H. Transplantation of the neonatal suprachiasmatic nuclei into rats with complete bilateral suprachiasmatic lesions. Neurosci Res 1984;1:67–72.
20. Ralph MR, Foster RG, Davis FC, et al. Transplanted suprachiasmatic nucleus determines circadian period. Science 1990;247:975–8.
21. Sollars PJ, Kimble DP, Pickard GE. Restoration of circadian behavior by anterior hypothalamic heterografts. J Neurosci 1995;15:2109–22.
22. Sujino M, Masumoto K-H, Yamaguchi S, et al. Suprachiasmatic nucleus grafts restore circadian behavioral rhythms of genetically arrhythmic mice. Curr Biol 2003;13:664–8.
23. Balsalobre A, Damiola F, Schibler U. A serum shock induces circadian gene expression in mammalian tissue culture cells. Cell 1998;93:929–37.
24. Welsh DK, Yoo SH, Liu AC, et al. Bioluminescence imagining of individual fibroblasts reveals persistent, independently phased circadian rhythms of clock gene expression. Curr Biol 2004;14:2289–95.
25. Mohawk JA, Green CB, Takahashi JS. Central and peripheral circadian clocks in mammals. Annu Rev Neurosci 2012;35:445–62.
26. Konopka RJ, Benzer S. Clock mutants of Drosophila melanogaster. Proc Natl Acad Sci U S A 1971;68:2112–6.
27. Sun ZS, Albrecht U, Zhuchenko O, et al. RIGUI, a putative mammalian ortholog of the Drosophila period gene. Cell 1997;90:1003–11.
28. Tei H, Okamura H, Shigeyoshi Y, et al. Circadian oscillation of a mammalian homologue of the Drosophila period gene. Nature 1997;389:512–6.
29. Partch CL, Green CB, Takahashi JS. Molecular architecture of the mammalian circadian clock. Trends Cell Biol 2014;24:90–9.
30. Sato T, Kawamura H. Circadian rhythms in multiple unit activity inside and outside the suprachiasmatic nucleus in the diurnal chipmunk (Eutamias sibiricus). Neurosci Res 1984;1:45–52.

31. Welsh DK, Logothetis DE, Meister M, et al. Individual neurons dissociated from rat suprachiasmatic nucleus express independently phased circadian firing rhythms. Neuron 1995;14:697–706.
32. Meijer JH, Watanabe K, Schapp J, et al. Light responsiveness of the suprachiasmatic nucleus: long-term multiunit and single-unit recordings in freely moving rats. J Neurosci 1998;18:9078–87.
33. Kuhlman SJ, McMahon DG. Encoding the ins and outs of circadian pacemaking. J Biol Rhythms 2006;21:470–81.
34. Branaccio M, Enoki R, Mazuski CN, et al. Network-mediated encoding of circadian time: the suprachiasmatic nucleus (SCN) from genes to neurons to circuits, and back. J Neurosci 2014;34:15192–9.
35. Kuhlman SJ, Quintero JE, McMahon DG. GFP fluorescence reports Period 1 circadian gene regulation in the mammalian biological clock. Neuroreport 2000;11:1479–82.
36. Quintero JE, Kuhlman SJ, McMahon DG. The biological clock nucleus: a multiphasic oscillator network regulated by light. J Neurosci 2003;23:8070–6.
37. Ko GYP, Shi L, Ko M. Circadian regulation of ion channels and their functions. J Neurochem 2009;110:1150–69.
38. Colwell CS. Linking neural activity and molecular oscillations in the SCN. Nat Rev Neurosci 2011;12:553–69.
39. Nitabach MN, Blau J, Holmes TC. Electrical silencing of Drosophila pacemaker neurons stops the free-running circadian clock. Cell 2002;109:485–95.
40. Nitabach MN, Sheeba V, Vera DA, et al. Membrane electrical excitability is necessary for the free-running larval Drosophila circadian clock. J Neurobiol 2005;62:1–13.
41. Lundkvist GB, Block GD. Role of neuronal membrane events in circadian rhythm generation. Methods Enzymol 2005;393:623–42.
42. Depetris-Chauvin A, Berni J, Aranovich EJ, et al. Adult-specific electrical silencing of pacemaker neurons uncouples molecular clock from circadian outputs. Curr Biol 2011;21:1783–93.
43. Schwartz W, Gross R, Morton M. The suprachiasmatic nuclei contain a tetrodotoxin-resistant circadian pacemaker. Proc Natl Acad Sci U S A 1987;84:1694–8.
44. Dunlap JC, Loros JJ, DeCoursey PJ. Chronobiology: biological timekeeping. Sunderland (MA): Sinauer; 2004.
45. Pittendrigh CS, Daan S. A functional analysis of circadian pacemakers in nocturnal rodents. IV. Entrainment: pacemaker as clock. J Comp Physiol 1976;106:291–331.
46. Elliott JA. Circadian rhythms and photoperiodic time measurement in mammals. Fed Proc 1976;35:2339–46.
47. Pittendrigh CS, Daan S. A functional analysis of circadian pacemakers in nocturnal rodents. I. The stability and liability of spontaneous period. J Comp Physiol 1976;106:223–52.
48. DeCoursey PJ. LD ratios and the entrainment of circadian activity in a nocturnal and diurnal rodent. J Comp Physiol 1972;78:221–35.
49. Earnest DJ, Turek FW. Effect of one second light pulses on testicular function and locomotor activity in the golden hamster. Biol Reprod 1983;28:557–65.
50. Czeizler C, Duffy J, Shanahan T, et al. Stability, precision, and near-24-hour period of the human circadian pacemaker. Science 1999;284:2177–81.
51. Hilaire M, Gooley J, Khalsa S, et al. Human phase response curve to a 1h pulse of bright white light. J Physiol 2012;590:3035–45.

52. Cajal S. Les nouvelles idees sur la sctructure du systeme nerveux chez l'Homme at chez les Vertebres. Paris: Reinwald; 1984.
53. Keeler CE. Iris movements in blind mice. Am J Physiol 1927;81:107–12.
54. Keeler CE. The inheritance of a retinal abnormality in white mice. Proc Natl Acad Sci U S A 1924;10:329–33.
55. Ebihara S, Tsuji K. Entrainment of the circadian activity rhythm to the light cycle: effective light intensity for a Zeitgeber in the retinal degenerate C3H mouse and the normal C57BL mouse. Physiol Behav 1980;24:523–7.
56. Foster RG, Provencio I, Hudson D, et al. Circadian photoreception in the retinally degenerate mouse (rd/rd). J Comp Physiol A 1991;169:39–50.
57. Freedman MS, Lucas RJ, Soni B, et al. Regulation of mammalian circadian behavior by non-rod, non-cone, ocular photoreceptors. Science 1999;284:502–4.
58. Lucas RJ, Reddman MS, Munoz M, et al. Regulation of mammalian pineal by non-rod, non-cone, ocular photoreceptors. Science 1999;284:505–7.
59. Yoshimura T, Ebihara S. Spectral sensitivity of photoreceptors mediating phase-shifts of circadian rhythms in retinally degenerate CBA/J (rd/rd) and normal CBA/N (+/+) mice. J Comp Physiol 1996;178:797–802.
60. Lucas RJ, Douglas RH, Foster RG. Characterization of an ocular photopigment capable of driving pupillary constriction in mice. Nat Neurosci 2001;4:621–6.
61. Brainard GC, Hanifin JP, Rollag MD, et al. Human melatonin regulation is not mediated by the three cone photopic visual system. J Clin Endocrinol Metab 2001;86:433–6.
62. Thapan K, Arendt J, Skene DJ. An action spectrum for melatonin suppression: evidence for a novel non-rod, non-cone photoreceptor system in humans. J Physiol 2001;535:261–7.
63. Pickard GE, Sollars PJ. Intrinsically photosensitive retinal ganglion cells. Rev Physiol Biochem Pharmacol 2012;162:59–90.
64. Provencio I, Jiang G, DeGrip WJ, et al. Melanopsin: an opsin in melanophores, brain and eye. Proc Natl Acad Sci U S A 1998;95:340–5.
65. Provencio I, Rodriguez IR, Jiang G, et al. A novel human opsin in the inner retina. J Neurosci 2000;20:600–5.
66. Gooley JJ, Lu J, Chou TC, et al. Melanopsin in cells of origin of the retinohypothalamic tract. Nat Neurosci 2001;4:1165.
67. Berson DM, Dunn FA, Takao M. Phototransduction by retinal ganglion cells that set the circadian clock. Science 2002;295:1070–3.
68. Hattar S, Liao HW, Takao M, et al. Melanopsin-containing retinal ganglion cells: Architecture, projections, and intrinsic photosensitivity. Science 2002;295:1065–70.
69. Do MT, Yau KW. Intrinsically photosensitive retinal ganglion cells. Physiol Rev 2010;90:1547–81.
70. Sand A, Schmidt TM, Kofuji P. Diverse types of ganglion cell photoreceptors in the mammalian retina. Prog Retin Eye Res 2012;31:287–302.
71. Lucas RJ. Mammalian inner retinal photoreception. Curr Biol 2013;23:R125–33.
72. Cui Q, Ren C, Sollars PJ, et al. The injury resistant ability of melanopsin-expressing intrinsically photosensitive retinal ganglion cells. Neurosci 2015;284:845–53.
73. Baver SB, Pickard GE, Sollars PJ, et al. Two types of melanopsin retinal ganglion cell differentially innervate the hypothalamic suprachiasmatic nucleus and the olivary pretectal nucleus. Eur J Neurosci 2008;27:1763–70.
74. Chen S-K, Badea T, Hattar S. Photoentrainment and pupillary light reflex are mediated by distinct populations of ipRGCs. Nature 2011;476:92–5.

75. Pickard GE, Ralph M, Menaker M. The intergeniculate leaflet partially mediates the effects of light on circadian rhythms. J Biol Rhythms 1987;2:35–56.
76. Morin LP, Blanchard JH, Provencio I. Retinal ganglion cell projections to the hamster suprachiasmatic nucleus, intergeniculate leaflet, and visual midbrain: bifurcation and melanopsin immunoreactivity. J Comp Neurol 2003;465:401–16.
77. Hattar S, Kumar M, Park A, et al. Central projections of melanopsin-expressing retinal ganglion cells in the mouse. J Comp Neurol 2006;497:326–49.
78. Meijer JH, Schwartz WJ. In search of the pathways for light-induced pacemaker resetting in the suprachiasmatic nucleus. J Biol Rhythm 2003;18:235–49.
79. Berson D. Strange vision: ganglion cells as circadian photoreceptors. Trends Neurosci 2003;26:314–20.
80. Morin LP, Allen CN. The circadian visual system. Brain Res Rev 2006;51:1–60.
81. Pennartz CM, de Jeu MT, Geurtsen AM. Enhanced NMDA receptor activity in retinal inputs to the rat suprachiasmatic nucleus during the subjective night. J Physiol 2001;532:181–94.
82. Michel S, Itri J, Colwell CS. Excitatory mechanisms in the suprachiasmatic nucleus: the role of AMPA/KA glutamate receptors. J Neurophysiol 2002;88: 817–28.
83. Hannibal J, Kankipati L, Strang CE, et al. Central projections of intrinsically photosensitive retinal ganglion cells in the macaque monkey. J Comp Neurol 2014;522:2231–48.
84. Hannibal J. Roles of PACAP-containing retinal ganglion cells in circadian timing. Int Rev Cytol 2006;251:1–39.
85. Purrier N, Engeland W, Kofuji P. Mice deficient of glutamatergic signaling from intrinsically photosensitive retinal ganglion cells exhibit abnormal circadian photoentrainment. PLoS One 2014;9:1–10.
86. Delwig A, Majumdar S, Ahern K, et al. Glutamatergic neurotransmission from melanopsin retinal ganglion cells is required for neonatal photoaversion but not adult pupillary light reflex. PLoS One 2013;8:1–8.
87. Engelund A, Fahrenkrug J, Harrison A, et al. Vesicular glutamate transporter 2 (VGLUT2) is co-stored with PACAP in projections from the rat melanopsin-containing retinal ganglion cells. Cell Tissue Res 2010;340:243–55.
88. Obrietan K, Impey S, Storm DR. Light and circadian rhythmicity regulate MAP kinase activation in the suprachiasmatic nuclei. Nat Neurosci 1998;1:693–700.
89. Butcher G, Dziema H, Collamore M, et al. The p42/44 mitogen-activated protein kinase pathway couples photic input to circadian clock entrainment. J Biol Chem 2002;277:29519–25.
90. Dziema H, Oatis B, Butcher G, et al. The ERK/MAP kinase pathway couples light to immediate early gene expression in the suprachiasmatic nucleus. Eur J Neurosci 2003;17:1617–27.
91. Coogan AN, Piggins HD. Circadian and photic regulation of phosphorylation of ERK1/2 and Elk-1 in the suprachiasmatic nuclei of the Syrian hamster. J Neurosci 2003;23:3085–93.
92. Butcher G, Lee B, Cheng H, et al. Light stimulates MSK1 activation in the suprachiasmatic nucleus via a PACAP-ERK/MAP kinase-dependent mechanism. J Neurosci 2005;25:5305–13.
93. Cheng H-YM, Dziema H, Papp J, et al. The molecular gatekeeper dexras1 sculpts the photic responsiveness of the mammalian circadian clock. J Neurosci 2006;26:12984–95.
94. Rea MA. Light increases Fos-related protein immunoreactivity in the rat suprachiasmatic nuclei. Brain Res Bull 1989;23:577–81.

95. Kornhauser JM, Nelson DE, Mayo KE, et al. Photic and circadian regulation of c-fos gene expression in the hamster suprachiasmatic nucleus. Neuron 1990; 5:127–34.
96. Shigeyoshi Y, Taguchi K, Yamamoto S, et al. Light-induced resetting of a mammalian circadian clock is associated with rapid induction of the mPer1 transcript. Cell 1997;91:1043–53.
97. Albrecht U, Sun Z, Eichele Z, et al. A differential response of two putative mammalian circadian regulators, mper1 and mper2, to light. Cell 1997;91: 1055–64.
98. Daan S, Albrecht U, van der Horst G, et al. Assembling a clock for all seasons: are there M and E oscillators in the genes? J Biol Rhythm 2001;16:105–16.
99. Spoelstra K, Albrecht U, van der Horst GTJ, et al. Phase responses to light pulses in mice lacking functional per and cry genes. J Biol Rhythms 2004;19: 518–29.
100. Diekman CO, Belle MD, Irwin RP, et al. Causes and consequences of hyperexcitation in central clock neurons. PLoS Comput Biol 2013;9:e1003196.
101. Irwin RP, Allen CN. Calcium response to retinohypothalamic synaptic transmission in the suprachiasmatic nucleus. J Neurosci 2007;27:11748–57.
102. Block GD, Khalsa SBS, McMahon DG, et al. Biological clocks in the retina: cellular mechanisms of biological time-keeping. Int Rev Cytol 1993;146:83–144.
103. Kiessling S, Sollars P, Pickard G. Light stimulates the mouse adrenal through a retinohypothalamic pathway independent of an effect on the clock in the suprachiasmatic nucleus. PLoS One 2014;9:1–11.
104. Welsh DK, Takahashi JS, Kay SA. Suprachiasmatic nucleus: cell autonomy and network properties. Annu Rev Physiol 2010;72:551–77.
105. Pickard GE, Turek FW. Splitting of the circadian rhythm of activity is abolished by unilateral lesions of the suprachiasmatic nuclei. Science 1982;215:1119–21.
106. de la Iglesia HO, Meyer J, Carpino A Jr, et al. Antiphase oscillation of the left and right suprachiasmatic nuclei. Science 2000;290:799–801.
107. Moore RY. The suprachiasmatic nucleus and the circadian timing system. Prog Mol Biol Transl Sci 2013;119:1–28.
108. Doi M, Ishida A, Miyake A, et al. Circadian regulation of intracellular G-protein signaling mediates intercellular synchrony and rhythmicity in the suprachiasmatic nucleus. Nat Comm 2011;327:1–9.
109. Enoki R, Kuroda S, Ono D, et al. Topological specificity and hierarchical network of the circadian calcium rhythm in the suprachiasmatic nucleus. Proc Natl Acad Sci U S A 2012;109:21498–503.
110. Evans JA, Leise TL, Castanon-Cervantes O, et al. Dynamic interactions mediated by nonredundant signaling mechanisms couple circadian clock neurons. Neuron 2013;80:973–83.
111. Fan J, Zeng H, Olson DP, et al. Vasoactive intestinal polypeptide (VIP)-expressing neurons in the suprachiasmatic nucleus provide sparse GABAergic outputs to local neurons with circadian regulation occurring distal to the opening of post-synaptic $GABA_A$ ionotropic receptors. J Neurosci 2015;35:1905–20.
112. Wagner S, Castel M, Gainer H, et al. GABA in the mammalian suprachiasmatic nucleus and its role in diurnal rhythmicity. Nature 1997;387:598–603.
113. Albus H, Vansteensel MJ, Michel S, et al. A GABAergic mechanism is necessary for coupling dissociable ventral and dorsal regional oscillators within the circadian clock. Curr Biol 2005;15:886–93.
114. Choi HJ, Lee CJ, Schroeder A, et al. Excitatory actions of GABA in the suprachiasmatic nucleus. J Neurosci 2008;28:5450–9.

115. Rivera C, Voipio J, Payne JA, et al. The K+/Cl- co-transporter KCC2 renders GABA hyperpolarizing during neuronal maturation. Nature 1999;397:251–5.

116. Belenky MA, Yarom Y, Pickard GE. Heterogeneous expression of gamma-aminobutyric acid and gamma-aminobutyric acid-associated receptors and transporters in the rat suprachiasmatic nucleus. J Comp Neurol 2008;506:708–32.

117. Belenky MA, Sollars PJ, Mount DB, et al. Cell-type specific distribution of chloride transporters in the rat suprachiasmatic nucleus. Neurosci 2010;165: 1519–37.

118. Alessi DR, Zhang J, Khanna A, et al. The WNK-SPAK/ORS1 pathway: master regulator of cation-chloride cotransporters. Sci Signal 2014;7:re3.

119. Farajnia S, van Westering TLE, Meijer JH, et al. Seasonal induction of GABAergic excitation in the central mammalian clock. Proc Natl Acad Sci U S A 2014; 111:9627–32.

120. Pickard GE. The afferent connections of the suprachiasmatic nucleus of the golden hamster with emphasis on the retinohypothalamic projection. J Comp Neurol 1982;211:65–83.

121. Morin LP, Blanchard JH. Depletion of brain serotonin by 5,7-DHT modifies hamster circadian responses to light. Brain Res 1991;566:173–85.

122. Pickard GE, Weber ET, Scott PA, et al. 5-HT1B receptor agonists inhibit light-induced phase shifts of behavioral circadian rhythms and expression of the immediate-early gene c-fos in the suprachiasmatic nucleus. J Neurosci 1996; 16:8208–20.

123. Pickard GE, Smith BN, Belenky M, et al. 5-HT1B receptor-mediated presynaptic inhibition of retinal input to the suprachiasmatic nucleus. J Neurosci 1999;19: 4034–45.

124. Rea MA, Pickard GE. A 5-HT1B receptor agonist inhibits light-induced suppression of pineal melatonin production. Brain Res 2000;858:424–8.

125. Smith BN, Sollars PJ, Dudek FE, et al. Serotonergic modulation of retinal input to the mouse suprachiasmatic nucleus mediated by 5-HT$_{1B}$ and 5-HT$_7$ receptors. J Biol Rhythms 2001;16:25–38.

126. Shimazoe T, Nakamura S, Kobayashi K, et al. Role of 5-HT$_{1B}$ receptors in entrainment disorder of Otsuka long evans tokushima fatty (OLETF) rats. Neurosci 2004;123:201–5.

127. Sollars PJ, Simpson AM, Ogilvie MD, et al. Light-induced fos expression is attenuated in the suprachiasmatic nucleus of serotonin 1B receptor knockout mice. Neurosci Lett 2006;401:209–13.

128. Bramley JR, Sollars PJ, Pickard GE, et al. 5-HT$_{1B}$ receptor-mediated presynaptic inhibition of GABA release in the suprachiasmatic nucleus. J Neurophysiol 2005;93:3157–64.

129. Moldavan MG, Allen CN. GABA$_B$ receptor-mediated frequency-dependent and circadian changes in synaptic plasticity modulate retinal input to the suprachiasmatic nucleus. J Physiol 2013;591:2475–90.

130. Sollars PJ, Ogilvie MD, Simpson AM, et al. Photic entrainment is altered in the 5-HT$_{1B}$ receptor knockout mouse. J Biol Rhythms 2006;17:428–37.

131. Terman M, Terman JS. Light therapy. In: Kryger MH, Roth T, Dement WC, editors. Principles and practice of sleep medicine. 4th edition. Philadelphia: Elsevier; 2005. p. 1424–42.

132. Svenningsson P, Chergui K, Rachleff I, et al. Alterations in 5-HT$_{1B}$ receptor function by p11 in depression-like states. Science 2006;311:77–80.

133. Svenningsson P, Kim Y, Warner-Schmidt J, et al. p11 and its role in depression and therapeutic responses to antidepressants. Nat Rev Neurosci 2013;14:673–80.

134. Saper CB, Lu J, Chou TC, et al. The hypothalamic integrator for circadian rhythms. Trends Neurosci 2005;28:152–7.

135. Sylvester CM, Krout KE, Loewy AD. Suprachiasmatic nucleus projection to the medial prefrontal cortex: a viral transneuronal tracing study. Neurosci 2002; 114:1071–80.

136. Watts AG, Swanson LW, Sanchez-Watts G. Efferent projections of the suprachiasmatic nucleus; I. Studies using anterograde transport of Phaseolus vulgaris leucoagglutinin in the rat. J Comp Neurol 1987;258:204–29.

137. Aston-Jones G, Chen S, Zhu Y, et al. A neural circuit for circadian regulation of arousal. Nat Neurosci 2001;4:732–8.

138. Schwartz MD, Kilduff TS. The Neurobiology of Sleep and Wakefulness. Psychiatr Clin N Am 2015, in press.

139. Pickard GE, Turek FW. The hypothalamic paraventricular nucleus (PVN) mediates the photoperiodic control of reproduction but not the effects of light on the circadian rhythm of activity. Neurosci Lett 1983;43:67–72.

140. Klein DC, Smoot R, Weller JL, et al. Lesions of the paraventricular nucleus area of the hypothalamus disrupt the suprachiasmatic leads to spinal cord circuit in the melatonin rhythm generating system. Brain Res Bull 1983;10: 647–52.

141. Todd WD, Gall AJ, Weiner JA, et al. Distinct retinohypothalamic innervation patterns predict the developmental emergence of species-typical circadian phase preference in nocturnal Norway rats and diurnal nile grass rats. J Comp Neurol 2012;520:3277–92.

142. Hut RA, Pilorz V, Boerema AS, et al. Working for food shifts nocturnal mouse activity into the day. PLoS One 2011;6:e17527.

143. Hut RA, Kronfeld-Schor N, van der Vinne V, et al. In search of a temporal niche: environmental factors. Prog Brain Res 2012;199:281–302.

144. Pickard GE, Turek FW. Effects of partial destruction of the suprachiasmatic nuclei on two circadian parameters: wheel-running activity and short-day induced testicular regression. J Comp Physiol A 1985;156:803–15.

145. Lu J, Zhang YH, Chou TG, et al. Contrasting effects of ibotenate lesions of the paraventricular nucleus and subparaventricular zone on sleep-wake cycle and temperature regulation. J Neurosci 2001;21:4864–74.

146. Vujovic N, Gooley JJ, Jhou TC, et al. Projections from the subparaventricular zone define four channels of output from the circadian timing system. J Comp Neurol 2015. [Epub ahead of print].

147. Canteras NS, Ribeiro-Barbosa ER, Goto M, et al. The retinohypothalamic tract: comparison of axonal projection patterns from four major targets. Brain Res Rev 2011;65:150–83.

148. Abizaid A, Horvath B, Keefe DL, et al. Direct visual and circadian pathways target neuroendocrine cells in primates. Eur J Neurosci 2004;20:2767–76.

149. Abe M, Herzog ED, Yamazaki S, et al. Circadian rhythms in isolated brain regions. J Neurosci 2002;22:350–6.

150. Amir S, Lamont EW, Robinson B, et al. A circadian rhythm in the expression of PERIOD2 protein reveals a novel-SCN-controlled oscillator in the oval nucleus of the bed nucleus of the stria terminalis. J Neurosci 2004;24:781–90.

151. Granados-Fuentes D, Sazena MT, prolo LM, et al. Olfactory bulb neurons express functional, entrainable circadian rhythms. Eur J Neurosci 2004;19: 898–906.

152. Cermakian N, Boivin DB. The regulation of central and peripheral circadian clocks in humans. Obes Rev 2009;10:25–36.

153. Dibner C, Schibler U, Albrecht U. The mammalian circadian timing system: organization and coordination of central and peripheral clocks. Annu Rev Physiol 2010;72:517–49.
154. Storch KF, Lipan O, Leykin I, et al. Extensive and divergent circadian gene expression in liver and heart. Nature 2002;417:78–83.
155. Buhr ED, Yoo S-H, Takahashi JS. Temperature as a universal resetting cue for mammalian circadian oscillators. Science 2010;330:379–85.
156. Morf J, Schibler U. Body temperature cycles. Cell Cycle 2013;12:539–40.
157. Stokkan KA, Yamazaki S, Tei H, et al. Entrainment of the circadian clock in liver by feeding. Science 2001;291:490–3.
158. Balsalobre A, Brown SA, Marcacci L, et al. Resetting of circadian time in peripheral tissues by glucocorticoid signaling. Science 2000;289:2344–7.
159. Stavreva DA, Wiench M, John S, et al. Ultratradian hormone stimulation induces glucocorticoid receptor-mediated pulses of gene transcription. Nat Chem Biol 2009;11:1093–102.
160. Lightman SL, Conway-Campbell BL. The crucial role of pulsatile activity of the HPA axis for continuous dynamic equilibration. Nat Rev Neurosci 2010;11:710–8.
161. Ford GK, Al-Barazanji KA, Wilson S, et al. Orexin expression and function: glucocorticoid manipulation, stress, and feeding studies. Endocrinology 2005; 146:3724–31.
162. Lamont EW, Robinson B, Stewart J, et al. The central and basolateral nuclei of the amygdala exhibit opposite diurnal rhythms of expression of the clock protein Period 2. Proc Natl Acad Sci U S A 2005;102:4180–4.
163. Yoshida M, Koyanagi S, Matsuo A, et al. Glucocorticoid hormone regulates the circadian coordination of μ-opioid receptor expression in mouse brainstem. J Pharmacol Exp Ther 2005;315:1119–24.
164. Malek ZS, Sage D, Pévet P, et al. Daily rhythm of tryptophan hydroxylase-2 messenger ribonucleic acid within raphe neurons is induced by corticoid daily surge and modulated by enhanced locomotor activity. Endocrinol 2007;148: 5165–72.
165. Minton GO, Young AH, McQuade R, et al. Profound changes in dopaminergic neurotransmission in the prefrontal cortex in response to flattening of the diurnal glucocorticoid rhythm: Implications for bipolar disorder. Neuropsychopharmacology 2009;34:2265–74.
166. Gilhooley MJ, Pinnock SB. Herbert J Rhythmic expression of per1 in the dentate gyrus is suppressed by corticosterone: Implications for neurogenesis. Neurosci Lett 2011;489:177–81.
167. Sage D, Ganem J, Guillaumond F, et al. Influence of the corticosterone rhythm on photic entrainment of locomotor activity in rats. J Biol Rhythms 2004;19: 144–56.
168. Kiessling S, Eichele G, Oster H. Adrenal glucocorticoids have a key role in circadian resynchronization in a mouse model of jet lag. J Clin Invest 2010;120: 2600–9.
169. McClung CA. How might circadian rhythms control mood? Let me count the ways. Biol Psychiatry 2013;74:242–9.
170. Clark JA, Flick RB, Pai L-Y, et al. Glucocorticoid modulation of tryptophan hydroxylase-2 protein in raphe nuclei and 5-hydroxytryptophan concentrations in frontal cortex of C57/Bl6 mice. Mol Psychiatry 2008;13:498–506.
171. Linkowski P, Mendlewicz J, Leclercq R, et al. The 24-hour profile of adrenocorticotropin and cortisol in major depressive illness. J Clin Endocrinol Metab 1984; 61:429–38.

172. Deuschle M, Schweiger U, Weber B, et al. Diurnal activity and pulsatility of the hypothalamus-pituitary-adrenal system in male depressed patients and healthy controls. J Clin Endocrinol Metab 1997;82:234–8.
173. Posener JA, DeBattista C, Williams GH, et al. 24-hour monitoring of cortisol and corticotrophin secretion in psychotic and nonpsychotic major depression. Arch Gen Psychiatry 2000;57:755–60.
174. Wong ML, Kling MA, Munson PJ, et al. Pronounced and sustained central hyper-noradrenergic function in major depression with melancholic features: relation to hyper-cortisolism and corticotrophin-releasing hormone. Proc Natl Acad Sci U S A 2000;97:325–30.
175. Avery DH, Dahl K, Savage MV, et al. Circadian temperature and cortisol rhythms during a constant routine are phase-delayed in hypersomic winter depression. Biol Psychiatry 1997;41:1109–23.
176. Sollars PJ, Weiser MJ, Kudwa AE, et al. Altered entrainment to the day/night cycle attenuates the daily rise in circulating corticosterone in the mouse. PLoS One 2014;9:e111944.

Genetics of Sleep Disorders

Philip R. Gehrman, PhD[a],*, Brendan T. Keenan, MS[b],
Enda M. Byrne, PhD[b,c], Allan I. Pack, MBChB, PhD, FRCP[d]

KEYWORDS

- Sleep disorder • Genetics • Insomnia • Sleep apnea • Narcolepsy
- Restless legs syndrome

KEY POINTS

- Past genetic studies have been hampered by methodological limitations, in particular small sample sizes.
- Genetic studies of narcolepsy highlight the important role of human leukocyte antigen variants in disease risk.
- Genes that confer risk for sleep apnea may do so through their influence on intermediate traits, such as obesity or craniofacial features.
- For insomnia, early work suggests that genetic factors may overlap with those for psychiatric disorders.
- There is a need to apply modern genetic approaches to the study of sleep disorders.

INTRODUCTION

There is growing evidence that adequate sleep quantity and quality is important for mental health. In psychiatric populations, sleep disorders are highly prevalent, including insomnia, obstructive sleep apnea, and circadian rhythm sleep disorders. The pathophysiology of these sleep disorders is likely complex, having components shared with those for psychiatric disorders as well as elements specific to sleep disturbance. Genetic factors are known to play a role in both psychiatric and sleep disorders, but causal genetic variants are only beginning to be discovered. This article reviews the current understanding of the genetic basis for sleep disorders and suggests possible links with mental health and illness.

Disclosures: None.
[a] Department of Psychiatry, Perelman School of Medicine, University of Pennsylvania, 3535 Market Street, Suite 670, Philadelphia, PA 19104, USA; [b] Center for Sleep and Circadian Neurobiology, Perelman School of Medicine, University of Pennsylvania, 125 South 31st Street, Suite 2100, Philadelphia, PA 19104-3403, USA; [c] Queensland Brain Institute, Brisbane QLD 4072, Australia; [d] Division of Sleep Medicine, Department of Medicine, Center for Sleep and Circadian Neurobiology, Perelman School of Medicine, University of Pennsylvania, 125 South 31st Street, Suite 2100, Philadelphia, PA 19104-3403, USA
* Corresponding author.
E-mail address: gehrman@exchange.upenn.edu

Psychiatr Clin N Am 38 (2015) 667–681
http://dx.doi.org/10.1016/j.psc.2015.07.004
0193-953X/15/$ – see front matter Published by Elsevier Inc.

Abbreviations	
AHI	Apnea-Hypopnea Index
ARNTL2	Aryl hydrocarbon receptor nuclear translocator–like 2
ASPS	Advanced sleep phase syndrome
BMAL	Brain and muscle aryl hydrocarbon receptor nuclear translocator–like
BTB	BR-C, ttk and bab
BTBD9	BTB/POZ domain-containing protein
CACNA1C	Calcium channel, voltage-dependent, L type, alpha1C subunit
CK	Casein kinase
CLOCK	Circadian locomotor output cycles kaput
CRSD	Circadian rhythm sleep disorder
CRY	Cryptochrome
EEG	Electroencephalogram
GWAS	Genome-wide association study
h^2	Heritability
HLA	Human leukocyte antigen
LOD	Logarithm of the odds
LPAR1	Lysophosphatidic acid receptor I
MAP2K5	Mitogen-activated protein kinase 5
MEIS1	Myeloid ecotropic viral integration site 1 homolog
nNOS	Neuronal nitric oxide synthase
OSA	Obstructive sleep apnea
PER	Period
P2RY11	Purinergic receptor subtype P2Y$_{11}$
POZ	Pox virus and Zinc finger
PTPRD	Protein tyrosine phosphatase receptor type delta
RLS	Restless legs syndrome
SKOR1	SKI family transcriptional corepressor 1
SNP	Single-nucleotide polymorphism
VNTR	Variable number tandem repeat

METHODS FOR IDENTIFYING GENETIC VARIANTS

The goals of research on the genetic basis for sleep disorders are to identify genetic variants that confer risk for disease and to understand how these variants affect the function of biological systems. Like psychiatric phenotypes, sleep disorders are complex traits that are likely to be influenced by a large number of gene variants, including regulatory portions of DNA. The proportion of variation in risk for a disease or trait in the population that can be attributed to genetic variation is known as the heritability. There are now a large number of studies showing that sleep disorders are heritable; that is, genetic factors play a substantial role in their pathophysiology. This statement is also true for normal variation in sleep/wake traits. Despite the established genetic heritability, only a small number of validated genetic risk variants have been discovered for sleep-related traits. There are several reasons for this lack of discovery, including low statistical power caused by inadequate sample sizes, phenotypes that are assessed with considerable variability, and the heterogeneous nature of many disorders and disease pathways.

Heritability analyses represent the first step in understanding the genetic basis for sleep disorders. These analyses determine the extent to which genetic factors explain the variance in a given trait. Heritability is usually established using twin or family studies, with the underlying rationale that individuals who are more similar genetically should also be more similar phenotypically compared with individuals with less genetic similarity. The goal of these analyses is to use different types of relatedness to isolate genetic effects from those of a shared environment. If a sleep disorder, for example, is not heritable then this suggests that genetic factors do not play a strong role in disease cause and there is no need to search for involved genes. In contrast, evidence that a trait is heritable suggests there are underlying variants affecting disease risk. Many sleep parameters and sleep-related disorders have been shown over the last few decades to be heritable, including sleep duration,[1–3] chronotype,[4–7] restless legs syndrome (RLS),[8–10] insomnia,[1,11–13] parasomnia,[14] obstructive sleep apnea (OSA),[15–21] and the neurobehavioral response to sleep deprivation.[22] Among behavioral traits, some of the most heritable are the spectral characteristics of the electroencephalogram (EEG) during sleep.[23]

Once it is established that a disorder is heritable, there are several approaches to determine the specific genes or, more generally, chromosomal regions that harbor genetic variants that influence the trait of interest. This task is much more challenging. One approach is to perform a genetic linkage analysis, which relies on the inheritance structure associated with family pedigrees. Genetic linkage analysis capitalizes on the observation that genes in close proximity to one another on a chromosome are more likely to get passed down to offspring than genes that are further away.[24–30] At their most basic level, linkage studies involve comparing chromosomal regions between affected and unaffected individuals (ie, cases and controls) in order to identify those DNA segments that are more commonly shared between affected relatives, and not between affected and unaffected individuals.[25,26]

A maximum likelihood logarithm of the odds (LOD) score is computed for each location examined, with higher LOD scores indicating greater association with the phenotype. Lander and Kruglyak[25] provided LOD score thresholds for statistical significance in complex traits, with an LOD greater than or equal to 3.3 for genome-wide significant linkage (corresponding with a $P = 4.9 \times 10^{-5}$) and an LOD greater than or equal to 1.9 for suggestive linkage ($P = 1.7 \times 10^{-3}$). Although suggestive signals are of interest, they should be interpreted with caution because they could be false-positives and many are not likely to be replicated in independent samples.

Linkage analysis can be used to identify the chromosomal region that may contain a causal variant, but often does not have the resolution to narrow down to the specific variant. Linkage analysis proved to be an important tool for mapping the variants underlying many single-gene disorders, such as Huntington disease and cystic fibrosis. However, this approach has not proved a successful strategy for complex disorders, in which hundreds of variants likely contribute to risk at the population level. For these and other reasons, linkage analysis has now largely been replaced by association-based methods, including candidate gene and genome-wide association studies.

Although linkage analysis provides a scan of the entire genome, an alternative approach is to focus more selectively on candidate genes that are a priori hypothesized to be of relevance to a phenotype of interest.[26,31] Candidate genes may be chosen in several ways, including from the results of prior genetic studies or from existing knowledge about the biological mechanisms involved in the pathophysiology of a disorder. In general, association studies using candidate genes are no different than typical epidemiologic studies examining the relationship between nongenetic risk factors and a phenotype of interest. Once candidate genes have been established, standard statistical modeling can be used to assess the correlation between the candidate alleles in these genes and the phenotype of interest. Compared with linkage analysis, candidate gene studies have been shown to have stronger statistical power for complex disease traits, because they can identify genes or gene variants with smaller effects.[31,32] As with many types of association analyses, initial candidate gene studies are prone to overestimates of the true association (also referred to as winner's curse)[33–35] and, as a result, are often not replicated in subsequent studies. Perhaps the biggest limitation of candidate gene studies is that they require making assumptions about which genes are most likely to be associated with a phenotype, and thus are limited by current understanding of the mechanisms underlying a particular disorder.

With the completion of the Human Genome Project and subsequent sequencing projects, the genetic variation that exists among individuals has been characterized in increasing detail. This characterization has allowed unbiased genome-wide genotyping to examine the association between a phenotype and genetic variants across the genome, rather than specifying candidate genes a priori. An initial hypothesis-free approach is referred to as a genome-wide association study (GWAS). Since the initial GWAS analyses, thousands of genetic loci have been associated with complex traits, as detailed by the National Human Genome Research Institute GWAS Catalog (available at http://www.genome.gov/gwastudies/).[36,37] These analyses are typically restricted to common genetic variants (ie, with minor alleles occurring in more than 5% of the population), many of which have small, but significant, effects on complex diseases such as sleep-related disorders. The statistical analysis for GWAS is similar to that for candidate gene studies, but is performed on a much larger scale, examining hundreds of thousands, or more, of genetic variants. Because of the large number of tests resulting from all single-nucleotide polymorphisms (SNPs) being examined individually, a multiple comparisons correction is necessary to determine statistical significance and protect against false-positive associations. The standard for genome-wide significance is typically 5×10^{-8}, reflecting a Bonferroni correction for 1 million independent tests of the hypothesis that SNPs are associated with a phenotype.[38–41] With such a stringent threshold for statistical significance, and the small effect sizes typical of common genetic variants in complex diseases, GWASs require sample sizes on the order of several thousand individuals, at a minimum. Moreover, there is a continued need for replication of GWAS results, because initial variants are often not confirmed in independent follow-up studies.

The identification of common genetic variants using GWAS can be complemented by searching for rare variants, namely those with less than 5% minor allele frequency in the population. Thus, for rare variants, most individuals in the population share the same allele, but a small proportion have the rarer allele. Information about SNPs of this frequency is typically obtained using sequencing analyses, which can be performed either in selected candidate regions or across the genome using whole-exome or whole-genome sequencing methodologies.[42] Exome sequencing focuses on variants only in protein coding regions of the genome, where mutations are more likely to have a significant impact on biological function and hence large phenotypic effects. Just as in GWAS, rare variant analysis may examine the relationships between individual variants and a given phenotype. However, because there are far fewer individuals in samples with the minor allele, statistical power for identifying single rare variants is often low. More complex statistical approaches that examine the combined effect of rare variants within a single gene or in a given genomic region have been developed to address this limitation, but are beyond the scope of this article. Although rare variant analysis is a newer field, there has already been success in identifying rare variants in the *HBLEH41* gene (also known as *DEC2*) that have been shown to affect sleep duration in humans.[43,44]

Although these are the most common approaches that have been used to investigate the genetic basis for sleep disorders, this is a rapidly evolving field with new approaches being developed continuously. In coming years, there is sure to be fruitful research using novel approaches.

GENETICS OF CIRCADIAN RHYTHM SLEEP DISORDERS

Circadian rhythm sleep disorders (CRSDs) are logical candidates for identification of genetic mechanisms considering the progress that has been made in understanding the molecular basis for the circadian clock.[45] Within each cell of the body, there is a molecular circadian clock consisting of an autoregulatory negative feedback loop comprising the *Period* (*PER1*, *PER2*, and *PER3*) and *Cryptochrome* (*CRY1* and *CRY2*) genes.[46] Other genes involved in the molecular generation of circadian rhythms include *casein kinase 1δ* (*CK1δ*) and *casein kinase 1ε* (*CK1ε*), *CLOCK* (circadian locomotor output cycles kaput), *NPAS1*, *NPAS2*, *DEC2*, *BMAL1* (brain and muscle aryl hydrocarbon receptor nuclear translocator–like 1), and *BMAL2*. There have been a few family studies of CRSDs, mostly focusing on familial advanced sleep phase syndrome (ASPS), a sleep disorder characterized by a circadian phase that is earlier (ie, advanced) relative to the desired sleep period. These individuals typically have difficulty staying awake until the desired bedtime and wake up earlier than intended in the morning. In one family study, 3 members with strong advanced sleep phase were found to have a shorter intrinsic period of their endogenous rhythm, suggesting that a shared genetic factor may play a role.[47] Other studies have sought to use affected families to identify specific genetic variants that segregate with ASPS. A serine to glycine mutation in the casein kinase epsilon–binding region of the *PER2* gene has been reported,[48] but this was not the basis in 2 ASPS pedigrees in Japan.[49] A missense mutation in the *CK1δ* gene was identified as the causal variant in another pedigree.[49] A strength of this study was the use of functional assays in transgenic *Drosophila* and mice, although this led to opposing phenotypes of longer and shorter circadian periods in these model systems, respectively.

A trait that is related to CRSDs is chronotype, which is an individual's circadian tendency, ranging from morningness in those with advanced rhythms to eveningness in those considered so-called night owls. Twin and family studies have estimated the heritability of chronotype, rather than examining CRSD, using self-report questionnaires such as the Horne-Ostberg Morningness-Eveningness Questionnaire.[50] In twin studies the heritability of chronotype was estimated to be 54% in the United States[5] and 44% in the Netherlands.[6] Family-based studies of Hutterites[7] and in the Amazon[4] give lower estimates of heritability, with estimates of 14% and 23%, respectively. These studies suggest that chronotype is moderately heritable, with genetic factors potentially explaining as much as 50% of the variability within populations.

Candidate gene studies have been conducted to examine the association between genes that are core components of the molecular clock and either chronotype or CRSD. Eveningness was associated with the 3111C allele of the *CLOCK* gene, as well as polymorphisms in the *PER3* gene, in some[51,52] but not all[53–55] studies. Polymorphisms in the clock genes *PER1* and *PER2* have been associated with morningness in other studies.[56,57] Polymorphisms in the *PER3* and *ARNTL2* (aryl hydrocarbon receptor nuclear translocator–like 2) genes were associated with chronotype in a sample of 966 British adults.[58] In terms of CRSDs, associations have been found between delayed sleep phase syndrome and the *PER3 VNTR* (variable number tandem repeat) polymorphism[59–61] and the 3111C allele of the *CLOCK* gene.[51] The results of these studies are mixed, likely because of the small sample sizes in these studies (n<450). The overall pattern suggests that circadian genes play an important role in chronotype and possibly CRSDs, although for the latter there are too few studies with significant power to draw any firm conclusions.

GENETICS OF INSOMNIA

Insomnia is the most prevalent sleep disorder, but it has largely been ignored in genetic studies. However, there has been some interest in recent years. Clinically, insomnia is defined as difficulty initiating or maintaining sleep that is associated with significant distress or daytime consequences. As such, case-control designs could be used for genetic studies by defining the presence or absence of the clinical phenotype. Alternatively, insomnia could be treated as a quantitative trait using 1 or more sleep parameters based on questionnaires or sleep diaries, such as sleep latency or time spent awake during the night. Examining quantitative traits has the advantage of greater statistical power and provides a better characterization of the variability in many sleep parameters seen in the population. Rather than relying on self-report measures to quantify insomnia, an objective assessment of sleep using actigraphy or polysomnography could also be used. These assessment methods are not subject to the biases inherent in self-reports. EEG-based parameters are also some of the most heritable traits, with estimates of greater than 90% for some features.[23] However, objective assessment of insomnia has the limitation of frequently differing from self-reports, making it difficult to know which method is correct.

The heritability of insomnia has been estimated in a series of family and twin studies that relied on self-report measures of insomnia traits. An Australian twin registry study assessed sleep quality, disturbance, and overall patterns in 1792 monozygotic and 2101 dizygotic twin pairs.[1] Moderate genetic influences were found for sleep quality (h^2 [heritability] = 0.32), initial insomnia (h^2 = 0.32), sleep latency (h^2 = 0.44 for men and 0.32 for women), so-called anxious insomnia (h^2 = 0.36), and so-called depressed insomnia (h^2 = 0.33). In the Vietnam Era Twin Registry,[13] moderate heritability was again found for trouble falling asleep (h^2 = 0.28), trouble staying asleep (h^2 = 0.42), waking up several times per night (h^2 = 0.26), waking up feeling tired and worn out (h^2 = 0.21), and a composite sleep score (h^2 = 0.28). In a larger cohort study,[12] rates of positive family history of insomnia were not significantly different in those categorized as good sleepers, those with symptoms of insomnia, and those meeting criteria for a full insomnia syndrome (32.7%, 36.7%, and 38.1%, respectively). Significant differences were only found when accounting for personal history of insomnia in the good sleepers. Those without a personal history had a significantly lower rate of family history (29.0%) than those without a past history (48.9%), indicating that the sometimes transient nature of insomnia needs to be taken into consideration in phenotypic assessment. These studies suggest that self-reported insomnia traits are moderately heritable, with 30% to 40% of the variance attributable to genetic factors.

Only 2 GWAS analyses have been conducted in patients with insomnia. A case-control study of 10,038 individuals in Korea found an association between insomnia and the *ROR1* (receptor tyrosine kinase–like orphan receptor 1) gene, which modulates synapse formation, although this association did not reach genome-wide significance.[62] A second GWAS conducted in 2323 Australian twins failed to find any SNPs that reached genome-wide significance, but the strongest associations were between sleep latency and a group of SNPs in the third intron of the *CACNA1C* (calcium channel, voltage-dependent, L type, alpha1C subunit) gene ($P = 1.3 \times 10^{-6}$), a gene associated with bipolar disorder and schizophrenia in multiple studies.[63] Replication was not supported in a second cohort, but a separate report did find evidence of replication in an independent European cohort.[64]

NARCOLEPSY

Narcolepsy represents the greatest success in finding a genetic basis for a sleep disorder. It has been known since 1984 that narcolepsy is associated with specific human leukocyte antigens (HLAs),[65] which are expressed in immune cells and are involved in presenting foreign peptides to receptors on T cells. The risk allele for narcolepsy is DQB1*0602 in Japanese people and those of European descent, which occurs together with DQA1*0102 on a haplotype.[66] There are differences in African Americans.[67] The association with DQB1*0602 is particularly strong in patients who present with cataplexy.[68] Recent data from the European Narcolepsy Study found an aggregate odds ratio of 251 for DQB1*0602, indicating an extremely strong effect. Some HLA class II haplotypes are also protective against narcolepsy. A protective variant near HLA-DQA2 was identified in a GWAS in European individuals.[69] In the future, it may be possible to use HLA antigen profiles in suspected cases of narcolepsy for clinical purposes, although this remains to be shown.

Of note, the DQB1*0602 variant is common in many individuals without narcolepsy. The frequency of this varies by ethnic group, with a 12% frequency in Japanese and 38% frequency in African Americans.[66] Thus, the presence of this variant is not sufficient to develop narcolepsy even in homozygotes. This finding suggests that narcolepsy is a complex disorder with multiple gene variants other than DQB1*0602 involved and/or that the DQB1*0602 variant may require an environmental trigger to lead to the clinical disorder. To examine the first possibility, a GWAS was conducted by including only individuals positive for DQB1*0602 in both cases and controls to remove the effects of this variant.[70] Three SNPs within the T-cell receptor alpha locus were then identified that were significantly associated with narcolepsy. This association has been replicated in the European narcolepsy study[71] and a study in China.[72]

Another GWAS study in narcolepsy with cataplexy has identified an SNP in the purinergic receptor subtype P2Y$_{11}$ (P2RY11) gene.[73] This variant may also play a role in the immune system because it is associated with reduced expression of P2RY11 in CD^{4+} T lymphocytes and natural killer cells. Narcolepsy is a complex disorder, but all genetic variants identified to date implicate the immune system as playing a pivotal role in the pathophysiology of the disorder. Thus, it is likely an autoimmune disease.

RESTLESS LEGS SYNDROME

Another sleep disorder in which there has been considerable success in identifying genetic mechanisms is RLS. Research in this area was initially stimulated by the finding that a large proportion of patients with RLS have positive family histories.[74–76] Twin studies confirmed heritability.[8–10] The high familial aggregation led to the use of linkage analyses within large family pedigrees in several parts of the world, including French Canada, northern Italy, North America, and southern Tyrol. Several different linkage regions that were genome-wide significant were found, but no specific gene variants were identified until case-control association analyses of SNPs in these linkage regions were performed. The first linkage region to be investigated in this way was RLS-1 on chromosome 12.[77] A case-control association analysis was conducted with

1536 SNPs in this region and a significant association with an SNP in neuronal nitric oxide synthase was identified that was protective.[77]

The RLS-3 region on chromosome 9 was investigated using a similar strategy, with 3270 SNPs in the discovery phase and 8 in an independent replication sample.[78] Two different SNPs in the protein tyrosine phosphatase receptor type delta (PTPRD) gene were significantly associated with RLS. PTPRD knockout mice show impairment in long-term potentiation in memory formation and abnormal axon targeting to motoneurons during development.[79,80] This developmental role could explain the importance of this gene in RLS, but the mechanisms are currently unknown.

The seminal event in RLS genetics was the direct, simultaneous publication of 2 independent successful GWASs.[81,82] The first study, conducted in Germans and French Canadians,[81] used a questionnaire-based case definition. There was a discovery phase, with 2 independent case-control samples for replication that identified 3 different loci: 2 SNPs in MEIS1 (myeloid ecotropic viral integration site 1 homolog) on chromosome 2; 5 SNPs in BTBD9 (BTB/POZ domain-containing protein) on chromosome 6p; and 7 SNPs in chromosome 15q in the MAP2K5 (mitogen-activated protein kinase 5) gene and the adjacent SKOR1 (SKI family transcriptional corepressor 1) gene. MEIS1[83] and SKOR1[84] play a role in development. The other study used a discovery sample in Iceland and 2 independent replication case-control samples in Iceland and the United States.[82] Rather than using questionnaires, phenotyping was done using actigraphy of the legs to assess the frequency of periodic limb movements over several nights. They found an association with the same SNP for BTBD9, but this was limited to patients with periodic limb movements and not in patients with only sensory symptoms. Thus, this specific gene variant likely contributes to the motor manifestations of RLS. This SNP was associated with ferritin levels in this study, which is noteworthy given that alterations in iron metabolism can play a role in the pathogenesis of RLS.[85] However, BTBD9 does not seem to play a key role in iron metabolism.[86] The association of MEIS1 and BTBD9 has been confirmed in 1 study[87] and all 3 identified loci in other studies.[88–90]

These findings are exciting, but the variants so far identified account for only around 3% of the heritability of RLS,[91] which is all too common for complex traits.[92] Studies have begun to search for rare variants involved in RLS, but are in their infancy. Early results suggest that individuals with RLS have an excess of rare variants of MEIS1 compared with controls.[93] Exome sequencing has also started to be applied.[94] A variant of PCDHA3 was identified in a family with RLS but was absent in 500 controls. This gene is expressed in neurons and is present at synaptic junctions, where it plays a role in neural cell-cell interaction.[95] Given the large number of carefully assembled case-control and family-based cohorts in RLS, it is likely that there will be significant progress in this area in the near future.

GENETICS OF OBSTRUCTIVE SLEEP APNEA

OSA is a common sleep disorder in which there is partial or complete blockage of the airway during sleep that leads to a repetitive reduction is blood oxygen saturation.[96] OSA aggregates in families. The initial indication that OSA has a major genetic component is from a single family with a high prevalence of OSA.[21] Symptoms of OSA such as habitual snoring, excessive sleepiness, snoring, gasping, and witnessed apneas also aggregate in families.[20] Anatomic OSA risk factors, including soft tissue sizes and craniofacial dimensions, have also been shown to be heritable.[97,98] A significant confound in this area is obesity, which is a major risk factor for OSA that is itself heritable.[99–102] The Cleveland Family Study addressed this issue and assessed increased relative risk of OSA in first-degree family members. This increased risk was not affected after controlling for body mass index.[19] Thus, family aggregation is unlikely to be explained solely by obesity.

Although family aggregation has been known for more than 20 years, there has been little progress in identifying relevant gene variants. Linkage studies that have been conducted have typically been underpowered, did not find genome-wide significant linkages, and did not use fine mapping to confirm the peak and narrow the linkage region.[103–105] Candidate gene studies examining multiple candidate SNPs did not include replication samples[106] and have been significantly underpowered for common variants.[107] Meta-analyses of candidate gene studies failed to find any evidence that reported associations are replicable.[107,108] The 1 exception is for a polymorphism in the tumor necrosis factor alpha promoter.[109] Association with this SNP and OSA has been identified in European and Indian populations.[110] In a pediatric population with OSA, this SNP was associated more with sleepiness than OSA,[111] suggesting that it may contribute to one of the key consequences of OSA that patients recognize, rather than the disorder itself.

The most convincing evidence of a relevant gene variant comes from a study combining subjects from the Cleveland Family Study and the Sleep Heart Health Study[112] with replication samples from the Western Australia Sleep Health Study and, for African Americans, the Cleveland Sleep Apnea Study and Case Transdisciplinary Research in Energetics and Cancer Colon Polyp Study. More than 2000 candidate genes were chosen because of their potential relevance to heart, lung, blood, and sleep disorders.[113]

In African Americans, 1 SNP in the lysophosphatidic acid receptor I (LPAR1) gene showed a genome-wide association with a quantitative measure of OSA severity, the Apnea-Hypopnea Index (AHI). The association was greater in nonobese compared with obese subjects. In European samples, this SNP also showed evidence of association with an apnea phenotype and a trend for association with AHI. The gene is thought to play a proinflammatory role[114,115] and is expressed in the developing cerebral cortex.[116] A mouse knockout results in craniofacial abnormalities,[117] so the connection with OSA might be related to effects on neural mechanisms of airway control or craniofacial features.

There are likely different phenotypic pathways to OSA, including obesity, neuronal control of respiration, and craniofacial features, each with distinct genetic contributions. The multiple pathways highlight the difficulty in determining genetic variants conferring risk or protection for OSA in the general population. They also suggest that the search for genetic factors may be most fruitful if it is focused on each of the relevant intermediate traits.

SUMMARY

The genetics of sleep disorders is still in its infancy. Much of the work that has been done has been plagued by issues of study design, in particular inadequate sample size and lack of replication. Discoveries in the genetics of narcolepsy and RLS are the most advanced, in part because of clearer phenotyping strategies and large sample sizes. In the case of OSA, the most relevant phenotype may not be a diagnosis of sleep apnea but rather intermediate traits that are related to the pathophysiology of the disorder and have also been shown to be heritable. Insomnia is a more difficult disorder to phenotype because the underlying mechanisms remain unknown, and thus intermediate phenotypes for genetic investigation remain to be uncovered.

With the genetic variants identified to date for sleep disorders, the proportion of heritability explained remains low, which suggests that there are several variants still to be discovered. However, rapid advances are being made in genotyping methods and statistical genetics that permit novel approaches to studying the genetics of sleep disorders. Moreover, the rapid reduction in cost for whole-exome and whole-genome sequencing has made the identification of rare variants more feasible. Ultimately, there is a significant need for functional studies in model systems to better understand the biology of how each of the genetic variants so far identified contributes to the clinical phenotype.

REFERENCES

1. Heath AC, Kendler KS, Eaves LJ, et al. Evidence for genetic influences on sleep disturbance and sleep pattern in twins. Sleep 1990;13(4):318–35.
2. Partinen M, Kaprio J, Koskenvuo M, et al. Genetic and environmental determination of human sleep. Sleep 1983;6(3):179–85.
3. Watson NF, Buchwald D, Vitiello MV, et al. A twin study of sleep duration and body mass index. J Clin Sleep Med 2010;6(1):11–7.
4. Aguiar GF, da Silva HP, Marques N. Patterns of daily allocation of sleep periods: a case study in an Amazonian riverine community. Chronobiologia 1991;18(1): 9–19.
5. Hur YM, Bouchard TJ Jr, Lykken DT. Genetic and environmental influence on morningness-eveningness. Pers Individ Dif 1998;25(5):917–25.
6. Vink JM, Groot AS, Kerkhof GA, et al. Genetic analysis of morningness and eveningness. Chronobiol Int 2001;18(5):809–22.
7. Klei L, Reitz P, Miller M, et al. Heritability of morningness-eveningness and self-report sleep measures in a family-based sample of 521 Hutterites. Chronobiol Int 2005;22(6):1041–54.
8. Desai AV, Cherkas LF, Spector TD, et al. Genetic influences in self-reported symptoms of obstructive sleep apnoea and restless legs: a twin study. Twin Res 2004;7(6):589–95.
9. Xiong L, Jang K, Montplaisir J, et al. Canadian restless legs syndrome twin study. Neurology 2007;68(19):1631–3.
10. Ondo WG, Vuong KD, Wang Q. Restless legs syndrome in monozygotic twins: clinical correlates. Neurology 2000;55(9):1404–6.
11. Hauri P, Olmstead E. Childhood-onset insomnia. Sleep 1980;3(1):59–65.
12. Beaulieu-Bonneau S, LeBlanc M, Merette C, et al. Family history of insomnia in a population-based sample. Sleep 2007;30(12):1739–45.
13. McCarren M, Goldberg J, Ramakrishnan V, et al. Insomnia in Vietnam era veteran twins: influence of genes and combat experience. Sleep 1994;17(5): 456–61.
14. Hublin C, Kaprio J, Partinen M, et al. Prevalence and genetics of sleepwalking: a population-based twin study. Neurology 1997;48(1):177–81.
15. Gislason T, Johannsson JH, Haraldsson A, et al. Familial predisposition and cosegregation analysis of adult obstructive sleep apnea and the sudden infant death syndrome. Am J Respir Crit Care Med 2002;166(6):833–8.
16. Guilleminault C, Partinen M, Hollman K, et al. Familial aggregates in obstructive sleep apnea syndrome. Chest 1995;107(6):1545–51.
17. Mathur R, Douglas NJ. Family studies in patients with the sleep apnea-hypopnea syndrome. Ann Intern Med 1995;122(3):174–8.

18. Pillar G, Lavie P. Assessment of the role of inheritance in sleep apnea syndrome. Am J Respir Crit Care Med 1995;151(3 Pt 1):688–91.
19. Redline S, Tishler PV, Tosteson TD, et al. The familial aggregation of obstructive sleep apnea. Am J Respir Crit Care Med 1995;151(3 Pt 1):682–7.
20. Redline S, Tosteson T, Tishler PV, et al. Studies in the genetics of obstructive sleep apnea. Familial aggregation of symptoms associated with sleep-related breathing disturbances. Am Rev Respir Dis 1992;145(2 Pt 1):440–4.
21. Strohl KP, Saunders NA, Feldman NT, et al. Obstructive sleep apnea in family members. N Engl J Med 1978;299(18):969–73.
22. Kuna ST, Maislin G, Pack FM, et al. Heritability of performance deficit accumulation during acute sleep deprivation in twins. Sleep 2012;35(9):1223–33.
23. Ambrosius U, Lietzenmaier S, Wehrle R, et al. Heritability of sleep electroencephalogram. Biol Psychiatry 2008;64(4):344–8.
24. Palmer LJ, Schnell AH, Witte JS, et al. Parametric linkage analysis. Methods Mol Biol 2002;195:13–35.
25. Lander E, Kruglyak L. Genetic dissection of complex traits: guidelines for interpreting and reporting linkage results. Nat Genet 1995;11(3):241–7.
26. Lander ES, Schork NJ. Genetic dissection of complex traits. Science 1994; 265(5181):2037–48.
27. Almasy L, Blangero J. Multipoint quantitative-trait linkage analysis in general pedigrees. Am J Hum Genet 1998;62(5):1198–211.
28. Garner CP. Nonparametric linkage analysis. I. Haseman-Elston. Methods Mol Biol 2002;195:37–60.
29. Marlow AJ. Nonparametric linkage analysis. II. Variance components. Methods Mol Biol 2002;195:61–100.
30. Kruglyak L, Daly MJ, Reeve-Daly MP, et al. Parametric and nonparametric linkage analysis: a unified multipoint approach. Am J Hum Genet 1996;58(6): 1347–63.
31. Tabor HK, Risch NJ, Myers RM. Candidate-gene approaches for studying complex genetic traits: practical considerations. Nat Rev Genet 2002;3(5):391–7.
32. Risch N, Merikangas K. The future of genetic studies of complex human diseases. Science 1996;273(5281):1516–7.
33. Ioannidis JP. Why most discovered true associations are inflated. Epidemiology 2008;19(5):640–8.
34. Kraft P. Curses–winner's and otherwise–in genetic epidemiology. Epidemiology 2008;19(5):649–51 [discussion: 657–48].
35. Ioannidis JP, Ntzani EE, Trikalinos TA, et al. Replication validity of genetic association studies. Nat Genet 2001;29(3):306–9.
36. Welter D, MacArthur J, Morales J, et al. The NHGRI GWAS Catalog, a curated resource of SNP-trait associations. Nucleic Acids Res 2014;42(Database issue):D1001–6.
37. Visscher PM, Brown MA, McCarthy MI, et al. Five years of GWAS discovery. Am J Hum Genet 2012;90(1):7–24.
38. McCarthy MI, Abecasis GR, Cardon LR, et al. Genome-wide association studies for complex traits: consensus, uncertainty and challenges. Nat Rev Genet 2008; 9(5):356–69.
39. Pe'er I, Yelensky R, Altshuler D, et al. Estimation of the multiple testing burden for genomewide association studies of nearly all common variants. Genet Epidemiol 2008;32(4):381–5.
40. Altshuler D, Daly MJ, Lander ES. Genetic mapping in human disease. Science 2008;322(5903):881–8.

41. NCI-NHGRI Working Group on Replication in Association Studies, Chanock SJ, Manolio T, et al. Replicating genotype-phenotype associations. Nature 2007; 447(7145):655–60.
42. Cirulli ET, Goldstein DB. Uncovering the roles of rare variants in common disease through whole-genome sequencing. Nat Rev Genet 2010;11(6):415–25.
43. He Y, Jones CR, Fujiki N, et al. The transcriptional repressor DEC2 regulates sleep length in mammals. Science 2009;325(5942):866–70.
44. Pellegrino R, Kavakli IH, Goel N, et al. A novel BHLHE41 variant is associated with short sleep and resistance to sleep deprivation in humans. Sleep 2014; 37(8):1327–36.
45. Sollars PJ, Pickard GE. The neurobiology of circadian rhythms. Psychiatr Clin N Am 2015, in press.
46. Lowrey PL, Takahashi JS. Genetics of circadian rhythms in mammalian model organisms. Adv Genet 2011;74:175–230.
47. Jones CR, Campbell SS, Zone SE, et al. Familial advanced sleep-phase syndrome: a short-period circadian rhythm variant in humans. Nat Med 1999; 5(9):1062–5.
48. Toh KL, Jones CR, He Y, et al. An hPer2 phosphorylation site mutation in familial advanced sleep phase syndrome. Science 2001;291(5506):1040–3.
49. Xu Y, Padiath QS, Shapiro RE, et al. Functional consequences of a CKIdelta mutation causing familial advanced sleep phase syndrome. Nature 2005; 434(7033):640–4.
50. Horne JA, Ostberg O. A self-assessment questionnaire to determine morningness-eveningness in human circadian rhythms. Int J Chronobiol 1976; 4(2):97–110.
51. Katzenberg D, Young T, Finn L, et al. A CLOCK polymorphism associated with human diurnal preference. Sleep 1998;21(6):569–76.
52. Mishima K, Tozawa T, Satoh K, et al. The 3111T/C polymorphism of hClock is associated with evening preference and delayed sleep timing in a Japanese population sample. Am J Med Genet B Neuropsychiatr Genet 2005;133(1): 101–4.
53. Robilliard DL, Archer SN, Arendt J, et al. The 3111 Clock gene polymorphism is not associated with sleep and circadian rhythmicity in phenotypically characterized human subjects. J Sleep Res 2002;11(4):305–12.
54. Iwase T, Kajimura N, Uchiyama M, et al. Mutation screening of the human Clock gene in circadian rhythm sleep disorders. Psychiatry Res 2002;109(2):121–8.
55. Pedrazzoli M, Louzada FM, Pereira DS, et al. Clock polymorphisms and circadian rhythms phenotypes in a sample of the Brazilian population. Chronobiol Int 2007;24(1):1–8.
56. Carpen JD, Archer SN, Skene DJ, et al. A single-nucleotide polymorphism in the 5′-untranslated region of the hPER2 gene is associated with diurnal preference. J Sleep Res 2005;14(3):293–7.
57. Carpen JD, von Schantz M, Smits M, et al. A silent polymorphism in the PER1 gene associates with extreme diurnal preference in humans. J Hum Genet 2006;51(12):1122–5.
58. Parsons MJ, Lester KJ, Barclay NL, et al. Polymorphisms in the circadian expressed genes PER3 and ARNTL2 are associated with diurnal preference and GNbeta3 with sleep measures. J Sleep Res 2014;23(5):595–604.
59. Ebisawa T, Uchiyama M, Kajimura N, et al. Association of structural polymorphisms in the human period3 gene with delayed sleep phase syndrome. EMBO Rep 2001;2(4):342–6.

60. Pereira DS, Tufik S, Louzada FM, et al. Association of the length polymorphism in the human Per3 gene with the delayed sleep-phase syndrome: does latitude have an influence upon it? Sleep 2005;28(1):29–32.
61. Archer SN, Robilliard DL, Skene DJ, et al. A length polymorphism in the circadian clock gene Per3 is linked to delayed sleep phase syndrome and extreme diurnal preference. Sleep 2003;26(4):413–5.
62. Ban HJ, Kim SC, Seo J, et al. Genetic and metabolic characterization of insomnia. PLoS One 2011;6(4):e18455.
63. Byrne EM, Gehrman PR, Medland SE, et al. A genome-wide association study of sleep habits and insomnia. Am J Med Genet B Neuropsychiatr Genet 2013; 162B(5):439–51.
64. Parsons MJ, Lester KJ, Barclay NL, et al. Replication of genome-wide association studies (GWAS) loci for sleep in the British G1219 cohort. Am J Med Genet B Neuropsychiatr Genet 2013;162B(5):431–8.
65. Juji T, Satake M, Honda Y, et al. HLA antigens in Japanese patients with narcolepsy. All the patients were DR2 positive. Tissue Antigens 1984;24(5): 316–9.
66. Faraco J, Mignot E. Genetics of narcolepsy. Sleep Med Clin 2011;6(2):217–28.
67. Neely S, Rosenberg R, Spire JP, et al. HLA antigens in narcolepsy. Neurology 1987;37(12):1858–60.
68. Mignot E, Hayduk R, Black J, et al. HLA DQB1*0602 is associated with cataplexy in 509 narcoleptic patients. Sleep 1997;20(11):1012–20.
69. Hor H, Kutalik Z, Dauvilliers Y, et al. Genome-wide association study identifies new HLA class II haplotypes strongly protective against narcolepsy. Nat Genet 2010;42(9):786–9.
70. Hallmayer J, Faraco J, Lin L, et al. Narcolepsy is strongly associated with the T-cell receptor alpha locus. Nat Genet 2009;41(6):708–11.
71. Tafti M, Hor H, Dauvilliers Y, et al. DQB1 locus alone explains most of the risk and protection in narcolepsy with cataplexy in Europe. Sleep 2014;37(1):19–25.
72. Han F, Lin L, Li J, et al. TCRA, P2RY11, and CPT1B/CHKB associations in Chinese narcolepsy. Sleep Med 2012;13(3):269–72.
73. Kornum BR, Kawashima M, Faraco J, et al. Common variants in P2RY11 are associated with narcolepsy. Nat Genet 2011;43(1):66–71.
74. Walters AS, Hickey K, Maltzman J, et al. A questionnaire study of 138 patients with restless legs syndrome: the 'Night-Walkers' survey. Neurology 1996;46(1): 92–5.
75. Winkelmann J, Wetter TC, Collado-Seidel V, et al. Clinical characteristics and frequency of the hereditary restless legs syndrome in a population of 300 patients. Sleep 2000;23(5):597–602.
76. Montplaisir J, Boucher S, Poirier G, et al. Clinical, polysomnographic, and genetic characteristics of restless legs syndrome: a study of 133 patients diagnosed with new standard criteria. Mov Disord 1997;12(1):61–5.
77. Winkelmann J, Lichtner P, Schormair B, et al. Variants in the neuronal nitric oxide synthase (nNOS, NOS1) gene are associated with restless legs syndrome. Mov Disord 2008;23(3):350–8.
78. Schormair B, Kemlink D, Roeske D, et al. PTPRD (protein tyrosine phosphatase receptor type delta) is associated with restless legs syndrome. Nat Genet 2008; 40(8):946–8.
79. Uetani N, Kato K, Ogura H, et al. Impaired learning with enhanced hippocampal long-term potentiation in PTPdelta-deficient mice. EMBO J 2000;19(12): 2775–85.

80. Uetani N, Chagnon MJ, Kennedy TE, et al. Mammalian motoneuron axon targeting requires receptor protein tyrosine phosphatases sigma and delta. J Neurosci 2006;26(22):5872–80.
81. Winkelmann J, Schormair B, Lichtner P, et al. Genome-wide association study of restless legs syndrome identifies common variants in three genomic regions. Nat Genet 2007;39(8):1000–6.
82. Stefansson H, Rye DB, Hicks A, et al. A genetic risk factor for periodic limb movements in sleep. N Engl J Med 2007;357(7):639–47.
83. Maeda R, Mood K, Jones TL, et al. Xmeis1, a protooncogene involved in specifying neural crest cell fate in Xenopus embryos. Oncogene 2001;20(11):1329–42.
84. Mizuhara E, Nakatani T, Minaki Y, et al. Corl1, a novel neuronal lineage-specific transcriptional corepressor for the homeodomain transcription factor Lbx1. J Biol Chem 2005;280(5):3645–55.
85. Earley CJ, Connor J, Garcia-Borreguero D, et al. Altered brain iron homeostasis and dopaminergic function in restless legs syndrome (Willis-Ekbom disease). Sleep Med 2014;15(11):1288–301.
86. Oexle K, Ried JS, Hicks AA, et al. Novel association to the proprotein convertase PCSK7 gene locus revealed by analysing soluble transferrin receptor (sTfR) levels. Hum Mol Genet 2011;20(5):1042–7.
87. Vilarino-Guell C, Farrer MJ, Lin SC. A genetic risk factor for periodic limb movements in sleep. N Engl J Med 2008;358(4):425–7.
88. Kemlink D, Polo O, Frauscher B, et al. Replication of restless legs syndrome loci in three European populations. J Med Genet 2009;46(5):315–8.
89. Yang Q, Li L, Chen Q, et al. Association studies of variants in MEIS1, BTBD9, and MAP2K5/SKOR1 with restless legs syndrome in a US population. Sleep Med 2011;12(8):800–4.
90. Moore HT, Winkelmann J, Lin L, et al. Periodic leg movements during sleep are associated with polymorphisms in BTBD9, TOX3/BC034767, MEIS1, MAP2K5/SKOR1, and PTPRD. Sleep 2014;37(9):1535–42.
91. Schormair B, Winkelman J. Genetics of restless legs syndrome: mendelian, complex, and everything in between. Sleep Med Clin 2011;6:203–15.
92. Manolio TA, Collins FS, Cox NJ, et al. Finding the missing heritability of complex diseases. Nature 2009;461(7265):747–53.
93. Schulte EC, Kousi M, Tan PL, et al. Targeted resequencing and systematic in vivo functional testing identifies rare variants in MEIS1 as significant contributors to restless legs syndrome. Am J Hum Genet 2014;95(1):85–95.
94. Weissbach A, Siegesmund K, Bruggemann N, et al. Exome sequencing in a family with restless legs syndrome. Mov Disord 2012;27(13):1686–9.
95. Wu Q, Maniatis T. Large exons encoding multiple ectodomains are a characteristic feature of protocadherin genes. Proc Natl Acad Sci U S A 2000;97(7):3124–9.
96. Young T, Palta M, Dempsey J, et al. The occurrence of sleep-disordered breathing among middle-aged adults. N Engl J Med 1993;328(17):1230–5.
97. Chi L, Comyn FL, Keenan BT, et al. Heritability of craniofacial structures in normal subjects and patients with sleep apnea. Sleep 2014;37(10):1689–98.
98. Schwab RJ, Pasirstein M, Kaplan L, et al. Family aggregation of upper airway soft tissue structures in normal subjects and patients with sleep apnea. Am J Respir Crit Care Med 2006;173(4):453–63.
99. Stunkard AJ, Harris JR, Pedersen NL, et al. The body-mass index of twins who have been reared apart. N Engl J Med 1990;322(21):1483–7.

100. Comuzzie AG, Allison DB. The search for human obesity genes. Science 1998; 280(5368):1374–7.
101. Stunkard AJ, Foch TT, Hrubec Z. A twin study of human obesity. JAMA 1986; 256(1):51–4.
102. Maes HH, Neale MC, Eaves LJ. Genetic and environmental factors in relative body weight and human adiposity. Behav Genet 1997;27(4):325–51.
103. Palmer LJ, Buxbaum SG, Larkin E, et al. A whole-genome scan for obstructive sleep apnea and obesity. Am J Hum Genet 2003;72(2):340–50.
104. Palmer LJ, Buxbaum SG, Larkin EK, et al. Whole genome scan for obstructive sleep apnea and obesity in African-American families. Am J Respir Crit Care Med 2004;169(12):1314–21.
105. Larkin EK, Patel SR, Elston RC, et al. Using linkage analysis to identify quantitative trait loci for sleep apnea in relationship to body mass index. Ann Hum Genet 2008;72(Pt 6):762–73.
106. Larkin EK, Patel SR, Goodloe RJ, et al. A candidate gene study of obstructive sleep apnea in European-Americans and African-Americans. Am J Respir Crit Care Med 2010;182:947–53.
107. Varvarigou V, Dahabreh IJ, Malhotra A, et al. A review of genetic association studies of obstructive sleep apnea: field synopsis and meta-analysis. Sleep 2011;34(11):1461–8.
108. Thakre TP, Mamtani MR, Kulkarni H. Lack of association of the APOE epsilon 4 allele with the risk of obstructive sleep apnea: meta-analysis and meta-regression. Sleep 2009;32(11):1507–11.
109. Kroeger KM, Carville KS, Abraham LJ. The -308 tumor necrosis factor-alpha promoter polymorphism effects transcription. Mol Immunol 1997;34(5):391–9.
110. Bhushan B, Guleria R, Misra A, et al. TNF-alpha gene polymorphism and TNF-alpha levels in obese Asian Indians with obstructive sleep apnea. Respir Med 2009;103(3):386–92.
111. Khalyfa A, Serpero LD, Kheirandish-Gozal L, et al. TNF-alpha gene polymorphisms and excessive daytime sleepiness in pediatric obstructive sleep apnea. J Pediatr 2011;158(1):77–82.
112. Patel SR, Goodloe R, De G, et al. Association of genetic loci with sleep apnea in European Americans and African-Americans: the Candidate Gene Association Resource (CARe). PLoS One 2012;7(11):e48836.
113. Keating BJ, Tischfield S, Murray SS, et al. Concept, design and implementation of a cardiovascular gene-centric 50 k SNP array for large-scale genomic association studies. PLoS One 2008;3(10):e3583.
114. Ferreira MA, Hottenga JJ, Warrington NM, et al. Sequence variants in three loci influence monocyte counts and erythrocyte volume. Am J Hum Genet 2009; 85(5):745–9.
115. Maugeri N, Powell JE, t Hoen PA, et al. LPAR1 and ITGA4 regulate peripheral blood monocyte counts. Hum Mutat 2011;32(8):873–6.
116. Hecht JH, Weiner JA, Post SR, et al. Ventricular zone gene-1 (vzg-1) encodes a lysophosphatidic acid receptor expressed in neurogenic regions of the developing cerebral cortex. J Cell Biol 1996;135(4):1071–83.
117. Contos JJ, Fukushima N, Weiner JA, et al. Requirement for the lpA1 lysophosphatidic acid receptor gene in normal suckling behavior. Proc Natl Acad Sci U S A 2000;97(24):13384–9.

Primary Sleep Disorders

John Khoury, MD[a],*, Karl Doghramji, MD[b]

KEYWORDS

- Narcolepsy • Cataplexy • Insomnia • Restless leg syndrome
- Periodic limb movement disorder • Obstructive sleep apnea • Central sleep apnea
- Hypersomnolence

KEY POINTS

- Insomnia disorder is a primary sleep disorder and does not require a comorbid psychiatric condition.
- Restless legs syndrome is a clinical diagnosis of an abnormal sensation in the legs, inducing an urge to move the legs to get them comfortable.
- Periodic limb movement disorder is a polysomnographic diagnosis of twitches of the legs during sleep causing insomnia.
- Obstructive sleep apnea syndrome is a disorder of breathing during sleep causing collapse of the upper airways muscles, most commonly treated with positive airway pressure.
- Narcolepsy can exist with or without cataplexy and various treatment options are available. Hypersomnolence not categorized as narcolepsy is treated with the same agents as narcolepsy without cataplexy.

THE CLINICAL APPROACH TO SLEEP-RELATED COMPLAINTS

The 2 cardinal symptoms of sleep disorders are insomnia and excessive daytime sleepiness (EDS; also called excessive daytime somnolence).[1–4] Sleepiness refers to the increased likelihood of falling asleep. This is considered a normal biological need or drive; an apt analogy is sleep is to sleepiness as food is to hunger. Sleepiness is considered excessive when there is an increased likelihood of falling asleep at inappropriate times, such as when driving or in the middle of a conversation. Insomnia is the inability to fall asleep or stay asleep despite adequate opportunity to do so.

Disclosures: J. Khoury is on the Speakers Bureau for Merck Pharmaceuticals. K. Doghramji served as a (Prior 12 months) consultant to Teva, Merck, Jazz, Pernix, Pfizer, Xenoport, Stock: Merck.
[a] Sleep Disorders Center, Abington Neurological Associates, Abington Memorial Hospital (Jefferson Health), 2325 Maryland Road, Willow Grove, PA 19090, USA; [b] Fellowship in Sleep Medicine, Jefferson Sleep Disorders Center, Thomas Jefferson University, 211 South Ninth Street, Suite 500, Philadelphia, PA 19107, USA
* Corresponding author.
E-mail address: jskhoury@gmail.com

Psychiatr Clin N Am 38 (2015) 683–704
http://dx.doi.org/10.1016/j.psc.2015.08.002
0193-953X/15/$ – see front matter © 2015 Elsevier Inc. All rights reserved.

Abbreviations

AASM	American Academy of Sleep Medicine
AHI	Apnea–Hypopnea Index
CPAP	Continuous Positive Airway Pressure
CSA	Central Sleep Apnea
DSM	*Diagnostic and Statistical Manual of Mental Disorders*
EDS	Excessive Daytime Sleepiness
FDA	US Food and Drug Administration
ICSD	International Classification of Sleep Disorders
MSLT	Multiple Sleep Latency Test
OSA	Obstructive Sleep Apnea
PLMD	Periodic Limb Movement Disorder
PSG	Polysomnography
REM	Rapid Eye Movement
RLS	Restless Legs Syndrome

Unusual activity during sleep is another cardinal symptom of sleep disorders, such as the parasomnias. Although all these complaints can be primary disorders, the first task is to identify the underlying disorder(s) before undertaking symptomatic treatment. After the identification of a primary sleep disorder, specific treatment can be instituted with confidence.

The diagnostic process, summarized in **Box 1**,[5] begins with a thorough history, with particular attention directed toward the hallmark symptoms of the major sleep disorders as outlined. In most cases, it is beneficial to interview the bed partner, who is more likely than the patient to be aware of unusual events during sleep. If the presenting symptom is excessive daytime sleepiness, its severity should be evaluated

---

Box 1
The clinical evaluation of sleep disorders

1. Patient interview
   a. Chief complaint: insomnia, excessive daytime sleepiness, or parasomnia?
   b. History of present illness
   c. Sleep/wake habit history
   d. Sleep hygiene history: meal and exercise times, ambient noise, light and temperature, etc.
   e. Pattern of consumption of recreational substances (especially caffeine and alcohol) and medications
   f. Medication history for both medical, psychiatric and sleep disorder
   g. General medical, psychiatric, and surgical history

2. Sleep diary

3. Inventories for daytime sleepiness/alertness

4. Psychological inventories

5. Bed partner interview

6. Physical and mental status examination

7. Serum laboratory tests

8. Polysomnography

From Doghramji K, Choufani D. Taking a sleep history. In: Winkelman J, Plante D, editors. Foundations of psychiatric sleep medicine. Cambridge (MA): Cambridge University Press; 2010. p. 95–110; with permission.

carefully. Patients almost invariably misjudge the extent of sleepiness. Therefore, direct questioning regarding how sleepy an individual feels often is not helpful. The propensity for falling asleep is a more accurate measure; in severe cases, individuals fall asleep while actively engaged in complex tasks such as speaking, writing, or even eating. They may also experience sleep attacks, which mandates rapid clinical intervention. Milder levels of daytime sleepiness result in falling asleep in passive situations, such as while reading or watching television. The Epworth Sleepiness Scale[6] is a useful office-based test for daytime sleepiness.

If the history is positive for naps, the possibility that they are related to narcolepsy should be examined by determining whether they are refreshing, brief in duration, or accompanied by dreams. The timing of naps also should be determined, because this may alert the physician to the possibility of a circadian rhythm sleep disorder.

If the presenting symptom is insomnia, its duration should be determined. Disorders causing acute insomnia are usually transient in nature and more likely to resolve with conservative intervention and treatment with hypnotic agents. Chronic and unrelenting insomnia, which lasts more than a few months, usually requires a more careful investigation and complex treatment. A determination also should be made as to whether the patient's difficulty is in falling asleep or maintaining sleep. The former may be related to a circadian rhythm sleep disorder, whereas the latter is more consistent with gastroesophageal reflux disease, obstructive or central sleep apnea (CSA) syndrome, or periodic limb movement disorder (PLMD), among others.

Sleep habits should be reviewed carefully, including the patient's usual bedtime, time spent awake in bed before and after the onset of sleep, and final morning awakening and arising times. Sleep logs completed daily over 2 weeks before the evaluation often are more revealing and accurate in this regard. The history also should include the pattern of drug, medication, and recreational substance use, as well as potential sleep hygiene difficulties.

A physical examination should be performed to assess signs of specific sleep disorders; for example, a neck circumference of 16 inches or greater in women and 17 inches or greater in men is associated with an increased risk for sleep-related breathing disorders.[7] The examination can also reveal the potential for contributory medical and neurologic illnesses. A thorough psychiatric history and mental status examination are also important. Finally, serum laboratory tests, including thyroid function studies, should be considered if they have not been performed within 6 months before the evaluation.

If these office-based processes raise the possibility of an intrinsic sleep disorder, polysomnography (PSG) should be considered. Circumstances when PSG can be useful are outlined in **Box 2**.

Insufficient Sleep Syndrome

Although not classified in the *Diagnostic and Statistical Manual of Mental Disorders* (DSM)-5, insufficient sleep syndrome is recognized in the International Classification of Sleep Disorders (ICSD).[8] Insufficient sleep syndrome is often underrecognized as the most common cause of excessive daytime sleepiness worldwide. Persons affected with insufficient sleep syndrome curtail their time in bed, usually in response to social and occupational demands.[9] Sleep deprivation may be acute—lasting a few hours or days—or chronic—lasting many days, months, or years. It may also be total, encompassing the entire night, or partial, involving a few hours per night. The most common type is chronic and partial.[10] The National Sleep Foundation recently released normative sleep times by age (**Table 1**), which is a helpful guideline for

---

Box 2
Circumstances when appropriate to refer to a sleep disorders center

1. Need for nocturnal or daytime polysomnography in the following situations:
   a. Suspicion of a sleep-related breathing disorder
   b. Assessment of efficacy of treatment for a sleep-related breathing disorder
   c. Suspicion of periodic limb movement disorder or another sleep-related neuromuscular disorder that cannot be fully diagnosed by clinical interview
   d. Paroxysmal arousals or other sleep-related behaviors thought related to a seizure disorder and an electroencephalogram and clinical evaluation are inconclusive
   e. Suspicion of narcolepsy
   f. When the diagnosis of insomnia is uncertain, if previous treatments have failed, or if that patient experiences abrupt arousals associated with violent behavior (Littner, 2001)[86]

2. Need for a consultation by a physician specializing in sleep medicine

From Roberts LW, Hoop JG, Heinrich TW. Clinical psychiatry essentials. Philadelphia: Wolters Kluwer Health/Lippincott Williams & Wilkins; 2010. p. 607; with permission.

---

clinicians and patients. Sleep deprivation by as little as 1 hour per night over long periods of time can lead to debilitating EDS, which may necessitate long periods of recovery sleep. Sleep logs usually reveal curtailed bedtimes, occasionally with extended bedtime hours on weekends and holidays. Treatment with stimulant agents is rarely warranted, because no degree of chronic curtailment in sleep needs can be overcome soundly by the habitual use of stimulant agents. Instead, sufferers, usually younger adults, should be urged to extend bedtimes on a daily basis.

Table 1
National sleep foundation guidelines for sleep time

	Expert Panel Recommended Sleep Durations		
Age	Recommended (h)	May Be Appropriate (h)	Not Recommended (h)
Newborns (0–3 mo)	14–17	11–13 18–19	<11 >19
Infants (4–11 mo)	12–15	10–11 16–18	<10 >18
Toddlers (1–2 y)	11–14	9–10 15–16	<9 >16
Preschoolers (3–5 y)	10–13	8–9 14	<8 >14
School-aged children (6–13 y)	9–11	7–8 12	<7 >12
Teenagers (14–17 y)	8–10	7 11	<7 >11
Young adults (18–25 y)	7–9	6 10–11	<6 >11
Adults (26–64 y)	7–9	6 10	<6 >10
Older adults (≥65 y)	7–8	5–6 9	<5 >9

From Hirshkowitz M, Whiton K, Albert SM, et al. National sleep foundation's sleep time duration recommendations: Methodology and results summary. Sleep Health. J National Sleep Foundation 2015;1(1):40–33; with permission.

INADEQUATE SLEEP HYGIENE

This problem is also not classified as a disorder in DSM-5, but inadequate sleep hygiene bears mentioning, especially because identifying this issue as the basis for the problem with insomnia may also facilitate developing a behavioral approach to address the problem. This category encompasses behaviors and external factors that impair sleep quality and quantity (**Box 3**). From a therapeutic standpoint, proper sleep hygiene behaviors may be used to improve sleep, although these techniques are quite variable in methodology and there are limited data substantiating their efficacy.[11] However, these measures can help at home when given to patients complaining of insomnia or EDS.

INSOMNIA DISORDER

Insomnia disorder represents the second most commonly expressed complaint (after pain) in the clinical settings.[12] Insomnia includes the complaint of an inability to fall asleep, stay asleep, or experiencing frequent early morning awakenings without the ability to return to sleep. Patients often report that sleep is unrefreshing. The sleep

---

Box 3
Sleep hygiene measures

The dos of sleep hygiene

- Increase exposure to bright light during the day.
- Establish a daily activity routine.
- Exercise regularly in the morning and/or afternoon.
- Set aside a worry time.
- Establish a comfortable sleep environment.
- Do something relaxing before bedtime.
- Try a warm bath.

The don'ts of sleep hygiene

- Alcohol.
- Caffeine, nicotine, and other stimulants.
- Exposure to bright light during the night.
- Exercise within 3 h of bedtime.
- Heavy meals or drinking within 3 h of bedtime.
- Using your bed for things other than sleep (or sexual activity).
- Napping, unless a shiftworker.
- Watching the clock.
- Trying to sleep.
- Noise.
- Excessive heat/cold in room.

Adapted from American Academy of Sleep Medicine. International classification of sleep disorders: A diagnostic and coding manual. Third ed. Darien, IL: American Academy of Sleep Medicine; 2014.

disturbance should cause significant distress or impairment in social settings, occupational settings, or other important areas of function. The sleep difficulty should occur despite adequate time for sleep. DSM-5 no longer specifies whether this disorder is primary or secondary. However, the DSM-5 recommends that the insomnia be specified if it occurs with (1) nonsleep disorder mental comorbidity, including substance use disorders, (2) with other medical comorbidities, or (3) with another sleep disorder. It should be further documented as episodic (lasting 1–3 months), persistent (≥3 months), or recurrent (≥2 episodes within the space of 1 year). In the United States, 70 million people have 1 or more symptoms of insomnia,[13,14] but only 23.5 million (10% of the US population) meet the diagnostic criteria for insomnia[15] and about one-third of these patients use medications for insomnia.[16] In a 3-year longitudinal study, 74% of insomnia patients reported symptoms persisting for 1 year and 46% of patients stated that their symptoms had persisted for 3 years.[17]

Insomnia is more common in women by a factor of 1.5 to 1.[18] In women, its prevalence peaks during pregnancy and the perimenopausal and postmenopausal years. It is also more common in adolescents (ages 11–14) than in younger girls (30.4% vs 16.8%).[19] Its prevalence also increases with advancing age and affects more than one-third of the population age 65 and older. The risk of insomnia is based on levels of inactivity, dissatisfaction with social life, and the presence of organic and mental disorders, without which the risk of insomnia in healthy seniors is similar to that of younger individuals.[20]

Insomnia is more common in shift workers than in individuals working fixed schedules (20.1% vs 12.0%),[14] and its prevalence increases in proportion to the number of shifts worked.[21] Working the night or third shift may not only acutely cause insomnia, but may have a persistent deleterious effect on sleep quality even after the individual has reverted to working a day or evening shift.[22] Unemployment, lower socioeconomic status,[20,23] marital status (being divorced, widowed, or single),[23] poor mental and physical health,[24] noisy environments,[25] medical problems (eg, congestive heart failure, obstructive airway disease and other respiratory illnesses, back and hip problems, and prostate problems), and psychiatric disorders (eg, depressive disorders, anxiety disorders, substance use disorders, and schizophrenia) are also associated with an increased prevalence of insomnia.[26,27]

Seasonal differences have been reported in patients suffering from chronic insomnia In Norway, a survey done among a representative sample of 14,667 adults living in the municipality of Tromso, north of the Arctic Circle, revealed an increased incidence of complaints of insomnia during the dark period of the year compared with any other season.[28]

Insomnia sufferers place a significant burden on both the health care system and their employers, in both direct and indirect expenses, including medical expenses, ramifications of accidents, and reduced productivity owing to absenteeism and decreased work efficiency.[29] Insomnia costs the American public $92.5 to $107.5 billion annually in both direct and indirect expenses.[30]

CONDITIONED (PSYCHOPHYSIOLOGIC) INSOMNIA

Although insomnia may be initiated by a wide variety of stressors and conditions, it may persist well beyond the resolution of these factors owing to the emergence of perpetuating factors, such as learned mental associations ("I'll never be able to fall asleep") or somatized tension that, in turn, causes arousal and prevents sleep. Patients then develop an excessive concern about the inability to fall asleep, mostly felt as bedtime approaches, leading to anticipatory anxiety over the prospect of another night of sleeplessness followed by another day of fatigue. A vicious cycle is set up, therefore, where excessive focus on sleep and "trying" to sleep cause greater tension and diminished sleep.

The term "psychophysiological insomnia" is not contained in the DSM-5, but it is discussed briefly in the ICSD-3.[8] This insomnia is supported by a history of difficulty in falling asleep that is situational, usually occurring in the context of the patient's own bedroom. Sleep may be normal in other situations, such as hotel rooms. Patients also report that they can fall asleep when they are not trying to, such as when they are watching TV or reading. Patients also report approaching bedtimes at home with intense anxiety and dread. Although they may have "hard driving" personalities, psychiatric evaluation usually does not uncover diagnosable psychopathology. During the clinical examination, patients may seem to be tense. Although PSG is not usually necessary to confirm the diagnosis, it can be useful in ruling out other, concurrent, sleep disorders. Cognitive–behavioral and pharmacologic treatments are well-suited for this disorder.

NONPHARMACOLOGIC TREATMENTS OF INSOMNIA

Cognitive–behavioral therapies for insomnia are summarized in **Table 2**.[11,31] They include sleep hygiene education, as described, and stimulus control therapy. Patients are instructed to get out of bed after 15 to 20 minutes of sleeplessness while in bed, go to another room, engage in relaxing activities, but remain awake. They then return to bed only when sleepy. This therapy strives to reassociate the bedroom and bed with sleep and break the mental association between the bedroom and wakefulness. In addition, relaxation training strives to diminish tension and anxiety with various strategies, including progressive muscle relaxation, biofeedback, guided imagery, autogenic training, abdominal breathing exercises, and meditation.

Sleep restriction therapy strives to curtail sleep and is especially useful in patients with multiple awakenings during the evening. It works by producing a state of sleep debt, which aids in consolidating subsequent sleep. Patients are instructed initially

Table 2
Psychological and behavioral treatments for insomnia

Techniques	Method
Stimulus control therapy[a]	If unable to fall asleep within 20 minutes, get out of bed and repeat as necessary
Relaxation therapies[a]	Biofeedback, progressive muscle relaxation
Restriction of time in bed (sleep restriction)	Decrease time in bed to equal time actually asleep and increase as sleep efficiency improves
Cognitive therapy	Talk therapy to dispel unrealistic and exaggerated notions about sleep
Paradoxic intention	Try to stay awake
Sleep hygiene education	Promote habits that help sleep; eliminate habits that interfere with sleep
Cognitive-behavioral therapy[a]	Combines sleep restriction, stimulus control, and sleep hygiene education with cognitive therapy

[a] Standard Treatment according to American Academy of Sleep Medicine.
Adapted from Morgenthaler T, Kramer M, Alessi C, et al. Practice parameters for the psychological and behavioral treatment of insomnia: an update. An American Academy of Sleep Medicine Report. Sleep 2006;29(11):1415–9; and Bootzin RR, Perlis ML. Nonpharmacologic treatments of insomnia. J Clin Psychiatry 1992;53(Suppl):37–41.

to limit the time spent in bed to the amount of actual time they habitually sleep, as determined using sleep logs. Sleep efficiency for the patient, which is the ratio of actual sleep time to time spent in bed, is calculated over a 5-day period. When sleep efficiency increases to greater than 90%, patients are allowed 15 to 20 minutes of additional time in bed by going to bed earlier. If sleep efficiency decreases to below 85%, then their time in bed is further curtailed by a similar amount. Morning rising time is kept constant, and napping is disallowed. Over time, sleep becomes more consolidated and productive.

Cognitive therapy strives to identify and dispel thoughts that are tension producing and have a negative effect on sleep. Many individuals develop misperceptions about sleep, such as unrealistic expectations ("I must get 8 hours of sleep every night"), amplifications of consequences ("insomnia is incurable"), and sleep performance anxiety ("if I do not sleep well tonight, my performance tomorrow will be seriously jeopardized"). Once identified, misperceptions are challenged consciously, and positive perceptions about sleep are substituted. Paradoxic intention attempts to dissolve performance anxiety that prevents sleep by asking patients to stop trying to sleep and deliberately attempt to remain awake.

PHARMACOLOGIC THERAPY FOR INSOMNIA

A wide array of compounds has been used for their sleep-promoting qualities over the years. Alcohol may be one of the most widely used "self-prescribed" agents by patients with insomnia because it enhances sleepiness and decreases sleep latency. However, it is a poor choice because it is associated with increased nocturnal awakenings and greater daytime somnolence.[32,33] Alcohol can also result in further impairment in sleep-related respiration in patients with obstructive sleep apnea (OSA). Antihistamines and over-the-counter products cannot be wholeheartedly recommended both because they have unpredictable effects on sleep, and also because they can cause adverse systemic effects owing to their anticholinergic and sympathomimetic properties. Although barbiturates and barbiturate-like drugs (choral hydrate, glutethimide, and others) were used as hypnotics in the past, they are generally no longer recommended because they have a far greater potential for significant sedation and even death in overdoses when compared with benzodiazepine compounds.

Melatonin, a hormone released by the pineal gland whose secretion peaks during sleep, has long been suggested to be helpful for sleep. Melatonin has had significant popularity in recent years among patients with insomnia as an over-the-counter sleep aid. Unfortunately, the evidence to support the efficacy of melatonin as a general sleep aid is limited.[34] Melatonin may, however, be useful in affecting positive changes in circadian rhythm sleep disorders, although more definitive studies are needed. In addition, concerns exist regarding the purity of certain melatonin preparations, because over-the-counter herbal supplements are not regulated in the United States. Because of the lack of methodologically rigorous dose–response studies, the proper dosage of melatonin to be used in the treatment of insomnia is not well-delineated.

In 2008, the American Academy of Sleep Medicine (AASM) provided recommendations on available sleep medications in its practice parameters.[35] **Box 4** summarizes the most frequently prescribed drugs that are approved by the US Food and Drug Administration (FDA) for the treatment of insomnia.[9,36–38] The AASM review recommended that pharmacologic agents be supplemented with behavioral and cognitive therapies when possible, and recommended not using over-the-counter sleep aids. It came to a consensus on a treatment algorithm listed in **Box 5**. Note that the new agent suvorexant[37,39] (Belsomra), an orexin receptor antagonist, was not yet

---

Box 4
Prescribed medications for the treatment of Insomnia

1. Benzodiazepine–gamma-aminobutyric acid receptor agonists
   a. Benzodiazepines

      i. Long half-life: flurazepam (Dalmane) and quazepam (Doral)

      ii. Intermediate half-life: estazolam (ProSom) and temazepam (Restoril)

      iii. Short half-life: triazolam (Halcion)
   b. Nonbenzodiazepines that act at the benzodiazepine receptor

      i. Zolpidem (Ambien)

      ii. Zolpidem extended release (Ambien CR)

      iii. Zaleplon (Sonata)

      iv. Eszopiclone (Lunesta)

2. Melatonin receptor agonists
   a. Ramelteon (Rozerem)

3. Orexin Receptor Antagonists
   a. Suvorexant (Belsomra)

4. Histamine receptor antagonists
   a. Doxepin (Silenor)

Adapted from Roberts LW, Hoop JG, Heinrich TW. Clinical psychiatry essentials. Philadelphia: Wolters Kluwer Health/Lippincott Williams & Wilkins; 2010. p. 607; with permission.

Box 5
American Academy of Sleep Medicine treatment algorithm for insomnia

1. Short- and intermediate-acting benzodiazepine receptor agonists (benzodiazepine or newer benzodiazepine receptor agonists) or ramelteon; examples of these medications include zolpidem, eszopiclone, zaleplon, and temazepam.[a]

2. Alternate short- and intermediate-acting benzodiazepine receptor agonists or ramelteon if the initial agent has been unsuccessful.

3. Sedating antidepressants, especially when used in conjunction with treating comorbid depression/anxiety; examples include trazodone,[b] amitriptyline,[b] doxepin, and mirtazapine.[b]

4. Combined benzodiazepine receptor agonist or ramelteon and sedating antidepressant.

5. Other sedating agents; examples include antiepilepsy medications (gabapentin,[b] tiagabine[b]) and atypical antipsychotics (quetiapine[b] and olanzapine[b]). These medications may only be suitable for patients with comorbid insomnia who may benefit from the primary action of these drugs as well as from the sedating effect.

[a] Suvorexant and doxepin were not approved by the US Food and Drug Administration for insomnia at the time of the American Academy of Sleep Medicine publications, but could be considered in this step.
[b] Agents are not approved by the US Food and Drug Administration for insomnia.
Adapted from Schutte-Rodin S, Broch L, Buysse D, Dorsey C, Sateia M. Clinical guideline for the evaluation and management of chronic insomnia in adults. J Clin Sleep Med 2008;4(5):487–504.

approved by the FDA for sleep initiation and sleep maintenance therapy at the time of this publication, but it would likely be included as a first-line option today.[35] Additionally, after the AASM publication, low-dose doxepin (Silenor)[40,41] was approved by the FDA for sleep maintenance therapy.

OBSTRUCTIVE AND CENTRAL SLEEP APNEA

There are 2 types of sleep apnea syndromes, OSA and CSA. The defining pathologic events in OSA are apneas, or pauses in ventilation, and hypopneas (shallow breathing) during sleep that are owing to a closure of the upper airway. In CSA, apneas are owing to impaired inspiratory effort despite a patent upper airway. Isolated cases of pure CSA are rare, but can be seen in patients with heart failure and neuromuscular disease. More commonly, CSA coexists with OSA, in which case the latter is considered the primary pathologic entity.[9] DSM-5 also recognizes CSA as (1) idiopathic CSA, (2) Cheyne–Stokes breathing, or (3) CSA comorbid with opioid use.[42] OSA can only be diagnosed by means of PSG, which determines the apnea–hypopnea index (AHI) and is typically classified as mild (AHI 5–14), moderate (AHI 15–29), or severe (AHI ≥30).[10,42]

Upper airway closure in OSA is thought to occur because of the failure of the genioglossus and other upper airway dilator muscles. Apneas are accompanied by cyclic asphyxia (hypoxemia, hypercarbia, and acidosis) that, in turn, can cause cardiac arrhythmias, pulmonary and systemic hypertension, and a decrease in cardiac output, which increases to normal levels after the termination of apneas. Apneas are terminated by arousals, episodes of sudden brain activation that are reflected by an increase in electroencephalographic frequency to the alpha range during sleep; in turn, they cause sleep fragmentation and poor sleep quality, which is thought to be responsible for the excessive daytime sleepiness EDS and emotional consequences of the disorder.[43]

Patients commonly present for clinical attention at the behest of their bed partner, who may be concerned about sleep-related gaps in breathing or loud snoring, or because sleepiness interferes with daytime function. Because patients are unaware of their own snoring, bed partners and family members must be interviewed to provide collateral information regarding the patient's symptoms related to possible OSA. Snoring can be exacerbated by weight gain, alcohol ingestion near bedtime, and lying on one's back.[43] It is often a source of embarrassment and may place significant strain on interpersonal relationships, because spouses may resort to sleeping in separate beds or bedrooms. Bed partners also often observe whole body movements, occasionally violent, during apneic episodes. Patients may talk and yell during sleep and assume unusual body positions as they attempt to inspire; however, sleepwalking is uncommon. Despite obvious discontinuous sleep, it is striking that most patients report sleep to be continuous, with the notable exception of the elderly, who may report insomnia. The symptoms associated with OSA are consequences of the fragmented nocturnal sleep and asphyxia. Factors that predispose an individual to OSA are summarized in **Box 6**.[44,45] The Mallampati score grades the amount of space available in the oropharynx and can independently predict apnea risk. It is defined as: class I, soft palate, uvula, fauces, tonsillar pillars visible; class II, soft palate, uvula, fauces visible; class III, soft palate, base of uvula visible; and class IV, only hard palate visible. Historical risk factors include a history of snoring, breathing pauses during sleep, and EDS.

Approximately 25% of the prevalence of OSA is owing to genetic inheritance.[46–48] OSA is 3 times more likely in active smokers than in individuals who have never

---

Box 6
Predisposing factors for obstructive sleep apnea syndrome

1. Obesity (body mass index > 30 kg/m^2)

2. Neck circumference greater than 17 inches in men and greater than 16 inches in women

3. Upper airway occlusion as judged by the Mallampati score

4. Adenotonsillar hypertrophy

5. Large uvula

6. Low-lying soft palate

7. Tonsilar hypertrophy

8. Narrow or obstructed nasal passages

9. Retrognathia, micrognathia, and other craniofacial abnormalities

From Roberts LW, Hoop JG, Heinrich TW. Clinical psychiatry essentials. Philadelphia: Wolters Kluwer Health/Lippincott Williams & Wilkins; 2010. p. 607; with permission.

---

smoked.[49] Also, people with chronic nocturnal nasal congestion owing to any cause have a 2-fold higher prevalence of OSA.[45,50] A variety of medical conditions, such as diabetes mellitus, increase the risk.[51]

Symptoms of depression are more common in OSA patients as compared with the general community.[1] The severity of depression correlates with the severity of the OSA; therefore, OSA should be considered in the differential diagnosis of major depression. Treatment of OSA in patients with depression symptoms has been shown to improve those symptoms.[2] Sudden awakenings associated with intense anxiety have also been reported, as have lapses in memory and judgment, personality changes, irritability, and aggressiveness leading to violent outbursts.[52] Many patients misuse alcohol to control anxiety and stimulants to stay awake. Cognitive changes include deficiencies in attention, concentration, complex problem solving, and short-term recall.[53,54] Occupational and academic productivity is often impaired.[55] Inhibited sexual desire, impotence, and ejaculatory impairment are reported by approximately one-third of OSA patients.

Dull, frontal morning headaches are common complaints of patients with OSA and are thought to be a result of episodic asphyxia and consequent cerebral vasodilation. These headaches can last for 1 to 2 hours. Gastroesophageal reflux is a consequence of decreased intrathoracic pressure during apneas. Sleep-related enuresis is occasionally reported, and waking up to urinate is very common in patients with OSA. Sedating pharmacologic agents, including alcohol and anxiolytic agents such as diazepam and alprazolam, tend to increase the duration and frequency of apneas. Therefore, benzodiazepines are contraindicated for untreated patients.[10]

Treatment Options for Obstructive Sleep Apnea

The first-line treatment for OSA is continuous positive airway pressure (CPAP) owing to a high level of efficacy for many patients with OSA. CPAP is an ambulatory device that introduces room air at a high flow rate into the upper airway by a nasal mask and dissipates apneas by means of a "pneumatic splint" mechanism. The optimum pressure required to eliminate apneas is determined through PSG with a variable pressure device, after which patients use CPAP at a constant pressure at home while asleep. The primary complication in the use of CPAP is nonadherence; only one-half of patients prescribed CPAP actually use it regularly.[56–58] Reasons for noncompliance with CPAP include upper airway irritation, discomfort at the mask site, and feelings of suffocation, among others. Various methods can enhance adherence, including in-line air humidification, mask shapes and sizes that are tailored to patients' preferences, bilevel positive airway pressure devices that deliver lower pressures during expiration than inspiration, and demand-pressure devices that tailor the pressure delivered to the severity of apneas on an ongoing basis. New masks, new data card recorders, and now smart phone applications are all constantly being developed to help patients become more compliant with CPAP therapy.

Medical weight reduction should always be encouraged, although its results are often unpredictable. Therefore, it should not be relied on as the sole treatment modality for more severe cases, although it can be very effective for obese patients with mild disease. Oral appliances that prevent mandibular and tongue collapse during sleep have also seen a recent increase in popularity, although the efficacy rates with oral appliances are lower than with CPAP. Their side effects include excessive salivation and jaw pain. The AASM guidelines recommend that oral appliances are not as effective as CPAP, but may be used in patients with mild or moderate OSA or in patients who cannot tolerate CPAP.[59] If breathing disturbances are found to be more frequent in the supine position, positioning devices that promote sleep in the nonsupine position can be helpful in mild OSA cases. The Zzoma device is the only FDA-approved device for positional therapy related to sleep apnea.[60,61]

Uvulopalatopharyngoplasty surgery is an operative procedure performed under general anesthesia, where the uvula is partially removed along with tonsils and part of the soft palate. It is highly effective for the elimination of snoring, but suffers from lower efficacy than CPAP for more severe forms of apnea. Combining this with more invasive procedures, such as genioglossus advancement–hyoid myotomy and suspension, bimaxillary advancement, or maxillary and mandibular osteotomy, yields higher success rates. Tracheostomy has been performed in the past, before the advent of CPAP, but is now rarely performed. Nasal surgery can be helpful in patients with mild-to-moderate OSA who also have some degree of nasal airway compromise. Surgical intervention should be considered to be second-line therapy for OSA patients who cannot tolerate CPAP therapy.[59]

Pharmacologic agents have not been met with predictable success. Modafinil (Provigil) or Armodafinil (Nuvigil) are wake-promoting agents that may be used in treating residual EDS when the OSA is treated effectively by other methods.[62,63] Upper airway stimulation was approved by the FDA for treatment of refractory OSA.[64] Currently the Inspire device is FDA approved for patients with baseline AHIs of 20 to 60 events per hour. The neurostimulator delivers electrical stimulating pulses to the hypoglossal nerve through a lead that interfaces with the hypoglossal nerve, in synchrony with ventilator activity as detected by a sensing lead placed at the fourth intercostal muscle. The median reduction of apneas reported with neurostimulation was 68%, so the device may not be curative. Slightly lees than 2% of patients had a serious adverse side effect requiring neurostimulator repositioning, but most adverse events were simply postoperative events, including sore throat from intubation, pain at the incision site, and muscle soreness.[64]

NARCOLEPSY

The 5 major symptoms of narcolepsy are persistent daytime sleepiness, cataplexy, hypnagogic (or, less commonly, hypnopompic) hallucinations, sleep paralysis, and disturbed and restless sleep. Persistent daytime sleepiness is present in all patients with narcolepsy and is usually accompanied by daytime naps that, unlike in OSA, are brief (typically 15 minutes) and refreshing. Naps are often accompanied by vivid dreams.

Cataplexy, an abrupt paralysis or paresis of skeletal muscles, usually follows emotional experiences, such as anger, surprise, laughter, or physical exercise. Rarely, it can be generalized, in which case the patient may collapse, or, more commonly, it is isolated to an individual muscle group, resulting in a transient loss of function, such as a locked jaw, feeling weak at the knees, or legs buckling during an outburst of laughter. The episode typically lasts anywhere from a few seconds to a few minutes, during which the patient is awake. After its termination, the patient typically regains function without any residual impairment. Although cataplexy is the pathognomic symptom of narcolepsy, it can only be elicited in about 70% of patient interviews.[10] Cataplexy should not be confused with its near-homonym catalepsy, or waxy flexibility, an unrelated phenomenon noted in schizophrenia of the catatonic type.

Hypnagogic (or hypnopompic) hallucinations are vivid and often frightening dreams that occur shortly after falling asleep (or upon awakening). Sleep paralysis involves a transient global paralysis of voluntary muscles, which usually occurs shortly after falling asleep and lasts a few seconds or minutes. Cataplexy, hypnagogic hallucinations, and sleep paralysis are thought to be manifestations of an underlying aberration in the control of the timing of rapid eye movement (REM) sleep, which, in turn, results in "attacks" of REM sleep during wakefulness or partial wakefulness. Sleep in narcoleptics is also typically disturbed, characterized by numerous awakenings and arousals.

Narcolepsy is a lifelong condition. Its peak age of onset is during the second decade, yet diagnosis is established an average of 10 years later. People with narcolepsy develop significant psychosocial impairments as a result of EDS, such as job loss and interpersonal difficulties. They are also susceptible to car accidents and to sustaining injuries as a result of falling asleep in inappropriate situations. Many patients with narcolepsy develop depression, anxiety, and substance use difficulties. Twenty percent of narcoleptic patients develop social anxiety disorder,[65] and in a separate study, 23% of patients with narcolepsy and cataplexy had a clinical eating disorder.[66] Children with narcolepsy may develop encompassing depressive feelings, hyperactive/aggressive behavior, and psychotic features.[67,68]

Most cases of narcolepsy are idiopathic, but there are cases of secondary narcolepsy. A genetic factor is thought to be involved because 1% to 2% of first-degree relatives are affected by the disorder, a frequency which is 20 to 40 times higher than the population risk. However, most cases are sporadic, and only 17% to 36% of monozygotic twins are concordant for narcolepsy.[69] Therefore, it cannot be explained solely on the basis of genetic factors; environmental triggers are thought to be involved, such as head trauma, viral illness, exposure to toxins, sleep deprivation, change in the sleep–wake cycle, and developmental factors such as puberty and aging.

There is a strong association between narcolepsy and HLA. The first marker identified was HLA-DR2, occurring in 85% to 98% of all white patients with narcolepsy–cataplexy. The association is weaker in the African-American population. The strongest association across all ethnic groups has been found with HLA DQB1*0602, occurring in 85% to 100% of those affected.[69-72] Other HLA-associated disorders, such as multiple sclerosis, myasthenia gravis, and systemic lupus erythematosus, are autoimmune in nature, raising the suspicion of a similar etiology in narcolepsy.[73,74] Recently, abnormalities in hypocretin (orexin)-containing neurons were found in narcoleptic animals and humans, and cerebrospinal fluid hypocretin-1 levels were noted to be lower in narcoleptics than in normal controls and in patients with other neurologic conditions.[75] Hypocretin neuron cell bodies in the human brain are localized to the perifornical region of the posterior hypothalamus, extending into the lateral hypothalamus. These neurons densely innervate the hypothalamus, histaminergic tuberomammillary nucleus, noradrenergic locus coeruleus, serotonergic raphe nuclei, dopaminergic ventral tegmental area, midline thalamus, and nucleus of the diagonal band–nucleus basalis complex of the forebrain, and are thought to be important in maintaining wakefulness. Collectively, these findings suggest that narcolepsy is caused by an autoimmune destruction of wakefulness-controlling hypocretin cells.

Other than the obvious behavioral manifestations of EDS (yawning, drooping eyelids, psychomotor retardation), the physical examination of narcoleptic patients is typically unrevealing. The diagnosis must be confirmed by nocturnal PSG, followed by a multiple sleep latency test (MSLT). PSG is performed to ensure adequate nocturnal sleep and the lack of other intrinsic sleep disorders. The PSG often reveals a short REM latency and sleep fragmentation caused by numerous awakenings and arousals. To establish the diagnosis, the average MSLT sleep latency should be 8 minutes or less[76] and should reveal REM episodes during at least 2 nap opportunities or in 1 nap opportunity if the previous night PSG reveals the onset of REM sleep within 15 minutes.[8] The DSM-5 allows the diagnosis of narcolepsy to be established by the presence of any one of the following: cataplexy, hypocretin deficiency by cerebrospinal fluid analysis, or a positive PSG and MSLT (as defined). However, in the ICSD-3, if cerebrospinal fluid hypocretin testing is not performed, or not diagnostic for the disorder, a positive PSG with MSLT is required for the diagnosis of narcolepsy (regardless of the presence or absence of cataplexy).[8]

Antidepressant medications can cause REM suppression on electroencephalography, so these drugs may prevent sleep onset REM occurrences during the PSG and MSLT, making the diagnosis of narcolepsy more difficult to establish. For patients who are able to stop their antidepressant drug, they should do so at least 2 weeks before testing to prevent REM rebound during testing.

Treatment of narcolepsy is directed at daytime somnolence, REM-related aberrations, and psychosocial consequences. In milder cases, excessive sleepiness can be managed with conservative measures, such as spending an adequate time in bed, taking 2 or 3 short naps, and avoiding alcohol and other sedating agents. Even in more severe cases, judiciously timed naps can minimize the dosage of medication required to control symptoms. Commonly used medications for excessive sleepiness and cataplexy are described in **Table 3**. Tolerance may be minimized by prescribing

Table 3
Pharmacologic treatment of narcolepsy

For EDS	For Cataplexy	For Both EDS and Cataplexy
Methylphenidate	Protriptyline	Sodium oxybate (γ-hydroxybutyrate)[a]
Methamphetamine	Fluoxetine	—
Amphetamine	Venlafaxine	—
Modafinil[a]	Clomipramine	—
Armodafinil[a]	—	—

Abbreviation: EDS, excessive daytime sleepiness.
  [a] Agents are approved by the US Food and Drug Administration for treating the listed symptom.
  Adapted from Mignot E. Narcolepsy: pharmacology, pathophysiology, and genetics. In: Kryger M, Thomas R, Dement W, editors. Principles and practice of sleep medicine. Philadelphia: Elsevier Science, WB Saunders; 2005. p. 761–79.

the lowest effective dose and asking patients to take regular drug holidays on days when their need for alertness is lowest. The only drug approved by the FDA for treatment of cataplexy is sodium oxybate. It is also approved for the treatment of EDS in narcolepsy.

Common side effects of stimulant medications include palpitations, flushing, headache, nausea, and dizziness. Modafinil and armodafinil may both cause headache, rash, or rarely Stevens–Johnson syndrome. It is also important to note that these agents may decrease the efficacy of hormonal contraception, and that women should be counseled to use an alternative barrier protection. Sodium oxybate side effects include weight loss, parasomnias, dizziness, and diarrhea.[77]

Many patients with narcolepsy also require emotional support. Education plays a key role in management, because peers, parents, teachers, and patients themselves may confuse the effects of drowsiness with laziness or lack of motivation.

HYPERSOMNIA DISORDER

The DSM-V criteria for hypersomnia disorder are listed in **Box 7**. It should be specified if it occurs with a (1) mental disorder, (2) medical condition, or (3) another sleep disorder. It should be specified whether it is (1) acute (duration <1 month), (2) subacute (1–3 months), or (3) persistent (>3 months). It can further be classified as mild (difficulty maintaining alertness 1–2 days per week), moderate (3–4 days per week), or severe (5–7 days per week). Nocturnal PSG followed by MSLT will help make the diagnosis as the patient should have a mean sleep latency of less than 8 minutes and fewer than 2 sleep onset REM periods.[8]

Hypersomnia disorder can often be challenging to treat because there are no drugs approved by the FDA for the treatment of hypersomnia as a primary disorder. Medications used are, in general, the same as those used for narcolepsy except that there is no role for anticataplexy medications.

Box 7
DSM 5 criteria for hypersomnia disorder

1. Self-reported excessive sleepiness (hypersomnolence) despite a main sleep period lasting at least 7 hours, with at least one of the following symptoms:
   a. Recurrent periods of sleep or lapses into sleep within the same day.
   b. A prolonged main sleep episode of more than 9 hours per day that is nonrestorative (ie, unrefreshing).
   c. Difficulty being fully awake after abrupt awakening.

2. The hypersomnolence occurs at least 3 times per week, for at least 3 months.

3. The hypersomnolence is accompanied by significant distress or impairment in cognitive, social, occupational, or other important areas of functioning.

4. The hypersomnolence is not better explained by and does not occur exclusively during the course of another sleep disorder (eg, narcolepsy, breathing-related sleep disorder, circadian rhythm sleep disorder, or a parasomnia).

5. The hypersomnolence is not attributable to the physiologic effects of a substance (eg, a drug of abuse, a medication).

6. Coexisting mental and medical disorders do not adequately explain the predominant complaint of hypersomnolence.

Reprinted with permission from the Diagnostic and Statistical Manual of Mental Disorders, Fifth Edition, (Copyright © 2013). American Psychiatric Association. All Rights Reserved.

RESTLESS LEGS SYNDROME AND PERIODIC LIMB MOVEMENT DISORDER

PLMD is characterized by the repetitive (usually every 20–40 seconds) twitches of the legs and, less commonly, arms during sleep. Patients usually present with the complaint of unrelenting insomnia, most often characterized by repeated awakenings after sleep onset. Some patients with PLMD complain of EDS. In either case, the patient with PLMD is usually unaware of the movements and the brief arousals that follow, and has no lasting sensation in the extremities. PLMD is not defined as a disorder in the DSM-5, but is described in the ICSD-3.[8]

Also known as Willis–Ekbom's disease,[78] the hallmark symptom in restless legs syndrome (RLS) is an irresistible urge to move the extremities, typically the legs, but occasionally also the arms and other body parts. Patients with RLS often experience uncomfortable and unpleasant sensations in the extremities, which are described as creepy–crawly, painful, tugging, and tingling, among others. These symptoms begin, or are worsened, during periods of rest or inactivity, such as while attending the theater or reading quietly, and peak in the evening. As a result, patients commonly complain of difficulty in falling and staying asleep. Their symptoms are also typically partially or totally relieved by movement, such as walking or stretching, although relief is usually temporary. Many patients with RLS are depressed, irritable, and angry. Psychosocial impairments, such as job loss and relationship difficulties, are quite common. The 2 disorders are believed to be related. Approximately 80% of patients with RLS also have PLMD, yet only 30% of individuals who have PLMD also have RLS symptoms.

Both periodic leg movements during sleep and RLS are more common in middle and older age. The disorders can be primary (idiopathic), in which case the etiology is thought to be owing to an abnormality of brain dopamine receptors, although the etiology of the disorder is unknown. They can also be secondary, in which case they coexist with a wide variety of conditions (eg, pregnancy), the intake of certain drugs (eg, caffeine and various antidepressants), drug withdrawal states, iron deficiency, uremia, leukemia, neuropathy, and rheumatoid arthritis, as well as after gastric surgery. The symptoms are typically exacerbated by stress.

PSG is not necessary to establish the diagnosis in RLS; its diagnosis is based on symptoms alone. However, PSG is necessary to confirm the diagnosis of PLMD. The results of PSG testing in this case reveal periodic leg muscle bursts during quiet wakefulness and sleep, the latter associated with arousals and awakenings. RLS should be distinguished from nocturnal leg cramps, which involve pain in the deep muscles of the lower extremities and are independent of sleep and usually worsen with movement, and from akathesia, a motor restlessness that occurs in the context of treatment with neuroleptics and antidepressants.

Once the diagnosis is established, the first goal is to identify the underlying cause. To this end, a thorough physical examination, chemistry panel, complete blood count, and serum ferritin should be performed and underlying abnormalities treated. If the serum ferritin is <50 µg/L, supplementation with ferrous sulfate should be instituted and follow-up testing should be performed to avoid iron overload. Sleep hygiene principles should be followed. For the primary disorder, treatment choices involve the use of dopamine agonists, including pramipexole (Mirapex), ropinirole (Requip), and rotigotine (Neupro), which are all FDA approved for the treatment of RLS. Typical side effects include augmentation (worsening of symptoms despite escalating dose), postural hypotension, somnolence, and nausea. Additionally, compulsive behavior can be seen at higher doses. Pramipexole should be avoided in patients with renal disease, because it primarily excreted in the urine. Gabapentin-enacarbil (Horizant) is also FDA approved for the treatment of RLS and differs from traditional gabapentin in that the enacarbil moiety is a prodrug that allows for better gastrointestinal absorption and enhanced bioavailability. Typical side effects include sedation, dizziness, fatigue, and peripheral edema. For refractory patients, benzodiazapines or opiates, such as codeine, can be used for therapy, but these treatments are not FDA approved for this indication.[79,80] Levodopa with carbidopa is no longer used for RLS, because it seems to have a high propensity for augmentation.[81,82]

PARASOMNIAS

Parasomnias are disturbing events that occur during sleep or are aggravated by sleep. REM sleep behavior is of particular concern, because patients with this disorder have

Table 4
Features and treatments of common parasomnias

Parasomnia	Clinical Features	PSG Findings	Treatment
Sleep walking	Ambulation in sleep Age affected: prepubertal children Difficulty in arousal during episode Amnesia for the episode Episodes occur in the first one-third of night	Sleepwalking out of slow wave sleep	Prevention: removal of sharp objects, floor mattress; reassurance of parents, psychiatric evaluation for adults; benzodiazepines in refractory cases
Sleep terrors	Sudden, intense scream during sleep with evidence of intense fear; no dream recall	Sleep terror beginning during slow wave sleep	Reassurance in children Psychiatric evaluation for adults
Nightmare disorder	Sudden awakening with intense fear Recall of frightening dream content Full alertness on awakening Usually occur in latter one-half of night Frequent nightmares can be indicative of psychiatric conditions	Abrupt awakening from REM Tachycardia and tachypnea during episode	Psychotherapy Hypnosis Prasozin[87–90]
REM sleep behavior disorder	Violent or injurious behavior during sleep Body movement associated with dreams Dream recall present Dreams are enacted while they occur Neurologic evaluations with MRI of the brain and evoked potentials rarely reveal structural lesions May be a harbinger for a synucleinopathy	Excessive EMG tone or phasic twitching in REM	Clonazepam Melatonin Protective measures Psychotherapy
Sleep bruxism	Tooth grinding or clenching during sleep Tooth wear and jaw discomfort	Bursts of jaw EMG activity	Dental examination Mouth guards Relaxation training Psychotherapy

Abbreviations: EMG, electromyogram; PSG, polysomnography; REM, rapid eye movement.
From Roberts LW, Hoop JG, Heinrich TW. Clinical psychiatry essentials. Philadelphia: Wolters Kluwer Health/Lippincott Williams & Wilkins; 2010. p. 607; with permission.

a very high rate of developing Parkinson's disease or other α-synucleinopathies. Notably, 40% to 66% of patients with REM sleep behavior are symptomatic within 10 years. Identification will become more important in the future as trials for potential neuroprotective agents in Parkinson's disease begin.[83–85] Clinical aspects, including the description and treatment of the most common parasomnias, are summarized in **Table 4**.

SUMMARY

Disturbances in sleep and wakefulness in the psychiatric setting can be related to primary sleep disorders, whose identification and direct management can augment psychiatric care. It is important, therefore, for psychiatrists to develop strategies to recognize the disorders discussed in this article and either be comfortable treating them or recognize when to refer to a sleep disorders center and sleep specialist.

REFERENCES

1. BaHammam AS, Kendzerska T, Gupta R, et al. Comorbid depression in obstructive sleep apnea: an under-recognized association. Sleep Breath 2015. [Epub ahead of print].
2. Edwards C, Mukherjee S, Simpson L, et al. Depressive symptoms before and after treatment of obstructive sleep apnea in men and women. J Clin Sleep Med 2015. [Epub ahead of print].
3. Gupta MA, Simpson FC. Obstructive sleep apnea and psychiatric disorders: a systematic review. J Clin Sleep Med 2015;11(2):165–75.
4. Breslau N, Roth T, Rosenthal L, et al. Sleep disturbance and psychiatric disorders: a longitudinal epidemiological study of young adults. Biol Psychiatry 1996;39(6):411–8.
5. Doghramji K, Choufani D. Taking a sleep history. In: Winkelman J, Plante D, editors. Foundations of psychiatric sleep medicine. Cambridge (MA): Cambridge University Press; 2010. p. 95–110.
6. Johns MW. A new method for measuring daytime sleepiness: the Epworth Sleepiness Scale. Sleep 1991;14(6):540–5.
7. Chung F, Yegneswaran B, Liao P, et al. STOP questionnaire: a tool to screen patients for obstructive sleep apnea. Anesthesiology 2008;108(5):812–21.
8. American Academy of Sleep Medicine. International classification of sleep disorders: a diagnostic and coding manual. 3rd edition. Darien (IL): American Academy of Sleep Medicine; 2014.
9. Roberts LW, Hoop JG, Heinrich TW. Clinical psychiatry essentials. Philadelphia: Wolters Kluwer Health/Lippincott Williams & Wilkins; 2010. p. 607.
10. Kryger M, Roth T, Dement WC. Principles and practice of sleep medicine. 5th edition. Philadelphia: Elsevier Saunders; 2011.
11. Morgenthaler T, Kramer M, Alessi C, et al. Practice parameters for the psychological and behavioral treatment of insomnia: an update. An American Academy of Sleep Medicine report. Sleep 2006;29(11):1415–9.
12. Mahowald MW, Kader G, Schenck CH. Clinical categories of sleep disorders I. Continuum 1997;3(4):35–65.
13. Ohayon MM, Partinen M. Insomnia and global sleep dissatisfaction in Finland. J Sleep Res 2002;11(4):339–46.
14. Ohayon MM, Lemoine P, Arnaud-Briant V, et al. Prevalence and consequences of sleep disorders in a shift worker population. J Psychosom Res 2002;53(1): 577–83.

15. National Institutes of Health. National institutes of health state of the science conference statement on manifestations and management of chronic insomnia in adults, June 13–15, 2005. Sleep 2005;28(9):1049–57.

16. Bertisch SM, Herzig SJ, Winkelman JW, et al. National use of prescription medications for insomnia: NHANES 1999-2010. Sleep 2014;37(2):343–9.

17. Morin CM, Belanger L, LeBlanc M, et al. The natural history of insomnia: a population-based 3-year longitudinal study. Arch Intern Med 2009;169(5):447–53.

18. Sutton DA, Moldofsky H, Badley EM. Insomnia and health problems in Canadians. Sleep 2001;24(6):665–70.

19. Camhi SL, Morgan WJ, Pernisco N, et al. Factors affecting sleep disturbances in children and adolescents. Sleep Med 2000;1(2):117–23.

20. Ohayon MM, Zulley J, Guilleminault C, et al. How age and daytime activities are related to insomnia in the general population: consequences for older people. J Am Geriatr Soc 2001;49(4):360–6.

21. Harma M, Tenkanen L, Sjoblom T, et al. Combined effects of shift work and lifestyle on the prevalence of insomnia, sleep deprivation and daytime sleepiness. Scand J Work Environ Health 1998;24(4):300–7.

22. Dumont M, Montplaisir J, Infante-Rivard C. Sleep quality of former night-shift workers. Int J Occup Environ Health 1997;3(Supplement 2):S10–4.

23. Ohayon MM. Epidemiology of insomnia: what we know and what we still need to learn. Sleep Med Rev 2002;6(2):97–111.

24. Li RH, Wing YK, Ho SC, et al. Gender differences in insomnia–a study in the Hong Kong Chinese population. J Psychosom Res 2002;53(1):601–9.

25. Kageyama T, Kabuto M, Nitta H, et al. A population study on risk factors for insomnia among adult Japanese women: a possible effect of road traffic volume. Sleep 1997;20(11):963–71.

26. Ishigooka J, Suzuki M, Isawa S, et al. Epidemiological study on sleep habits and insomnia of new outpatients visiting general hospitals in japan. Psychiatry Clin Neurosci 1999;53(4):515–22.

27. Morgan K, Clarke D. Risk factors for late-life insomnia in a representative general practice sample. Br J Gen Pract 1997;47(416):166–9.

28. Pallesen S, Nordhus IH, Nielsen GH, et al. Prevalence of insomnia in the adult Norwegian population. Sleep 2001;24(7):771–9.

29. Walsh JK, Engelhardt CL. The direct economic costs of insomnia in the United States for 1995. Sleep 1999;22(Suppl 2):S386–93.

30. Stoller MK. Economic effects of insomnia. Clin Ther 1994;16(5):873–97 [discussion: 854].

31. Bootzin RR, Perlis ML. Nonpharmacologic treatments of insomnia. J Clin Psychiatry 1992;53(Suppl):37–41.

32. Johnson EO, Roehrs T, Roth T, et al. Epidemiology of alcohol and medication as aids to sleep in early adulthood. Sleep 1998;21(2):178–86.

33. Roehrs T, Roth T. Sleep, sleepiness and alcohol use. Alcohol Res Health 2001;25(2):101–9.

34. Stone BM, Turner C, Mills SL, et al. Hypnotic activity of melatonin. Sleep 2000;23(5):663–9.

35. Schutte-Rodin S, Broch L, Buysse D, et al. Clinical guideline for the evaluation and management of chronic insomnia in adults. J Clin Sleep Med 2008;4(5):487–504.

36. Markov D, Doghramji K. Doxepin for insomnia. Curr Psychiatry 2010;9(10):67–77.

37. Herring WJ, Connor KM, Ivgy-May N, et al. Suvorexant in patients with insomnia: results from two 3-month randomized controlled clinical trials. Biol Psychiatry 2014. [Epub ahead of print].

38. Bennett T, Bray D, Neville MW. Suvorexant, a dual orexin receptor antagonist for the management of insomnia. P T 2014;39(4):264–6.
39. Michelson D, Snyder E, Paradis E, et al. Safety and efficacy of suvorexant during 1-year treatment of insomnia with subsequent abrupt treatment discontinuation: a phase 3 randomised, double-blind, placebo-controlled trial. Lancet Neurol 2014; 13(5):461–71.
40. Krystal AD, Durrence HH, Scharf M, et al. Efficacy and safety of doxepin 1 mg and 3 mg in a 12-week sleep laboratory and outpatient trial of elderly subjects with chronic primary insomnia. Sleep 2010;33(11):1553–61.
41. Krystal AD, Lankford A, Durrence HH, et al. Efficacy and safety of doxepin 3 and 6 mg in a 35-day sleep laboratory trial in adults with chronic primary insomnia. Sleep 2011;34(10):1433–42.
42. American Psychiatric Association. Diagnostic and statistical manual of mental disorders: DSM-V. 5th edition. Arlington (VA): American Psychiatric Association; 2013.
43. Chokroverty S. Sleep disorders medicine: basic science, technical considerations, and clinical aspects. 3rd edition. Philadelphia: Saunders/Elsevier; 2009. p. 676.
44. Nuckton TJ, Glidden DV, Browner WS, et al. Physical examination: Mallampati score as an independent predictor of obstructive sleep apnea. Sleep 2006; 29(7):903–8.
45. Young T, Skatrud J, Peppard PE. Risk factors for obstructive sleep apnea in adults. JAMA 2004;291(16):2013–6.
46. Patel SR, Larkin EK, Redline S. Shared genetic basis for obstructive sleep apnea and adiposity measures. Int J Obes (Lond) 2008;32(5):795–800.
47. Palmer LJ, Redline S. Genomic approaches to understanding obstructive sleep apnea. Respir Physiolo Neurobiol 2003;135(2–3):187–205.
48. Palmer LJ, Buxbaum SG, Larkin EK, et al. Whole genome scan for obstructive sleep apnea and obesity in African-American families. Am J Respir Crit Care Med 2004;169(12):1314–21.
49. Zhang L, Samet J, Caffo B, et al. Cigarette smoking and nocturnal sleep architecture. Am J Epidemiol 2006;164(6):529–37.
50. Young T, Shahar E, Nieto FJ, et al. Predictors of sleep-disordered breathing in community-dwelling adults: the Sleep Heart Health Study. Arch Intern Med 2002;162(8):893–900.
51. West SD, Nicoll DJ, Stradling JR. Prevalence of obstructive sleep apnoea in men with type 2 diabetes. Thorax 2006;61(11):945–50.
52. Ohayon MM, Shapiro CM. Sleep disturbances and psychiatric disorders associated with posttraumatic stress disorder in the general population. Compr Psychiatry 2000;41(6):469–78.
53. Beebe DW, Groesz L, Wells C, et al. The neuropsychological effects of obstructive sleep apnea: a meta-analysis of norm-referenced and case-controlled data. Sleep 2003;26(3):298–307.
54. Findley LJ, Barth JT, Powers DC, et al. Cognitive impairment in patients with obstructive sleep apnea and associated hypoxemia. Chest 1986;90(5): 686–90.
55. Engleman H, Joffe D. Neuropsychological function in obstructive sleep apnoea. Sleep Med Rev 1999;3(1):59–78.
56. Wohlgemuth WK, Chirinos DA, Domingo S, et al. Attempters, adherers, and non-adherers: latent profile analysis of CPAP use with correlates. Sleep Med 2015; 16(3):336–42.

57. Weaver TE, Grunstein RR. Adherence to continuous positive airway pressure therapy: the challenge to effective treatment. Proc Am Thorac Soc 2008;5(2): 173–8.
58. Kribbs NB, Pack AI, Kline LR, et al. Objective measurement of patterns of nasal CPAP use by patients with obstructive sleep apnea. Am Rev Respir Dis 1993; 147(4):887–95.
59. Epstein LJ, Kristo D, Strollo PJ Jr, et al. Clinical guideline for the evaluation, management and long-term care of obstructive sleep apnea in adults. J Clin Sleep Med 2009;5(3):263–76.
60. Permut I, Diaz-Abad M, Chatila W, et al. Comparison of positional therapy to CPAP in patients with positional obstructive sleep apnea. J Clin Sleep Med 2010;6(3):238–43.
61. Available at: https://www.zzomaosa.com. Accessed July 10, 2015.
62. Ivanenko A, Tauman R, Gozal D. Modafinil in the treatment of excessive daytime sleepiness in children. Sleep Med 2003;4(6):579–82.
63. Roth T, White D, Schmidt-Nowara W, et al. Effects of armodafinil in the treatment of residual excessive sleepiness associated with obstructive sleep apnea/hypopnea syndrome: a 12-week, multicenter, double-blind, randomized, placebo-controlled study in nCPAP-adherent adults. Clin Ther 2006;28(5):689–706.
64. Strollo PJ Jr, Soose RJ, Maurer JT, et al. Upper-airway stimulation for obstructive sleep apnea. N Engl J Med 2014;370(2):139–49.
65. Ohayon MM. Narcolepsy is complicated by high medical and psychiatric comorbidities: a comparison with the general population. Sleep Med 2013;14(6): 488–92.
66. Fortuyn HA, Swinkels S, Buitelaar J, et al. High prevalence of eating disorders in narcolepsy with cataplexy: a case-control study. Sleep 2008;31(3):335–41.
67. Inocente CO, Gustin MP, Lavault S, et al. Depressive feelings in children with narcolepsy. Sleep Med 2014;15(3):309–14.
68. Inocente CO, Gustin MP, Lavault S, et al. Quality of life in children with narcolepsy. CNS Neurosci Ther 2014;20(8):763–71.
69. Mignot E. Genetic and familial aspects of narcolepsy. Neurology 1998;50(2 Suppl 1):S16–22.
70. Hayduk R, Flodman P, Spence MA, et al. HLA haplotypes, polysomnography, and pedigrees in a case series of patients with narcolepsy. Sleep 1997;20(10):850–7.
71. Taheri S, Mignot E. The genetics of sleep disorders. Lancet Neurol 2002;1(4): 242–50.
72. Taheri S, Zeitzer JM, Mignot E. The role of hypocretins (orexins) in sleep regulation and narcolepsy. Annu Rev Neurosci 2002;25:283–313.
73. Mignot E, Lammers GJ, Ripley B, et al. The role of cerebrospinal fluid hypocretin measurement in the diagnosis of narcolepsy and other hypersomnias. Arch Neurol 2002;59(10):1553–62.
74. Mignot E, Lin X, Arrigoni J, et al. DQB1*0602 and DQA1*0102 (DQ1) are better markers than DR2 for narcolepsy in Caucasian and black Americans. Sleep 1994;17(8 Suppl):S60–7.
75. Ripley B, Overeem S, Fujiki N, et al. CSF hypocretin/orexin levels in narcolepsy and other neurological conditions. Neurology 2001;57(12):2253–8.
76. Arand D, Bonnet M, Hurwitz T, et al. The clinical use of the MSLT and MWT. Sleep 2005;28(1):123–44.
77. Xyrem (sodium oxybate) prescribing information. 2015. Available at: http://www.xyrem.com/xyrem-pi.pdf. Accessed June 29, 2015.
78. EKBOM KA. Restless legs syndrome. Neurology 1960;10:868–73.

79. Aurora RN, Kristo DA, Bista SR, et al. The treatment of restless legs syndrome and periodic limb movement disorder in adults–an update for 2012: practice parameters with an evidence-based systematic review and meta-analyses: an American Academy of Sleep Medicine clinical practice guideline. Sleep 2012; 35(8):1039–62.
80. Aurora RN, Kristo DA, Bista SR, et al. Update to the AASM clinical practice guideline: "The treatment of restless legs syndrome and periodic limb movement disorder in adults-an update for 2012: practice parameters with an evidence-based systematic review and meta-analyses". Sleep 2012;35(8):1037.
81. Kurlan R, Richard IH, Deeley C. Medication tolerance and augmentation in restless legs syndrome: the need for drug class rotation. J Gen Intern Med 2006; 21(12):C1–4.
82. Earley CJ, Allen RP. Pergolide and carbidopa/levodopa treatment of the restless legs syndrome and periodic leg movements in sleep in a consecutive series of patients. Sleep 1996;19(10):801–10.
83. Postuma RB, Gagnon JF, Bertrand JA, et al. Parkinson risk in idiopathic REM sleep behavior disorder: preparing for neuroprotective trials. Neurology 2015; 84(11):1104–13.
84. Postuma RB, Bertrand JA, Montplaisir J, et al. Rapid eye movement sleep behavior disorder and risk of dementia in Parkinson's disease: a prospective study. Mov Disord 2012;27(6):720–6.
85. Britton TC, Chaudhuri KR. REM sleep behavior disorder and the risk of developing Parkinson disease or dementia. Neurology 2009;72(15):1294–5.
86. Littner M, Johnson SF, McCall WV, et al. Practice parameters for the treatment of narcolepsy: an update for 2000. Sleep 2001;24(4):451–66.
87. Racin PR, Bellonci C, Coffey DB. Expanded usage of prazosin in pre-pubertal children with nightmares resulting from posttraumatic stress disorder. J Child Adolesc Psychopharmacol 2014;24(8):458–61.
88. Nadorff MR, Lambdin KK, Germain A. Pharmacological and non-pharmacological treatments for nightmare disorder. Int Rev Psychiatry 2014;26(2):225–36.
89. Writer BW, Meyer EG, Schillerstrom JE. Prazosin for military combat-related PTSD nightmares: a critical review. J Neuropsychiatry Clin Neurosci 2014;26(1):24–33.
90. Green B. Prazosin in the treatment of PTSD. J Psychiatr Pract 2014;20(4):253–9.

Sleep Disturbances and Behavioral Disturbances in Children and Adolescents

Shirshendu Sinha, MBBS[a],*, Ronak Jhaveri, MD[b],
Alok Banga, MD, MPH, MS[c]

KEYWORDS

- RLS • PLMD • OSA • Parasomnias • Hypersomnias • Polysomnography
- Electroencephalogram

KEY POINTS

- Normal sleep–wake function evolves from infancy to adolescence.
- Sleep complaints are common in the pediatric population.
- Sleep disturbances can often lead to neurocognitive and psychosocial impairments.
- Sleep disturbances in children and adolescents should be appropriately diagnosed and treated with behavioral and pharmacologic interventions as indicated.

INTRODUCTION

Sleep is an essential component of development and is required for physical and mental health. Unfortunately, sleep deprivation and sleep disorders are prevalent among children and adolescents (0–19 years). Cross-sectional surveys of Canadian high school students reported that up to 70% of students get less than the recommended amount of sleep for their age.[1] In addition, 25% to 50% of youth are affected by some type of sleep disorder during infancy, childhood, and/or adolescence.[2] Inadequate sleep has a pervasive negative impact on the health, cognitive function, and quality of life of children and adolescents, which in turn causes significant economic and social costs.[1,2]

Disclosures: Dr S. Sinha is the recipient of 2014 Janssen Academic Research Mentorship Award (Research and travel support) and 2015 American Society of Clinical Psychopharmacology (ASCP) Clinical Trial Fellowship Award (travel support). Drs R. Jhaveri and A. Banga have no disclosures.
[a] Department of Psychiatry and Psychology, Mayo School of Graduate Medical Education, Mayo Clinic College of Medicine, 200 First Street SW, Rochester, MN 55905, USA; [b] Department of Psychiatry, University of Connecticut School of Medicine, 263 Farmington Avenue, Farmington, CT 06030, USA; [c] Sierra Vista Hospital, 8001 Bruceville Road, Sacramento, CA 95823, USA
* Corresponding author.
E-mail address: Sinha.shirshendu@mayo.edu

Psychiatr Clin N Am 38 (2015) 705–721
http://dx.doi.org/10.1016/j.psc.2015.07.009
0193-953X/15/$ – see front matter © 2015 Elsevier Inc. All rights reserved.

psych.theclinics.com

Abbreviations

ADHD	Attention deficit hyperactive disorder
EDS	Excessive daytime sleepiness
FDA	Food and Drug Administration
MSLT	Multiple sleep latency test
NREM	Non–rapid eye movement
OSA	Obstructive sleep apnea
PLMD	Periodic Limb Movement Disorder
PLMS	Periodic limb movement during sleep
PSG	Polysomnography or nocturnal polysomnography
REM	Rapid eye movement
RLS	Restless legs syndrome

This article addresses developmental aspects of sleep in children and adolescents, the assessment of sleep deprivation, counseling strategies, and evidence-based practice guidelines with regard to the evaluation and treatment of pediatric sleep disorders.

THE NORMAL DEVELOPMENT OF SLEEP

Whether a person is awake or asleep at any given time depends on the net balance between the circadian drive, which facilitates wakefulness, and the homeostatic drive, which facilitates sleep.[3] These processes interact to determine sleep quality, quantity, and timing. Developmental stages in physiologic, chronobiological, neurologic, and social/environmental factors impact the pattern of sleep in various ways.

Changes in the polysomnographic (PSG) assessment of sleep can be seen across the lifespan and evolve throughout the developmental years.[4] In a fetus, cyclical patterns of quiet sleep and active sleep have been identified and reflect non–rapid eye movement (NREM) and rapid eye movement (REM) sleep, respectively.[5] Quiet sleep presents as minimal movement with rhythmic breathing, whereas active sleep is associated with irregular breathing patterns, orofacial movements, and gross motor movements. Intermediate sleep is defined as sleep that cannot be distinctly identified as quiet sleep or active sleep.[6] Cerebral blood flow and metabolism are increased during active sleep.[7]

By weeks 32 to 34 after conception, cortical synaptic functioning continues to mature and a continuous PSG pattern is evident, with bursts of tracings being synchronized across the 2 hemispheres. At this point, 80% of sleep is active sleep and 20% is quiet sleep.[8] By week 40 after conception, active sleep comprises 50% of total sleep and is evident in neonates as periods of REM, notable motor activity, and periodic breathing with apneic episodes.[7] Quiet sleep in the neonate is observed as the child lying calmly with limited muscle tone, rhythmic respirations, and rare eye movements.[9] A neonate sleeps approximately 16 hours a day.[10]

In a 1-month-old infant, sleep progressively shifts toward night time. However, a 24-hour circadian rhythm is not yet present, and infants are unable to respond to external cues to regulate sleep cycles.[11] As the brain develops between ages 3 and 6 months, evidence of NREM sleep appears and a temporal pattern of sleep begins to form, with response to external cues.[11,12] NREM and REM patterns are divided evenly until about 6 months of age, after which REM sleep periods are more present in the later third of the night, resembling the pattern of adult sleep architecture.[13] By 6 months of age, infants sleep predominantly at night, with discrete naps during the day. Sleep onset at 6 months begins to occur through NREM as opposed to REM periods. REM periods exhibit muscle paralysis by 6 months of age.[12]

Children between the ages of 1 and 5 years progressively decrease their hours of sleep from 15 to 12 hours per day and have fewer naps.[10] They also spend less time in REM and stage 4 NREM.[12] In early preadolescence, sleep onset generally occurs around 8:00 PM, with a progressive and gradual drift to a later time with increasing age. The drift in sleep onset progresses to a 2- to 3-hour physiologic delay in sleep onset during adolescence.[14] Adolescents also have a decrease in stages 3 and 4 NREM sleep, although total REM sleep time is unchanged.[9] It is imperative to teach good sleep hygiene to teenagers, and to promote a soothing environment in an effort to reduce disruptive night awakenings.[15]

SLEEP DEPRIVATION IN CHILDREN AND ADOLESCENTS

Sleep deprivation refers to the inability to obtain a sufficient amount of sleep.[16] Data from the National Sleep Foundation indicate that 34% of toddlers, 32% of preschoolers, and 27% of school-age children sleep fewer hours than their parents think that they need.[17,18] Fatigue or sleepiness in sleep-deprived children and adolescents can manifest as increased sleepiness and "sleepy behavior," such as yawning or rubbing eyes, "paradoxic" hyperactivity, aggression, moodiness, irritability, poor frustration tolerance, inattention, difficulty following through, and noncompliance.[19]

Causes of Sleep Deprivation

A number of lifestyle and environmental factors influence the amount and quality of sleep in children and adolescents, affecting the sleep–wake cycle and promoting later bedtimes. Longer hours of nighttime arousal can disrupt the quality and duration of sleep. Many behavioral factors contribute to disruption of sleep and to sleep deprivation in adolescents, including the use of electronic media in the bedroom at night, consumption of caffeinated beverages and energy drinks, as well as environmental conditions that are not conducive to effective sleep patterns, including noisy environments, uncomfortable room temperature, as well as a variety of other potentially interfering environmental variables.

Prevention of Sleep Deprivation

The clinician should emphasize the benefits of healthy sleep to parents and their children, and help them to identify unhealthy lifestyle patterns and environmental factors that contribute to sleep deprivation. It is imperative for families to be involved in the plan of care. Gruber and colleagues[20] proposed a personalized sleep "prescription" for children to be used at home.

Child Sleep Prescription

For school-age and adolescent children, emphasis is placed on good sleep hygiene practices, guided by the approach of stimulus control (eg, minimizing the use of electronic media in the late evening, avoidance of evening caffeinated drinks), regular exercise earlier in the day, avoidance of late-evening caffeinated drinks, and promotion of regular nocturnal sleep habits with the implementation of consistent meal-time and bed-time rituals.[20]

ASSESSMENT OF PEDIATRIC SLEEP DISORDERS

Between 25% and 50% of youth are affected by some type of sleep disorder during infancy, childhood, and adolescence.[2] Pediatric sleep disorders are underdiagnosed and undertreated. The differential diagnosis of pediatric sleep disorders necessitates a multidimensional approach, with consideration of coexisting medical and neurologic conditions. Coexisting clinical conditions are the rule, not the exception. This section provides an overview of comprehensive methods for the assessment of pediatric sleep disorders.

Sleep History

A thorough sleep and medical history, conducted with an understanding of normal sleep physiology, provides the foundation for the diagnosis and management of sleep disorders in children. Informants include the child and at least one parent. Sleep complaints in children are categorized into 1 or more of the following categories[21]:

1. Difficulty initiating or maintaining sleep;
2. Excessive daytime sleepiness (EDS);
3. Snoring or other breathing problems during sleep; and
4. Abnormal movements or behaviors during sleep.

The history includes details with regard to the onset, duration, pervasive nature, and variability of the sleep-related complaints.

For adolescents, it is important to assess behavioral, physiologic, environmental, and psychosocial factors, including afterschool activities, rigorous exercise, consumption of heavy meals, caffeine, tobacco and other illicit drugs, exposure to bright light through use of electronic devices, inconsistent bedtime routine, presence of parenteral discord, or the possibility of physical, emotional, or sexual abuse, which all may interfere with reasonable bedtime rituals.[8,21] Difficulty initiating or maintaining sleep in children could be an early sign of a mental health disorder, such as an anxiety disorder, a mood disorder or attention deficit hyperactive disorder (ADHD).[20]

Symptoms of EDS in children could be owing to a number of factors. Questions should be asked to assess the presence of involuntary naps in the afternoon, cataplexy, and hypnagogic hallucinations to explore the possibility of narcolepsy. The impact of the sleepiness on the activities of daily living (eg, missing school days, and academic performance) must be evaluated for risk stratification and to help identify therapeutic interventions.[21] EDS must be differentiated from chronic fatigue and from other secondary effects of a primary medical or psychiatric comorbidity, as discussed elsewhere in this article.

Sleep-related breathing disorders may be associated with snoring and other sounds while sleeping. Nocturnal signs of obstructive sleep apnea (OSA) syndrome may include difficulty breathing, paradoxic chest–abdominal movements, retractions, restless sleep, excessive sweating, and cyanosis. Daytime symptoms include nasal obstruction, mouth breathing, poor attentiveness, irritability, behavioral problems, fatigue, and sleepiness.[22]

Children with abnormal limb movements associated with restless legs syndrome (RLS) may present with a history of an urge to move their limbs, which is exacerbated at rest and relieved with movement.

The clinician should also perform a thorough medical review. Special attention must be paid to possible neurodevelopmental or medical problems. Chronic medical disorders, such as reactive airway disease, gastroesophageal reflux, congenital heart disease, and conditions associated with chronic pain, predispose a child to sleep problems. Neurodevelopmental disorders such as cerebral palsy, nocturnal seizures, developmental delay, and autism spectrum disorder also frequently present with sleep disorders.[22]

A careful review of the child's medication history should also be obtained. Psychostimulants may cause some degree of insomnia, whereas sedating antidepressants and antipsychotics can cause daytime somnolence, which could interfere with the child's quality of life.[21]

For adolescents, clinicians should inquire about any substance use. Substances such as alcohol or marijuana can produce an hypnotic effect. In contrast, stimulants such as diet pills or inappropriate use of diverted psychostimulants can cause wakefulness at night.[20] The evaluation should also include completion of a sleep log, consisting of both a parent report and a child self-report sleep log during the 2 weeks before the evaluation. These logs provide valuable information with regard to sleep–wake patterns for the child and other nocturnal events.[21]

Rating Scales

The Pediatric Daytime Sleepiness Scale is a simple, validated questionnaire that can be administered to children in the 11- to 14-year-old age group to assess daytime sleepiness.[23] It has 8 items, with each rated on a scale of 0 to 4. The scale provides a numerical score for sleepiness: the 50th percentile score on the Pediatric Daytime Sleepiness Scale is 16, the 75th percentile is 20, and the 90th percentile is 23.

Another common screening tool that can be used in clinical practice is the Children's Sleep Habits Questionnaire.[24] This scale is a 45-item, validated questionnaire that is completed by parents of 4- to 11-year-old children. The questions address sleep–wake function in the preceding 2 weeks, such as the "child sleeps too little" or "the child suddenly falls asleep in the middle of active behavior." The items represent several domains of sleep complaints, such as bedtime resistance, sleep-onset delay, sleep duration, sleep anxiety, night awakenings, parasomnias, breathing disturbance, and daytime sleepiness. Responses are rated as occurring rarely (0–1 time/wk; 1 point), sometimes (2–4 nights/wk; 2 points), or usually (5–7 nights/wk; 3 points). Scores of 41 or greater correlate with presence of a sleep disorder.

The Adolescent Sleep Hygiene Scale is a 28-item, self-report questionnaire to measure sleep hygiene appropriate for use with children older than 12 years of age.[25] This self-report questionnaire assesses sleep-facilitating and inhibiting practices in adolescents along 9 domains: physiologic, cognitive, emotional, sleep environment, daytime sleep, substance use, bedtime routine, sleep stability, and bed/bedroom sharing. Scores are reported on 6-point scale and a higher score indicates better sleep hygiene.

Physical Examination

The physical examination is critical to establishing an understanding of the etiology of a sleep disorder, as well as providing a foundation to anticipate the sequelae associated with the sleep disturbance. The clinician should carefully assess the child's level of alertness. Repetitive yawning, droopy eyelids, a blank facial expression, frequent changes in position, overactivity, and irritability are consistent with EDS.[22] The general examination should include assessment of dysmorphic features that may be present in children with genetic disorders, such as trisomy 21 and Prader–Willi syndromes, craniofacial anomalies, or abnormalities of head size (ie, macrocephaly or microcephaly). Inspection for signs of scoliosis and neuromuscular disease should be performed.[22] Neuromuscular disorders such as myotonic dystrophy can be associated with chronic obstructive hypoventilation from a combination of palatal muscle weakness, high arched palate, and diminished chest wall–abdominal excursion.[26] Developmental milestones should be obtained as part of the initial evaluation.

Evaluation of growth parameters including body mass index (calculated as weight in kilograms divided by the square of height in meters) may indicate failure to thrive in infancy or obesity.[21] OSA may be associated with failure to thrive in infancy and with obesity in adolescence. Blood pressure should be measured because long-standing and severe OSA may be associated with hypertension. Patients with OSA may show craniofacial abnormalities, such as micrognathia, dental malocclusion, macroglossia, myopathic face and midface hypoplasia, deviated nasal septum, swollen inferior turbinates, tonsillar hypertrophy, and mouth breathing.[27]

Bulbar dysfunction can manifest with decreased or absent gag reflex, poor movement of the soft palate, or swallowing problems.[21] Persistent mouth breathing or noisy breathing may indicate nasal obstruction. Clubbing, cyanosis, or edema may indicate heart failure, whereas lung examination may reveal clinical signs of chronic lung disease or reactive airways disease.[21]

Careful observation of the parent–child interaction may provide invaluable information with regard to parenteral behaviors toward setting limits to certain behaviors that can contribute to insomnia, as well as providing clues for child maltreatment syndrome. Home videos may aid in the assessment of abnormal movements and behaviors during sleep, such as periodic limb movements, nocturnal seizures, and parasomnias.

Sleep Laboratory Investigations

Sleep laboratory tests (PSGs) provide objective measures of physiologic events and activity patterns during sleep, and the multiple sleep latency test (MSLT) provides an objective measure of daytime sleepiness.

Polysomnography

A PSG is performed to characterize sleep architecture and sleep pathology, including sleep-related respiratory disturbances and periodic limb movements during sleep.[21] Recordings include a combination of the electroencephalogram, electrooculogram (eye movements), and submental muscle tone via electromyography to characterize sleep/wake states, arousals and awakenings, and sleep architecture.[28] Respiratory function is assessed using registration of air flow at the nose and mouth, respiratory movements of the chest and abdomen, and oximetry. The electrocardiogram measures heart rate and rhythm, and limb movements are monitored using limb electromyography sensors. Audio recordings detect sounds such as snoring and video recordings help to characterize movements or behaviors during sleep.[27] A standardized scoring manual provides guidelines and criteria for analysis of PSG results in adults and children, with separate guidelines being available for infants.[20,27] PSG monitoring to aid in the diagnosis and treatment of primary sleep disorders in children and adolescents is indicated for suspected OSA, periodic limb movement during sleep (PLMS), narcolepsy, and a variety of other sleep disorders that may be present in the child/adolescent population.

PSG assessment in children and adolescents is not indicated for evaluation of insomnia, in cases of circadian rhythm sleep disorders, for nonepileptic seizures, chronic lung disease, and bruxism, or in cases of behavior-based sleep disorders.

Actigraphy

Sleep–wake patterns and circadian rhythms can be investigated by assessing movement through actigraphy.[29] Its use in clinical practice depends on the availability of the equipment and expertise. This method is used to evaluate insomnia, circadian rhythm sleep disorders, and excessive sleepiness, and to assess the effectiveness of treatments.[21]

COMMON PEDIATRIC SLEEP DISORDERS
Sleep-Related Breathing Disorders

The sleep-disordered breathing disorders in childhood include snoring without sleep disruption (primary snoring), upper airway resistance syndrome (snoring that disrupts sleep continuity but without apnea or oxygen desaturation), classic OSA, and obstructive hypoventilation (apnea, oxygen desaturation, plus hypercarbia).[8]

Primary snoring

Snoring without associated apnea and oxygen desaturation is called primary snoring.[8] Studies indicate that about 10% to 12% of children snore on a habitual basis.[30] The consequences of primary snoring include worse performance on neuropsychological measures of attention. Compared with age-matched nonsnoring children, children with primary snoring seem to have more social problems and anxious or depressive symptoms.[31]

Obstructive sleep apnea

OSA is characterized by partial or complete upper airway occlusion, with associated impairment of air exchange despite persistence of thoracic and abdominal respiratory effort. The duration of the obstructive apnea events should be 5 seconds or more.[32] A 3% oxygen desaturation threshold is used when scoring childhood obstructive apnea events.[33] It is estimated that 1% to 4% of otherwise healthy children are affected by OSA, with a greater prevalence in children with underlying medical issues such as obesity or genetic disorders.[34] A recent systematic review has found a prevalence ranging from 0% to 5.7% in the general pediatric population.[35] Infants with OSA often present with stridor and laryngomalacia and may have a higher incidence of congenital anomalies of the upper airway, such as choanal atresia.[8] The metabolic syndrome may develop as a consequence of OSA.

Diagnosis of childhood obstructive sleep apnea Nocturnal PSG is not needed to confirm the diagnosis in patients who present with the classic symptoms of OSA with marked tonsillar hypertrophy. Instead, overnight oximetry at home indicating recurrent oxygen desaturation is sufficient for the diagnosis in these patients.[36] PSG is indicated in cases of uncertain diagnosis, as well as when OSA is suspected in presence of a neurologically compromised situation such as in patients with Down syndrome or cerebral palsy.[8] For therapeutic purposes, PSG is performed when a nonsurgical treatment is contemplated, such as the use of continuous positive airway pressure device.[8]

Treatment of childhood obstructive sleep apnea Treatment is based on the severity of OSA as stratified by the apnea–hypopnea index. Treatment options for OSA in children include the use of topical nasal corticosteroids for mild OSA, operative procedures, including adrenotonsillectomy and/or supraglottoplasty (done in infancy), the use of continuous positive airway pressure in various delivery options, orthodontic devices to help maintain a patent oropharyngeal passageway, and a weight reduction regimen, which is advisable for overweight/obese youths with OSA.

Central hypoventilation syndromes

This category of disorders is characterized by a defect in the automatic control of breathing during sleep as a result of brainstem dysfunction. It can be present in infancy and childhood. Diagnosis is obtained by means of PSG, which is suggestive of central sleep apnea, as indicated by oxygen desaturation, shallow respiratory effort, and increased levels of end-tidal CO_2.[8] Surgical decompression is indicated in patients with Chiari malformation and syringobulbia. For children with central hypoventilation syndrome, management is similar to that of primary congenital central alveolar hypoventilation.[8]

Congenital central alveolar hypoventilation syndrome

This is a disorder with no obvious brainstem structural explanation for defective central control of breathing during sleep.[37,38] Symptoms usually start during infancy or early childhood. In addition, 15% to 20% of patients also carry the diagnosis of Hirschsprung disease or neural crest tumors such as neuroblastoma or ganglioneuroma.[39,40] Congenital central alveolar hypoventilation syndrome is caused by a genetic mutation in PHOX2B gene, which is transmitted in an autosomal-dominant manner.[41,42] Treatment with acetazolamide and theophylline has limited value and the patient may die in infancy or childhood.[8,43] The American Thoracic Society guidelines recommend that patients with congenital central alveolar hypoventilation syndrome undergo an annual comprehensive, multidisciplinary evaluation.

Central sleep apnea
Central sleep apnea is characterized by central nervous system dysfunction that results in diminished or absent respiratory effort that occurs in an intermittent or a cyclical fashion. Central sleep apnea may be associated with anatomic or genetic abnormalities, or environmental causes.[29] It is relatively rare in children.[20]

Apnea of prematurity
Apnea of prematurity is a developmental disorder that occurs in extremely preterm infants characterized by respiratory pauses of 20 seconds or longer.[29] Treatment generally includes caffeine and watchful waiting because spontaneous resolution develops over time.

Obesity hypoventilation syndrome
Patients with obesity hypoventilation syndrome present with a combination of obesity and chronic hypercapnia.[44] Obesity hypoventilation syndrome is associated with increased levels of carbon dioxide in the blood without an underlying cardiorespiratory condition, and is often associated with some form of sleep-disordered breathing (ie, apnea/hypopnea or sustained periods of hypoventilation). This disorder is increasingly recognized among the obese pediatric population.

Hypersomnia

These disorders are characterized by EDS or prolonged night time sleep, which has occurred for at least 3 months.[45] Common manifestations of hypersomnia are seen in youths with narcolepsy, idiopathic hypersomnolence and in periodic hypersomnia (ie, Klein–Levin syndrome).

Narcolepsy
Narcolepsy is characterized by EDS, fragmented sleep at night, sleep-onset paralysis, hypnagogic hallucinations, and cataplexy.[8] Cataplexy presents as a sudden attack of atonia lasting seconds to minutes with preserved consciousness that typically occurs in response to an emotionally charged experience.[46,47] Narcolepsy–cataplexy is linked to a hypothalamic hypocretin (orexin) deficiency and is associated with the HLA DBQ1*0602 gene allele in more than 90% of individuals with narcolepsy, indicating a possible underlying autoimmune pathophysiology.[48] The most accepted method of diagnosing narcolepsy is by means of the MSLT to document quantitatively the extent of EDS and to determine the presence of short REM onsets during the four to five 20-minute nap opportunities that are evaluated as part of the MSLT procedure. Conventionally, the MSLT is conducted on the day after an overnight PSG evaluation to document a night of adequate sleep before the MSLT, as well as to rule out the presence of another primary sleep disorder that might account for the presence of EDS. A low level of orexin A in the cerebrospinal fluid has become an additional diagnostic criterion for narcolepsy according to the *International Classification of Sleep Disorders–second edition*.

Treatment of narcolepsy The treatment of narcolepsy involves a combination of non-pharmacologic preventative measures and pharmacologic treatment interventions to address both daytime sleepiness and cataplexy. Pharmacologic treatment interventions have traditionally involved the administration of stimulant compounds, such as dextroamphetamine to target reduction of daytime sleepiness and to suppress sleep attacks. In recent years, the nonstimulant compounds modafinil and armodafinil have become widely accepted as alternative therapeutic options to the stimulants as "wake-prompting" compounds, although they have limited efficacy to alleviate episodes of cataplexy. To obtain control of cataplexy in children with narcolepsy, the addition of an antidepressant drug with potent REM suppressant effects may be used. Fluoxetine has been studied most extensively among the antidepressant drugs for use in children. A recently developed pharmacologic option that has been approved for use in adults with narcolepsy who experience prominent disruption of sleep at night is sodium oxybate, which is marketed for the treatment of sleep disturbance in narcolepsy patients as Xyrem. To date, no studies have examined the efficacy and safety of sodium oxybate in children with narcolepsy. Behavioral approaches for children with narcolepsy include the use of scheduled naps to mitigate EDS and attention to maintaining a regular sleep–wake schedule augmented by regular physical exercise.

Idiopathic Hypersomnia

Idiopathic hypersomnia presents as EDS similar to narcolepsy.[49] However, individuals with idiopathic hypersomnia do not experience cataplexy, hypnagogic hallucinations, or sleep paralysis. Additionally, they can have long nocturnal sleep intervals lasting more than 10 hours.[50] Many children have periods of "sleep drunkenness," during which they engage in automatic behaviors. Idiopathic hypersomnia is a diagnosis of exclusion, and PSG is used to rule out other diagnoses. The MSLT results in children with idiopathic hypersomnia demonstrating sleep latencies of less than 8 minutes without sleep-onset REM periods, thus distinguishing it from narcolepsy.[51] Treatment for idiopathic hypersomnia is similar to narcolepsy in that it requires planned naps, regular exercise, and medication management for EDS.[8]

Periodic Hypersomnia (Kleine–Levin Syndrome)

Periodic hypersomnia is characterized by relapsing and remitting episodes of hypersomnia, apathy, cognitive limitations, and derealization lasting 10 to 14 days, during which time a child will sleep 18 to 20 hours per day.[52] Kleine–Levin syndrome typically occurs in adolescents, with a 4:1 male predominance. It also has an association with HLA DQB1 *0201.[53] The PSG in children with Kleine–Levin syndrome demonstrates decreased sleep efficiency, decreased REM latency, and decreased time spent in stage 3 sleep. The MSLT shows shortened sleep latency but fewer than 2 short-onset REM periods, thus differentiating it from narcolepsy. There are no treatment modalities that are recommended for Kleine–Levin syndrome, but modafinil may decrease the duration of symptomatic episodes.[54]

Circadian Rhythm Sleep Disorders

Delayed sleep phase syndrome is the most common circadian rhythm sleep disorder in children (see Chapter 12). It presents with stably delayed sleep and wake times compared with social/occupational expectations.[55] Delayed sleep phase syndrome typically has onset in adolescence.[15] It tends to run in families with a male predominance, and is speculated to occur as the result of an abnormal feedback loop between CLOCK and BMAL1 genes; period genes Per1, Per2, Per3; and cytochrome genes

Cyr1, Cyr2.[56] Sleep logs and wrist actigraphy are used in conjunction with a clinical interview to establish the diagnosis. As a result of the growing body of data on the importance of sleep for children and adolescents, school districts have begun to push back school start times to allow children to have extra time for sleep in the morning.[57]

Treatment approaches for youths with delayed sleep phase syndrome can include an emphasis on good sleep hygiene, associated with positive lifestyle changes, restricting bright light exposure in the late evening, and the use of light therapy (phototherapy) in the morning, immediately upon awakening. The use of melatonin in the evening to promote earlier sleep onset and the administration of modafinil in the morning to enhance wakefulness represent plausible, although not evidence-supported, therapeutic options for this population.

Parasomnias

Parasomnias are episodic behaviors that occur during sleep and generally do not impact sleep quality. They are most likely to occur in preschool-aged children, and they typically decrease in frequency over the first decade of life.[58] Manifestations of parasomnias in children can include sleep walking, nightmares, sleep terrors, confusional arousals, and nocturnal enuresis.

Non–Rapid Eye Movement Parasomnias

NREM parasomnias occur in about 15% of the population and peek between the ages of 8 and 12.[59] Nocturnal seizures can mimic NREM parasomnias owing to disorganized movements, unresponsiveness, vocalizations, and confused behavior.[60] Electroencephalogram recordings demonstrate activity in the 2- to 6-Hz range, indicating partial arousal from slow-wave sleep.[61] Common NREM parasomnias include confusional arousals, which typically occur 2 to 3 hours after sleep onset; sleep terrors, which usually arise abruptly in the first third of the night; and sleep walking. Treatment begins with educating caregivers that parasomnias are benign and self-limiting, and will likely resolve by adolescence. Safety in the home should be discussed with the parents if the child is sleepwalking. If other measures fail and the parasomnias are problematic, a low dose of imipramine or clonazepam (0.25–0.5 mg at bedtime) can prevent most NREM parasomnias.

Rapid Eye Movement Parasomnias

Nightmares represent the most common REM parasomnia. They typically present in the last third of the night.[61] Because the child can recall the event, providing reassurance and rescripting the event can help to provide comfort. If nightmares persist and continue to be distressing, psychological evaluation should considered.

Nocturnal Enuresis

Nocturnal enuresis occurs when a child over the age of 5 has incontinence during sleep at least twice per week.[62] It can occur during both REM and NREM sleep, and can be disruptive to both the child and the family. Continence training is the most effective method of treatment.

Sleep-related Movement Disorders

Sleep-related movement disorders are characterized by simple stereotyped movements that disturb sleep. Nocturnal high-amplitude movements may present a significant risk of injury to the child.[63] Video recording of the clinical events such as abnormal movement can provide useful information.

Periodic limb movements disorder

Periodic limb movement disorder (PLMD) is a disorder characterized by repetitive, highly stereotyped PLMS.[64] Studies indicates a 5% to 25% prevalence rate of PLMD in children referred for evaluation of a sleep disorder.[65] Children with PLMD report greater difficulty falling asleep, maintaining sleep, a higher frequency of nocturnal awakening, and increased difficulty falling back to sleep after waking up during the night. There is considerable overlap between PLMD and RLS. Recent genetic research suggests that PLMS characterizes a common endophenotype for RLS.[65] Children with PLMS greater than 5 per hour and hypersomnia should be evaluated for narcolepsy, because PLMS are found commonly in narcolepsy and moderate to severe daytime sleepiness is uncommon in children with PLMD.[66]

Restless leg syndrome

RLS is an autosomal-dominant, sensorimotor disorder in which the patient complains of a peculiar creepy or crawling feeling in the extremities.[67,68] The undesirable sensation is worse or only occurs in the evening or at night, is exacerbated by keeping the limbs still, and is relieved or partially relieved by movement. The symptoms interfere with initiation and maintenance of sleep. The diagnosis of RLS is clinical, based solely on reported symptoms or symptoms observed in the patient. The symptoms of RLS cause significant distress or impairment in social, occupational, educational, or other important areas of functioning by the impact on sleep, energy/vitality, daily activities, behavior, cognition, or mood. Epidemiologic studies indicate that 1.9% to 2% of children and adolescents in the United States and UK have pediatric RLS, with between 25% and 50% reporting moderate to severe symptoms. The symptoms of RLS interfere with sleep initiation and maintenance. On nocturnal PSG, patients may show PLMS.[8]

Pharmacologic agents such pramipexole and ropinirole are the Food and Drug Administration (FDA)–approved first-line agents for the treatment of RLS in adults.[66] Pramipexole and ropirinole are dopamine receptor agonists and their therapeutic role suggests possibility of underlying dopamine deficiency in the central nervous system.[8] Patients with RLS often have iron deficiency with a low level of serum ferritin. Iron is a cofactor for tyrosine hydroxylase, which is essential for dopamine synthesis.[8] Underlying dopamine deficiency could explain the reported association of pediatric RLS with ADHD. In addition to dopamine receptor agonists, oral iron, clonazepam, gabapentin, gabapentin, enacrabil, and pregabalin have also been reported to have therapeutic roles for the treatment of RLS, but the safety and efficacy of these agents (except iron) has not been established in the pediatric population.

THE RELATIONSHIP OF SLEEP DISTURBANCES TO BEHAVIORAL AND PSYCHIATRIC DISORDERS

A higher prevalence of sleep complaints has been reported in pediatric populations with psychiatric conditions compared with nonpsychiatric controls.[69]

Attention-Deficit Hyperactive Disorder

ADHD is among the most prevalent childhood psychiatric conditions, estimated to occur in 3% to 7.5% of school-aged children.[70] Sleep complaints affect as many as 25% to 50% of children and adolescents with ADHD. Stimulant medications that are used for treatment of ADHD have been associated with sleep complaints, but the effects of the stimulant medications do not account fully for the sleep disturbances observed in patients with ADHD.[51] Chronic sleep disturbances in children with ADHD have a negative impact on the mood, attention, and behavior of the affected children, which in turn adversely affect their day time functioning. Chronic sleep disturbances in children and adolescents also affect the health and well-being of the family members.

There are no pharmacologic agents currently approved to treat sleep disturbances in ADHD. A recently published study of eszopiclone as a treatment for insomnia in children with ADHD failed to show any improvement in insomnia with either low- or high-dose eszopiclone administration.[17] The results of this study are consistent with a 2009 publication in which zolpidem failed to separate from placebo in children with ADHD-related insomnia.[18] Clinically, ADHD patients with sleep disturbances are often treated with α-2 adrenergic receptor agonists such as clonidine and guanfacine, although none of these agents have received FDA approval for this indication. Another clinical option involves administration of melatonin about 5 to 5.5 hours before bedtime in a dose of 0.5 to 1 mg in patients with ADHD and sleep-onset insomnia.[8] Behavioral interventions such as consistent bedtime rituals, sleep hygiene, and cognitive–behavioral therapy have also been reported to have a positive role in the treatment of insomnia in this population.[20]

Affective Disorders

Sleep complaints are common in pediatric populations with affective disorders including major depressive disorder and bipolar disorder.[71] Major depressive disorder is prevalent in 2% of children and 8% of adolescents, and often recurrent in nature. Sleep problems have been reported to occur in about 70% of depressed children and adolescents. Sleep disturbances include insomnia related to sleep initiation and maintenance in 53% and hypersomnia in approximately 10% of youths with major depressive disorder. Depressed children with sleep disturbances have a greater severity of depression and higher rates of comorbid anxiety disorders. Treatment of depression and comorbid insomnia in these patients requires a dual approach that includes cognitive–behavioral therapy in conjunction with an antidepressant medication, especially one with sedating properties such as mirtazapine, amitriptyline, or the addition of low-dose trazodone or melatonin to a nonsedating antidepressant.[21]

In pediatric bipolar disorder, sleep disturbances are predominant features associated with the state of mania or hypomania. Stabilizing mania or hypomania with appropriate pharmacotherapy often treats the sleep disturbances in these patients, but the possibility of adding a hypnotic medication to adequately control an unresolved sleep disturbance may need to be considered in some cases.[8]

Anxiety Disorders

Anxiety disorders are common in pediatric populations, with prevalence rates between 12% and 20%.[72] Anxiety disorders in this population include separation anxiety disorder, generalized anxiety disorder, social phobia, specific phobias, panic disorder, and agoraphobia.[71] Successful treatment of anxiety disorders with cognitive behavioral therapy and evidenced-based pharmacotherapy when indicated is often associated with improvement in sleep complaints in pediatric populations with anxiety disorders.[8]

Behavioral Insomnia of Childhood

Behavioral insomnia of childhood is common, affecting 20% to 30% of infants and toddlers.[73] Behavioral insomnia often presents with bedtime refusal, delayed onset of sleep, and/or prolonged night-time waking that requires parenteral intervention. Behavioral intervention is the mainstay of treatment of behavioral insomnia of childhood.

Off-Label Use of Prescription Hypnotics

Prescription hypnotics do not have an FDA-approved indication for adolescents younger than 18 years. The American Academy of Sleep Medicine recommends against the use of hypnotics to treat childhood insomnia, stating that most childhood insomnia arises from parent–child interactions and should therefore be treated with a behavioral intervention.[74] Basic environmental approaches, modified sleep scheduling to enhance sleep hygiene, sleep practice, and physiologic features should be optimized before hypnotic use is considered for children. When necessary, short-acting hypnotics should be used short term, with caution and close monitoring with respect to efficacy and side effects.[75]

Posttraumatic Stress Disorder

Sleep disturbances in children with posttraumatic stress disorder can encompass various parasomnias, including night terrors, nightmares, sleep enuresis, and severe insomnia.[76] Nightmares, as a specific sleep disturbance, are uniquely frequent in children and adolescents suffering from traumatic events, such as sexual abuse.[77] Available data on the use of psychopharmacologic treatments (eg, prazosin, a selective α-1 antagonist) for nightmares and other sleep disturbances in pediatric patients with posttraumatic stress disorder are very limited.

Off-Label Use of Antipsychotic Drugs

Antipsychotic drugs such as risperidone, quetiapine, aripiprazole, and olanzapine are prescribed conventionally to treat several specific psychiatric disorders, such as schizophrenia and bipolar mania. Their off-label use in children with psychiatric or developmental disorders has been reported.[78] Antipsychotic drugs are often used off-label to treat insomnia in adults.[79] Although these medications may facilitate sleep, their routine use to treat sleep disorders in children is not recommended.[80]

SUMMARY

Pediatric sleep complaints can present as a primary sleep disorder or as a secondary consequence of an underlying medical or psychiatric disorder. Sleep disturbances in children and adolescents can affect social, academic, and neurobehavioral functioning. Obtaining a detailed and accurate sleep history followed by a comprehensive physical examination, including screening for developmental delays and cognitive dysfunction, represents a cornerstone for diagnosing pediatric sleep complaints. Assessment of lifestyle factors, such as substance use and the use of electronics, is important during the evaluation of sleep complaints, especially in adolescents. Behavioral interventions should be the mainstay of treatment for primary insomnia in children. Pharmacologic guidelines need to be developed for sleep disorders in children. Training programs should enhance clinicians' knowledge of the evidenced-based behavioral and pharmacologic options for the treatment of sleep disorders in pediatric populations.

REFERENCES

1. Gibson ES, Powles AC, Thabane L, et al. "Sleepiness" is serious in adolescence: two surveys of 3235 Canadian students. BMC Public Health 2006;6:116.
2. Davis KF, Parker KP, Montgomery GL. Sleep in infants and young children: Part two: Common sleep problems. J Pediatr Health Care 2004;18(3):130–7.
3. Czeisler CA, Allan JS, Strogatz SH, et al. Bright light resets the human circadian pacemaker independent of the timing of the sleep-wake cycle. Science 1986; 233(4764):667–71.

4. Carno M, Hoffman LA, Carcillo JA, et al. Developmental stages of sleep from birth to adolescence, common childhood sleep disorders: overview and nursing implications. J Pediatr Nurs 2003;18(4):274–83.
5. Groome L, Bentz LS, Singh K. Behavioral state organization in normal human term fetuses: The relationship between periods of undefined state and other characteristics of state control. Sleep 1995;18:77–81.
6. Sheldon SH. Sleep in infants and children. In: Lee-Chiong TL, Sateia MJ, Carskadon MA, editors. Sleep medicine. Philadelphia: Hanley & Belfus, Inc; 2002. p. 99–103.
7. Van Cauter E, Spiegel K, Tasali E, et al. Metabolic consequences of sleep and sleep loss. Sleep Med 2008;9(Suppl 1):S23–8.
8. Kotagal S, Chopra A. Pediatric sleep-wake disorders. Neurol Clin 2012;21: 1193–212.
9. Scher MS. Understanding sleep ontogeny to assess brain dysfunction in neonates and infants. J Child Neurol 1998;13:467–74.
10. Galland BC, Taylor BJ, Elder DE, et al. Normal sleep patterns in infants and children: a systematic review of observational studies. Sleep Med Rev 2012;16(3):213–22.
11. Mindell JA, Owens JA, Carskadon MA. Developmental features of sleep. Child Adolesc Psychiatr Clin N Am 1999;8:695–725.
12. Anders TF, Sadeh A, Appareddy V. Normal sleep in neonates and children. In: Ferber R, Kryger M, editors. Principles and practice of sleep medicine in the child. Philadelphia: W. B. Saunders Company; 1995. p. 7–18.
13. Sadeh A, Raviv A, Gruber R. Sleep patterns and sleep disruptions in school-age children. Dev Psychol 2000;36:291–301.
14. Carskadon MA, Wolfson AR, Acebo C, et al. Adolescent sleep patterns, circadian timing, and sleepiness at a transition to early school days. Sleep 1998;21:871.
15. Howard B, Wong J. Sleep disorders. Pediatr Rev 2001;22:327–41.
16. Pressman MR. Definition and consequences of sleep deprivation, from. 2014. Available at: http://www.uptodate.com/contents/definition-and-consequences-of-sleep-deprivation. Accessed June 1, 2015.
17. Sangal RB, Blumer JL, Lankford DA, et al. Eszopiclone for insomnia associated with Attention-Deficit/Hyperactivity Disorder. Pediatrics 2014;134(4):1095 103.
18. Blumer JL, Findling RL, Shih WJ, et al. Controlled clinical trial of zolpidem for the treatment of insomnia associated with attention-deficit/hyperactivity disorder in children 6 to 17 years of age. Pediatrics 2009;123:e770–6.
19. Dahl R. The impact of inadequate sleep on children's daytime cognitive function. Semin Pediatr Neurol 1996;3:44–50.
20. Gruber R, Carrey N, Weiss SK, et al. Position statement on pediatric sleep for psychiatrists. J Can Acad Child Adolesc Psychiatry 2014;23(3):174.
21. Wise MS, Glaze DG. Assessment of sleep disorders in children. 2013. Available at: http://www.uptodate.com/contents/assessment-of-sleep-disorders-in-children. Accessed June 1, 2015.
22. Brown LW, Maistros P, Guilleminault C. Sleep in children with neurological problems. In: Ferber R, Kryger M, editors. Principles and practice of sleep medicine in the child. Philadelphia: WB Saunders; 1995. p. 135.
23. Drake C, Nickel C, Burduvali E, et al. The Pediatric Daytime Sleepiness Scale (PDSS): sleep habits and school outcomes in middle school children. Sleep 2003;26:455–8.
24. Owens JA, Spirito A, McGuinn M. The Children's Sleep Habits Questionnaire (CHSQ): psychometric properties of a survey instrument for school-aged children. Sleep 2000;23:1043–51.

25. Storfer-Isser A, LeBourgeois MK, Harsh J, et al. Psychometric properties of the adolescent sleep hygiene scale. J Sleep Res 2013;22:707–16.
26. Mindell JA, Owens JA. A clinical guide to pediatric sleep, diagnosis and management of sleep problems. 2nd edition. Philadelphia: Wolters Kluwer; 2010.
27. American Academy of Sleep Medicine. International classification of sleep disorders: diagnostic and coding manual. 2nd edition. Westchester (IL): American Academy of Sleep Medicine; 2005.
28. Khoury J, Doghramji K. Primary Sleep Disorders. Psychiatr Clin N Am 2015, in press.
29. Littner M, Kushida CA, McDowell Anderson W, et al. Practice parameters for the role of actigraphy in the study of sleep and circadian rhythms: an update for 2002. Sleep 2003;26(3):337–41.
30. O'Brien LM, Holbrook CR, Mervis CB, et al. Sleep and neurobehavioral characteristics in 5–7 year old hyperactive children. Pediatrics 2003;111:554–63.
31. O'Brien LM, Mervis CB, Holbrook CR, et al. Neurobehavioral implications of habitual snoring in children. Pediatrics 2004;114:44–9.
32. Iber C, Ancoli-Israel S, Chesson A, et al. The AASM manual for the scoring of sleep and associated events: rules, terminology and technical specifications. 1st edition. Westchester (IL): American Academy of Sleep Medicine; 2007.
33. Goldstein NA, Stefanov DG, Graw-Panzer GD, et al. Validation of a clinical assessment score for pediatric sleep-disordered breathing. Laryngoscope 2012;122:2096–104.
34. Ofer D, Marcus CL. CPAP treatment in children. In: Kheirandish-Gozal L, Gozal D, editors. Sleep disordered breathing in children: a comprehensive clinical guide to evaluation and treatment (Respiratory medicine). New York: Humana Press; 2012. p. 531–40.
35. Marcus CL, Brooks LJ, Davidson-Ward S, et al. Diagnosis and management of childhood obstructive sleep apnea syndrome. Pediatrics 2012;130:e714–55.
36. Brouillette RT, Morielli A, Leimanis A, et al. Nocturnal pulse oximetry as an abbreviated testing modality for pediatric obstructive sleep apnea. Pediatrics 2000; 105:405–12.
37. Gozal D, Harper RM. Novel insights into congenital hypoventilation syndrome. Curr Opin Pulm Med 1999;5:335–8.
38. Gozal D. New concepts in abnormalities of respiratory control in children. Curr Opin Pediatr 2004;16:305–8.
39. Roshkow JE, Haller JO, Berdon WE, et al. Hirschsprung's disease, Ondine's curse, and neuroblastoma–manifestations of neurocristopathy. Pediatr Radiol 1988;19:45–9.
40. Swaminathan S, Gilsanz V, Atkinson J, et al. Congenital central hypoventilation syndrome associated with multiple ganglioneuromas. Chest 1989;96:423–4.
41. Trochet D, O'Brien LM, Gozal D, et al. PHOX2B genotype allows for prediction of tumor risk in congenital central hypoventilation syndrome. Am J Hum Genet 2005; 76:421–6.
42. Weese-Mayer DE, Berry-Kravis EM, Ceccherini I, et al. An official ATS clinical policy statement: congenital central hypoventilation syndrome: genetic basis, diagnosis, and management. Am J Respir Crit Care Med 2010;181:626–44.
43. Spitzer AR. Evidence-based methylxanthine use in the NICU. Clin Perinatol 2012; 39:137–48.
44. Berger KI, Goldring RM, Rapoport DM. Obesity hypoventilation syndrome. Semin Respir Crit Care Med 2009;30(3):253–61.

45. Dauvilliers Y. Differential diagnosis in hypersomnia. Curr Neurol Neurosci Rep 2006;6(2):156–62.
46. Challamel MJ, Mazzola ME, Nevsimalova S, et al. Narcolepsy in children. Sleep 1994;17:S17–20.
47. St Louis EK. Key sleep neurologic disorders: Narcolepsy, restless legs syndrome/ Willis-Ekbom disease, and REM sleep behavior disorder. Neurol Clin Pract 2014; 4(1):16–25.
48. Han F, Lin L, Warby SC, et al. Narcolepsy onset is seasonal and increased following the 2009 H1N1 pandemic in China. Ann Neurol 2011;70:410–7.
49. Frenette E, Kushida CA. Primary hypersomnias of central origin. Semin Neurol 2009;29:354–67.
50. Anderson KN, Pilsworth S, Sharples LD, et al. Idiopathic hypersomnia: a study of 77 cases. Sleep 2007;30(10):1274–81.
51. Konofal E, Lecendreux M, Cortese S. Sleep and ADHD. Sleep Med 2010;11(7): 652–8.
52. Arnulf I, Lin L, Gadoth N, et al. Kleine Levin syndrome: a systematic study of 108 patients. Ann Neurol 2008;63:482–93.
53. Dauvilliers Y, Mayer G, Lecendreux M, et al. Kleine Levin syndrome. An autoimmune hypothesis based on clinical and genetic analyses. Neurology 2002;59:1739–45.
54. Huang YS, Lakkis C, Guilleminault C. Kleine Levin syndrome: current status. Med Clin North Am 2010;94:557–62.
55. Morgenthaler TE, Lee-Chiong T, Alessi C, et al. Practice parameters for the clinical evaluation and treatment of circadian rhythm sleep disorders. Sleep 2007;30: 1445–59.
56. Wulff K, Porcheret K, Cussans E, et al. Sleep and circadian rhythm disturbances: multiple genes and multiple phenotypes. Curr Opin Genet Dev 2009;19:237–46.
57. Lamberg L. Sleep data lead large school system to push back high school start times. Psychiatr News 2011;50(3):24–5.
58. Furet O, Goodwin JL, Quan SF. Incidence and remission of parasomnias among adolescent children in the Tucson Children's Assessment of Sleep Apnea (Tu-CASA) study. Southwest J Pulm Crit Care 2011;2:93.
59. Tinuper P, Provini F, Bisulli F, et al. Movement disorders in sleep: guidelines for differentiating epileptic from non-epileptic motor phenomena arising from sleep. Sleep Med Rev 2007;11:255.
60. Provini F, Tinuper P, Bisulli F, et al. Arousal disorders. Sleep Med 2011;12(Suppl 2):S22.
61. Kotagal S. Parasomnias of childhood. Curr Opin Pediatr 2008;20:659.
62. Thiedke CC. Nocturnal enuresis. Am Fam Physician 2003;67(7):1499–506.
63. Gingras JL, Gaultney JF. Restless legs syndrome and periodic limb movement disorders: association with ADHD. In: Ivanenko A, editor. Sleep and psychiatric disorders in children and adolescents. 1st edition. New York: Informa Healthcare USA, Inc; 2008. p. 193–224.
64. Crabtree V, Ivanenko A, O'Brien L, et al. Periodic limb movement disorder of sleep in children. J Sleep Res 2003;12:73–81.
65. Winkelman JW. Periodic limb movements in sleep—endophenotype for restless legs syndrome? N Engl J Med 2007;357:703–5.
66. Picchietti DL, Rajendran RR, Wilson MP, et al. Pediatric restless legs syndrome and periodic limb movement disorder: parent–child pairs. Sleep Med 2009;10: 925–31.
67. Picchietti MA, Picchietti DL. Restless legs syndrome and periodic limb movement disorder in children and adolescents. Semin Pediatr Neurol 2008;15:91–9.

68. Sullivan SS. Current treatment of selected pediatric sleep disorders. Neurotherapeutics 2012;9(4):791–800.
69. Ivanenko A, Johnson K. Sleep disturbances in children with psychiatric disorders. Semin Pediatr Neurol 2008;15:70–80.
70. Sung V, Hiscock H, Sciberras E, et al. Sleep problems in children with attention deficit hyperactivity disorder: prevalence, and the effect on the child and family. Arch Pediatr Adolesc Med 2008;162:336–42.
71. Liu X, Buysse DJ, Gentzler AL, et al. Insomnia and hypersomnia associated with depressive phenomenology and comorbidity in childhood depression. Sleep 2007;30:83–90.
72. Costello EJ, Egger HL, Angold A. The developmental epidemiology of anxiety disorders: phenomenology, prevalence and comorbidity. Child Adolesc Psychiatr Clin N Am 2005;14:631–48.
73. Goodlin-Jones BL, Burnham MM, Gaylor EE, et al. Night waking, sleep-wake organization, and self-soothing in the first year of life. J Dev Behav Pediatr 2001;22: 226–33.
74. American Academy of Sleep Medicine. Five things physicians and patients should question released December 2, 2014. Available at: http://www.choosingwisely.org/societies/american-academy-of-sleep-medicine/. Accessed May 30, 2015.
75. Owens JA, Babcock D, Blumer J, et al. The use of pharmacotherapy in the treatment of pediatric insomnia in primary care: rational approaches. A consensus meeting summary. J Clin Sleep Med 2005;1(1):49–59.
76. Krakow B, Sandoval D, Schrader R, et al. Treatment of chronic nightmares in adjudicated adolescent girls in a residential facility. J Adolesc Health 2001; 29(2):94–100.
77. Raskind MA, Peskind ER, Hoff DJ, et al. A parallel group placebo controlled study of prazosin for trauma nightmares and sleep disturbance in combat veterans with post-traumatic stress disorder. Biol Psychiatry 2007;61(8):928–34.
78. Masi G, Cosenza A, Millepiedi S, et al. Aripiprazole monotherapy in children and young adolescents with pervasive developmental disorders: a retrospective study. CNS Drugs 2009;23:511–21.
79. Doan RJ. Risperidone for insomnia in PDDs. Can J Psychiatry 1998;43:1050–1.
80. Harrison-Woolrych M, Garcia-Quiroga J, Ashton J, et al. Safety and usage of atypical antipsychotic medications in children: a nationwide prospective cohort. Drug Saf 2007;30:569–79.

Sleep Disturbances in the Elderly

Kristina F. Zdanys, MD*, David C. Steffens, MD, MHS

KEYWORDS

- Geriatric • Old-age • Sleep disorders • Insomnia • Alzheimer's • Dementia
- Delirium • Melatonin

KEY POINTS

- Changes to circadian rhythm and sleep cycles have been observed in aging, but do not necessarily result in subjective sleep disturbance.
- Behavioral factors contribute to poor sleep and when addressed may improve sleep quality in older adults.
- Psychiatric, cognitive, and medical disorders often present with disturbed sleep in the elderly.
- First-line treatment of sleep disorders in the elderly is nonpharmacologic.
- When nonpharmacological treatment approaches are unsuccessful, pharmacologic treatments may be considered, although the elderly are at higher risk of side effects from sleeping medications.

Do not go gentle into that good night,
Old age should burn and rave at close of day...
—Dylan Thomas[1]

INTRODUCTION

Sleep problems are a common presenting symptom of elderly patients to primary care physicians and psychiatrists. It is estimated that more than half of older adults have at least one sleep complaint.[2] In older adults, poor sleep may result in increased risk of falls, lower quality of life, risk of nursing home placement, and mortality.[3] As individuals

Disclosures: None (K.F. Zdanys); Financial from the American Psychiatric Press for the American Psychiatric Press Textbook of Geriatric Psychiatry, Fifth Edition, 2015; Consultant to Janssen R&D (D.C. Steffens).
Department of Psychiatry, University of Connecticut Health Center, 263 Farmington Avenue, Farmington, CT 06030, USA
* Corresponding author.
E-mail address: zdanys@uchc.edu

Psychiatr Clin N Am 38 (2015) 723–741
http://dx.doi.org/10.1016/j.psc.2015.07.010
0193-953X/15/$ – see front matter Published by Elsevier Inc.

psych.theclinics.com

age, there are changes in the normal sleep cycle that may complicate the identification of sleep disturbances. Sleep disorders in the elderly involve medical, psychiatric, cognitive, behavioral, and environmental factors, which are summarized in **Box 1**. Older adults are also at higher risk of side effects from many commonly prescribed sleep medications. These complexities result in many challenges for diagnosis and treatment. This article explores these factors, discusses approaches to treatment, and highlights new research in the area of geriatric sleep disorders.

SLEEP CHANGES WITH AGING

As individuals age, their overall sleep efficiency decreases.[4] Circadian rhythms become "phase-advanced," such that wake time is earlier in relation to the nadir of circadian temperature fluctuation, although early awakening may not be solely attributable to phase advancement.[5,6] Other changes include increased sleep latency, increased nighttime arousals, reductions in rapid eye movement (REM) sleep, and decreased stages 3 and 4 sleep ("deep," non-REM, slow-wave sleep characterized by delta waves).[4,7,8] There may be gender differences among these age-related changes: in terms of circadian rhythm, older women tend to go to bed earlier and wake up earlier than older men[8] and men older than 70 appear to have a disproportionate reduction in stages 3 and 4 sleep relative to women of the same age.[7] It is important to distinguish between sleep changes and sleep problems: although sleep changes are an inherent part of the aging process, sleep problems are not. As such, an older adult presenting with a sleep concern should not merely be told he or she is experiencing "normal aging." Sleep changes, however, may contribute to development of sleep problems in combination with other factors discussed in this article.

SLEEP DISORDERS IN THE ELDERLY
Insomnia

According to the *Diagnostic and Statistical Manual of Mental Disorders, 5th Edition*, insomnia is defined as reported dissatisfaction with sleep quantity or quality and associated with difficulty with sleep initiation, maintenance, or early-morning awakening and that causes clinically significant distress or impairment, occurs at least 3 nights per week for 3 months, occurs despite adequate opportunity for sleep, and is not better explained by another disorder or substance abuse.[9] Older adults are at risk of insomnia as a consequence of medical and psychiatric comorbidities.[10] Behavioral factors, discussed later in this article, also may contribute. These underlying factors contributing to the patient's presentation should be identified and addressed. Nonpharmacological strategies are the first-line approach to the treatment of insomnia in the elderly given the high risk of side effects of sedative-hypnotic medications in this population, also discussed later in this article.

Obstructive Sleep Apnea

Obstructive sleep apnea (OSA) is a sleep disorder estimated to affect 3% to 7% of adult men and 2% to 5% of adult women that is characterized by repetitive partial or complete airway collapse during sleep, resulting in hypoxemia, sleep fragmentation, and poor sleep quality.[11] OSA is thought to be more common among the elderly, such that as many as 24% to 42% of elderly patients have 5 or more apneas per hour of sleep.[12] Traditional risk factors for OSA (such as obesity and large neck circumference) may be less significant among the elderly, making identification of those elderly at risk for OSA more challenging.[13] Among the most notable sequelae of OSA are its cardiovascular effects. OSA is associated with hypertension independent of obesity,

Box 1
Common factors affecting sleep in the elderly

Primary Sleep Disorder

Insomnia

Obstructive sleep apnea

Restless legs syndrome

Medical

Delirium

Parkinson disease

Nocturia

Chronic obstructive pulmonary disease

Pain

Psychiatric

Mood disorders

Anxiety

Posttraumatic stress disorder

Cognitive

Alzheimer disease

Lewy body dementia

Other neurocognitive disorders

Behavioral

Alcohol

Nicotine

Caffeine

Naps

Exercise

Environmental

Light

Noise

Heat

Pharmacologic

Cholinesterase inhibitors

Stimulants

Antihypertensives

Decongestants

Corticosteroids

Stimulating antidepressants

Diuretics

and treatment of sleep apnea has been associated with improvements in hypertension.[14] Associations have also been established between OSA and both clinical and subclinical coronary artery disease, including higher incidence of cardiovascular events and mortality.[15] The mechanisms by which sleep-disordered breathing may result in cardiovascular outcomes likely involve intermittent hypoxia, inflammation, sympathetic activation, and sleep fragmentation, which lead to endothelial cell dysfunction, hypercoagulability, vasoconstriction, and atherosclerosis.[14] Associations have also been established between OSA and metabolic syndrome, which also may contribute to cardiovascular mortality.[16] Neuropsychiatric symptoms, both cognitive and affective, may result from OSA and thus screening for sleep-related complaints is important, particularly among the elderly patient population.[17] Treatment for OSA includes positive airway pressure (PAP) as well as lifestyle changes, such as weight loss, blood pressure control, and avoidance of alcohol and sedative drugs.[3]

Restless Legs Syndrome

Restless legs syndrome (RLS) is a sleep-related disorder characterized by an urge to move the legs, often accompanied by an unpleasant sensation, which is aggravated by rest, alleviated by movement, and worsened at night.[18] Elderly age is a risk factor for RLS, with estimated prevalence of approximately 4% among individuals ages 70 to 89, with older adults comprising 9% to 20% of all reported cases.[19,20] Risk factors for RLS that pertain to older adults include low iron, low socioeconomic status, medical and psychiatric comorbidity, Parkinson disease, and end-stage renal disease.[21] The first-line pharmacologic approach to treatment of RLS involves the use of dopamine agonists. Other strategies include anticonvulsants, benzodiazepines, opioids, and dopaminergic agents,[21] although these secondary treatments may cause significant side effects in the elderly population. Nonpharmacological strategies, such as sleep hygiene, exercise, restriction of caffeinated beverages, and pneumatic compression stockings, may help treat symptoms.[21]

BEHAVIORS INFLUENCING SLEEP
Alcohol

It has long been established that consumption of alcohol before sleep affects sleep stages on polysomnography (PSG).[22] Alcohol intake before bed decreases sleep-onset latency, but increases arousals during the second half of the night in a dose-dependent manner.[23] Consumption of alcohol in the elderly before bed may have a particular negative impact on the quality of sleep. Chronic alcohol abuse in older men is associated with increased hypoxemia overnight.[24] This effect is sustained among elderly individuals with a history of chronic alcohol abuse who abstain from drinking.[25] Alcohol consumption has been correlated with lower self-reported sleep quality in patients with mild cognitive impairment.[26] Evaluation of alcohol consumption should always be included when evaluating sleep disorders in the elderly.

Exercise

Regular daytime exercise is routinely recommended as part of a comprehensive sleep hygiene strategy, and may be helpful for promoting modest improvements in sleep among individuals regardless of an existing sleep complaint.[23] Among older adults, regular exercise training over several weeks demonstrated moderate improvement in sleep quality.[27] Physically active older men have been shown to have shorter sleep onset latency, less wake time after onset, higher sleep efficiency, and more total slow wave sleep than sedentary older men.[28]

Naps

It is estimated that more than half of older adults take at least one nap per day.[29] Changes in sleep quantity and quality that occur with aging (discussed previously) may contribute to the increased likelihood that older adults take a nap. There is conflicting evidence regarding the potential detriments and benefits of napping. Although it has been observed that daytime naps decrease depth of subsequent sleep and increase latency to sleep onset, napping in older adults has been shown to have no negative effect on subsequent overnight sleep quality or duration, and increased total sleep time over a 24-hour period is associated with enhanced cognitive performance in older adults.[30,31] Although naps of less than 30 minutes have been associated with improved wakefulness, performance, and learning ability, frequent and long naps among the elderly are associated with higher morbidity and mortality.[32] Naps have been associated specifically with an increased risk of cardiac events, although the mechanisms of this association are not well understood.[33]

Caffeine

A dose of caffeine in an older adult may result in a higher plasma and tissue concentration relative to younger adults due to more adipose tissue, lower lean body mass, and impaired clearance of caffeine by the liver.[34,35] As adults age, their sleep becomes more sensitive to high doses of caffeine, including increased sleep latency, shortened sleep duration, and reduced sleep efficiency.[36] Consumption of caffeinated beverages is associated with sleep-disordered breathing.[37] Among patients with dementia, both daytime and evening consumption of caffeine may increase nighttime awakenings.[38]

Nicotine

Nicotine is known to have stimulantlike effects.[39] Smoking cigarettes has been associated with sleep disturbances including delayed sleep latency, reduced sleep duration, and lower sleep quality.[40,41] In the elderly, smoking is associated with longer daytime sleep, which could disrupt sleep patterns.[42] Smoking has also been linked to OSA.[43] Although the use of a transdermal nicotine patch is an effective treatment and generally well-tolerated in the elderly,[44] this population may also be sensitive to the side effects of nicotine replacement therapies, including those that affect sleep quality.[45]

SLEEP, MOOD, AND ANXIETY
Mood

Mood disorders are common in the elderly, with an estimated 11% of older adults suffering from either major or minor depression.[46] A bidirectional relationship between sleep and mood disorders has been reported in elderly individuals, such that poor sleep has been linked to the development of depression, and poor sleep is a common presenting symptom of depression.[47,48] In the elderly, this relationship can be confounded by comorbid medical illness for which poor sleep may also be an associated symptom, thereby leading to either underdiagnosis or overdiagnosis of depression.[49] Bereavement may present unique sleep difficulties in older adults, particularly those experiencing the loss of a life partner or complicated grief, often due to overlap with major depressive disorder or loss of a bedfellow.[50] Sleep disturbances seen among older patients with depression include impaired sleep continuity (eg, increased sleep latency, frequent or prolonged awakenings, and early-morning awakening), increased REM sleep, earlier onset of REM sleep, and reduced stage 3 and 4 ("deep") sleep.[48] Because many of these changes overlap with the sleep changes associated with aging described earlier in this article, it may be difficult to distinguish sleep symptoms of depression from normal sleep changes, and a full assessment of psychiatric and medical symptoms may help to clarify the diagnosis.

Anxiety

Although much research has been devoted to elucidating the relationship between mood disorders and sleep disturbance, few studies have examined the relationship of anxiety and sleep disturbance in older adults.[51] There is considerable overlap between anxiety and depression in the elderly, making a clear distinction between the two illnesses for the purposes of research quite challenging. Half or more of the older adult population may suffer from significant anxiety symptoms.[52] Sleep disturbances and anxiety are frequently comorbid, although (as with mood disorders) the nature and directionality of that relationship are complex.[53] Factors associated with insomnia and anxiety in the elderly include short sleep duration, other sleep disturbances (coughing, snoring, feeling cold, and nightmares), and daytime sleepiness.[54] The relationship between sleep and anxiety may also depend on the form of anxiety disorder. In older adults, sleep disturbances may be observed in generalized anxiety disorder[55]; sleep problems are twice as likely among patients with this diagnosis relative to individuals not meeting criteria for this disorder in a primary care setting.[56] Panic disorder has also been associated with sleep disturbance, and panic symptoms may improve with the use of continuous positive airway pressure among patients with a history of sleep apnea.[57] However, patients with a history of claustrophobia are less likely to adhere to continuous positive airway pressure, impacting their sleep quality.[58]

Posttraumatic Stress Disorder

Older adults may experience posttraumatic stress disorder (PTSD) as a consequence of remote trauma, such as combat, torture, physical abuse, or sexual abuse,[59–61] or may develop PTSD following more recent trauma, such as violence, natural disasters, or accidents.[62] PTSD related to remote trauma may be either chronic or delayed-onset, although there is some disagreement whether delayed-onset PTSD may have been previously subclinical or misdiagnosed, or whether cognitive changes predispose the individual to reemergence of symptoms.[63,64] Estimates of PTSD prevalence in an older adult population are highly varied depending on the population studied.[62] Sleep disturbance, including nightmares, is a common presenting symptom of PTSD in older adults.[56,61,65] There is evidence from studies involving small samples that the use of prazosin may be efficacious and well-tolerated in older adults for treatment of PTSD-related nightmares, although more research is needed to establish safety and efficacy.[59]

SLEEP AND NEUROCOGNITIVE DISORDERS

In the elderly, poor sleep may contribute to cognitive symptoms, and conversely different types of dementia may present with associated sleep disturbances. Studies suggest that sleep duration, sleep fragmentation, sleep-disordered breathing, and hypoxemia may contribute to cognitive impairment.[66,67] Mild cognitive impairment has been associated with difficulty initiating sleep, difficulty maintaining sleep, and early morning awakening.[68] Among forms of dementia, two with notable sleep disturbances are Alzheimer disease (AD) and Lewy Body Dementia (LBD), both of which are discussed here.

Alzheimer Disease

Recent evidence suggests that disruption of sleep-wake cycle and circadian rhythms previously thought to develop in later stages of AD may actually occur before the onset of cognitive symptoms.[69] Early sleep changes in AD include decreased stage 3 and 4 non-REM sleep, and loss of REM sleep as the disease progresses.[70] Other specific symptoms of sleep disorder in AD include abnormal timing and duration of sleep cycle, increased sleep latency, increased nocturnal awakenings, and increased daytime sleep.[71] An association has been demonstrated between higher daytime activity levels and lower nocturnal activity among patients with AD with better functional status and reported patient well-being,[72] suggesting that increased sleep fragmentation may worsen quality of life for patients with AD. Behavioral symptoms in AD also may be associated with poor sleep, including agitation, verbal outbursts, wandering, and aggressive behaviors.[73] Sundowning is a phenomenon frequently seen in moderate AD in which patients display increased behavioral symptoms in the afternoon and early evening. Sundowning is associated with increased rate of cognitive decline, increased caregiver stress, and increased likelihood of institutionalization.[74,75] It is thought that on a neurobiological level the degeneration of cholinergic neurons in the Nucleus basalis of Meynert and disruption of the suprachiasmatic nucleus may result in this rest-activity disturbance.[76,77]

Lewy Body Dementia

Sleep symptoms in LBD are common and considered to be a suggestive clinical feature when making the diagnosis, particularly REM sleep behavior disorder.[78] This disorder is characterized by the lack of muscle atonia that is typically observed during REM sleep, and dream enactment behavior (in which patients act out their dreams either vocally or physically and may risk injury to their bed partners) may occur.[79] The onset of REM sleep behavior disorder may be concurrent with cognitive or parkinsonian symptoms, although evidence suggests REM sleep behavior disorder may also precede either type of symptom by up to 20 years.[80] Other sleep symptoms seen in LBD include insomnia and excessive daytime sleepiness.[81]

SLEEP AND MEDICAL DISORDERS
Delirium

Among the critically ill, amplitude and phase of circadian rhythm may be disrupted.[82] Delirium in particular is characterized by disrupted sleep-wake cycles,[83] and disruption of sleep-wake cycles may also predispose patients to develop delirium.[84] In an acute hospital setting there are many factors that may contribute to the disruption of sleep-wake cycle, including persistent dim lighting in intensive care units,[85] lack of daylight,[86] noise,[87] medication administration, automatic blood pressure cuff inflation, mechanical ventilation, and other patient care interventions.[88] Interventions to reduce the negative impact of these factors, such as having windows in intensive care unit patient rooms, have been associated with lower incidence of delirium.[89,90] Brighter rooms have also been associated with lower mortality and length of stay in the intensive care setting.[91]

Parkinson Disease

Sleep disorders are common and disabling in Parkinson disease (PD), affecting up to 90% of patients and at times presenting even before the onset of motor symptoms.[92] The most frequent sleep disorders in patients with PD include insomnia, daytime sleepiness with sleep attacks, restless legs syndrome, and REM-sleep behavior disorder (RBD).[93] The role of dopamine in regulating sleep and circadian rhythms has been implicated in the development of sleep disturbances in PD.[92] Multiple other etiologies of sleep disturbances in PD have been proposed, including impairment of sleep architecture, impairment of the arousal system, impairment of the sleep-wake cycle, nocturnal motor and nonmotor symptoms, neuropsychiatric symptoms, sensory symptoms, comorbid primary sleep disorders, and medication side effects.[94] Poor sleep among patients with PD is associated with daytime fatigue, which is in turn associated with poorer quality of life, higher severity of depressive symptoms, and worse social and psychological behaviors.[95] It has been observed that patients with onset of PD at a younger age are less likely to experience insomnia, daytime sleepiness, nightmares, and general sleep restlessness than older patients with PD.[96]

Nocturia

Nocturia is a prevalent symptom among men and women of all ages, but particularly among the elderly. By definition, nocturia is considered to be two or more nocturnal voidings.[97] It is estimated that up to 60% of both men and women older than 70 void two or more times nightly.[98] Nocturia, and specifically number of episodes per night, is related to poor sleep quality.[99] Other associations include daytime fatigue, depression, and reduction in general health-related quality of life.[100] Benign prostatic hypertrophy (BPH) is a common etiology of nocturia among men. Other etiologies include overactive bladder, urinary tract infection, bladder hypersensitivity, calculi, cancer, neurogenic detrusor overactivity, hypercalcemia, diabetes, polydipsia, renal insufficiency, impaired circadian rhythm of arginine vasopressin secretion, diuretic use, and estrogen deficiency, among others.[98] Medical options for treatment of nocturia are limited in the elderly, as use of desmopressin increases risk of hyponatremia, and antimuscarinic agents, such as oxybutynin and tolterodine, have anticholinergic side effects.[97,101]

Chronic Obstructive Pulmonary Disease

Risk of developing chronic obstructive pulmonary disease (COPD) increases with age.[102] Patients with COPD are at higher risk of hypercapnia and hypoxemia during sleep.[103] It is estimated that more than half of patients with a diagnosis of moderate to severe COPD meet criteria for OSA, which may contribute to higher morbidity and mortality.[104] Sleep quality is decreased in patients with COPD, characterized by impaired sleep initiation and maintenance, daytime sleepiness, and consequently increased use of sedating medications.[105] Use of hypnotic medications among patients with COPD is potentially dangerous and may result in hypoventilation, worsened hypercapnia and hypoxemia, diminished arousal response, and increased frequency of apnea.[106] Melatonin receptor agonists,[107] cognitive behavioral therapy,[108] and noninvasive mechanical ventilation[109] may be helpful and safer alternatives to hypnotic medications among patients with COPD and sleep-disordered breathing.

Chronic Pain

Chronic pain is a common symptom in the elderly population and often is associated with peripheral neuropathy, arthritis, degenerative spine disease, and other bone and joint disorders.[110] Sleep disturbance is common among patients with chronic pain.[111] Patients with higher pain intensity report increased sleep latency, decreased sleep duration, and increased frequency of awakening relative to those with low pain intensity.[112] Among elderly patients, there tends to be an overlap among insomnia, chronic pain, and depression such that pain and depression contribute to insomnia, and insomnia may also worsen pain and depression.[113] Although chronic pain and depression are often comorbid, sleep disturbance in patients with chronic pain exists independent of mood disorder.[112] Treatment of chronic pain in the elderly is challenging given the risk of side effects from commonly prescribed pain medications,[101] but effective management of pain may improve sleep quality among elderly patients.

MEDICATIONS AFFECTING SLEEP

In addition to medical and psychiatric illnesses, medications used to treat these disorders may also disrupt sleep. A list of such medications commonly used in the elderly are included in **Box 1**. Acetylcholinesterase inhibitors are used for cognitive enhancement in patients with AD. A common adverse effect of this therapeutic class is vivid dreams or nightmares, which may be related to shortened REM latency,[114–116] increased REM density,[115,116] and increased time spent in REM sleep.[117] However, not all research has demonstrated a consistent impact of acetylcholinesterase inhibitors on sleep quality.[118] Beta-adrenergic receptor antagonists (beta-blockers) have been associated with the suppression of melatonin, which may cause insomnia.[119,120] Pseudoephedrine, a sympathomimetic amine used as a nasal decongestant for allergic rhinitis and the common cold, more frequently causes insomnia than other nondrowsy decongestants.[121] Corticosteroids, frequently prescribed in the elderly for respiratory, allergic, and immunologic illness, also contribute to insomnia as well as delirium.[122,123] Some antidepressants are activating and have been associated with insomnia in 30% to 40% of patients, including several tricyclic antidepressants (eg, protriptyline, desipramine), selective serotonin reuptake inhibitors (eg, fluoxetine, paroxetine), serotonin norepinephrine reuptake inhibitors (eg, venlafaxine), and bupropion.[124] Diuretics, although not directly affecting sleep architecture, have been associated with insomnia due to repeat awakenings to void throughout the night.[125]

NONPHARMACOLOGIC TREATMENT APPROACHES

Given risk of side effects and polypharmacy with medication management in the elderly population, nonpharmacologic treatment approaches are the first-line approach for treatment of sleep disorders. Both nonpharmacologic and pharmacologic approaches to treatment of sleep disorders are summarized in **Table 1**.

Cognitive Behavioral Therapy

Cognitive behavioral therapy for insomnia has been studied in older adults and is based on the premise that patients have a dysfunctional belief or attitude about sleep and its impact on daily living. The purpose of the therapy is to identify, challenge, and alter those dysfunctional beliefs, often through implementation of the strategies described as follows.[126]

Table 1 Treatment approaches to sleep disorders in the elderly	
Nonpharmacologic	**Pharmacologic**
Cognitive behavioral therapy	Melatonin
Sleep hygiene	Trazodone
Stimulus control	Benzodiazepines
Sleep restriction	Nonbenzodiazepine hypnotics
	Sedating antidepressants

Sleep Hygiene

Sleep hygiene is an educational technique in which patients are taught about the effects of environmental and behavioral factors on sleep, as well as reasonable expectations for sleep given the individual's age and comorbidities. Typical recommendations for sleep hygiene include avoidance of caffeine and nicotine for 6 hours prior to sleep, avoidance of alcohol at bedtime, avoidance of a heavy meal before sleep, avoidance of exercise close to bedtime, and minimization of noise, light, and heat during sleep.[127]

Stimulus Control

The purpose of stimulus control is to reestablish an association between bed and sleep. Approaches to stimulus control include using the bed only for sleep and sex, going to bed only when tired, getting out of bed if unable to sleep within 20 minutes, and awakening at the same time each day.[128]

Sleep Restriction

This approach to insomnia treatment involves limiting time spent in bed at night and sleep during the day.[129] By observing how much time spent in bed is actually asleep, patients adjust and maintain their sleep schedule.

PHARMACOLOGIC TREATMENT APPROACHES
Melatonin

In the elderly population, melatonin has been demonstrated to decrease sleep latency, awakenings per night, and movements per night.[130] Melatonin is considered second-line treatment for REM sleep behavior disorder after clonazepam.[131] There is evidence that use of melatonin in patients with a diagnosis of dementia may also improve sun-downing behavior.[77] The current recommendation for treatment of sleep disorders in the elderly with melatonin is to use the lowest possible dose of the immediate-release formulation so as to approximate normal physiologic pattern.[132]

Trazodone

Trazodone is a commonly used agent for the treatment of insomnia in both depressed and nondepressed patients.[133] Side effects of particular importance in the elderly include sedation, dizziness, orthostatic hypotension, arrhythmias, priapism, and psychomotor impairment.[134,135] However, trazodone is generally better tolerated in the elderly population than some other treatment strategies (such as tricyclic antidepressants, as described later in this article) given the lower risk of cardiac and anticholinergic side effects.[135]

Benzodiazepines

Although the use of benzodiazepines is common practice in the treatment of insomnia among adults of all ages, the elderly are more sensitive to the adverse effects of benzodiazepines, which may include tolerance, withdrawal, oversedation, cognitive impairment, and risk of falls.[136–138] Prescribing guidelines for benzodiazepine use in the elderly include short-term use, low dosage, and preference for shorter half-life medications.[139]

Nonbenzodiazepine Hypnotics

Nonbenzodiazepine hypnotics, including zolpidem, zaleplon, zopiclone, and eszopiclone, are frequently prescribed for adults of all ages to treat insomnia. Older adults may be more sensitive to the motor and cognitive side effects of these medications due to slower metabolism, medical problems, and polypharmacy.[140] There is a lack of studies investigating the efficacy and risks of these medications in the elderly. What data are available suggest that these medications improve sleep latency and quality in older adults, and are generally well-tolerated.[141]

Sedating Antidepressants

Sedating antidepressants are often considered as a treatment option for patients experiencing insomnia, particularly when insomnia overlaps with depression.[142] Tricyclic antidepressants are often used for this purpose; however, in an elderly population, this class of medication has a poor side-effect profile, including dry mouth, postural hypotension, cardiac arrhythmias, weight gain, and drowsiness.[143] Mirtazapine produces demonstrated improvement in sleep efficiency and total sleep time in depressed patients[144]; however, there is a lack of evidence for use of mirtazapine for treatment of sleep disorders in nondepressed patients.[145]

FUTURE TARGETS
Amyloid Beta and Circadian Rhythm

Understanding sleep disorders in the elderly may give insight into pathogenesis of late-life diseases. As an example, there may be a link between the development of amyloid beta plaques (a well-established pathologic finding in AD) and a disruption of circadian rhythms. Briefly, some studies in animal models as well as in humans have suggested that there is a diurnal variation in the concentration of amyloid beta protein levels as measured in brain interstitial fluid and cerebrospinal fluid.[146–148] Sleep deprivation appears to exacerbate amyloid beta pathology in mouse models of AD,[146,149] and also may contribute to neurodegeneration unrelated to amyloid beta deposition as well.[69]

Melatonin and Delirium

Four recent studies have examined the role of melatonin in the prevention of delirium among elderly patients, 3 of which found a lower incidence of delirium among patients who were treated with melatonin versus placebo.[150–152] The fourth did not find a statistically significant difference between melatonin and placebo groups. However, this study did report a shorter duration of delirium among patients treated with melatonin.[153] Although further research is needed, the use of this well-tolerated treatment intervention could prove useful in improving patient outcomes among critically ill patients during inpatient hospitalization.

SUMMARY

Sleep disorders in the elderly pose unique challenges for diagnosis and treatment. The elderly are at high risk for the development of sleep disorders given their propensity for changes in sleep architecture in combination with medical, psychiatric, cognitive, behavioral, and environmental factors. A thorough assessment of these components provides the physician with data to guide treatment, often by addressing the underlying problem. Management of sleep disorders is complicated by the risk of side effects of pharmacologic treatment approaches, and thus nonpharmacologic strategies are preferred when possible. Additionally, many of the pharmacologic strategies used in treating younger adults have not been studied adequately in the geriatric population, and more specifically in patients with underlying cognitive disorders, making treatment choices difficult. Sleep changes in the elderly may have a far broader impact on geriatric health than originally thought, with implications for AD and delirium, and further research is needed in these areas as well.

REFERENCES

1. Thomas D. Do not go gentle into that good night. In: Ferguson M, Salter M, Stallworthy J, editors. The Norton anthology of poetry. 5th edition. New York: W.W. Norton; 2004. p. 1572.
2. Foley DJ, Monjan AA, Brown SL, et al. Sleep complaints among elderly persons: an epidemiologic study of three communities. Sleep 1995;18(6):425–32.
3. Rodriguez JC, Dzierzewski JM, Alessi CA. Sleep problems in the elderly. Med Clin North Am 2015;99(2):431–9.
4. Fetveit A. Late-life insomnia: a review. Geriatr Gerontol Int 2009;9(3):220–34.
5. Duffy JF, Dijk DJ, Klerman EB, et al. Later endogenous circadian temperature nadir relative to an earlier wake time in older people. Am J Physiol 1998;275(5 Pt 2):R1478–87.
6. Yoon IY, Kripke DF, Elliott JA, et al. Age-related changes of circadian rhythms and sleep-wake cycles. J Am Geriatr Soc 2003;51(8):1085–91.
7. Redline S, Kirchner HL, Quan SF, et al. The effects of age, sex, ethnicity, and sleep-disordered breathing on sleep architecture. Arch Intern Med 2004;164:406–18.
8. Moe KE, Prinz PN, Vitiello MV, et al. Healthy elderly women and men have different entrained circadian temperature rhythms. J Am Geriatr Soc 1991;39:383–7.
9. American Psychiatric Association. Diagnostic and statistical manual of mental disorders. 5th edition. Washington, DC: American Psychiatric Association; 2013.
10. Vitiello MV, Moe KE, Prinz PN. Sleep complaints cosegregate with illness in older adults: clinical research informed by and informing epidemiological studies of sleep. J Psychosom Res 2002;53:555–9.
11. Lam JC, Sharma SK, Lam B. Obstructive sleep apnoea: definitions, epidemiology & natural history. Indian J Med Res 2010;131:165–70.
12. Ancoli-Israel S, Kripke DF. Prevalent sleep problems in the aged. Biofeedback Self Regul 1991;16(4):349–59.
13. Ganga H, Thangaraj Y, Puppala V, et al. Obstructive sleep apnea in the elderly population: atypical presentation and diagnostic challenges. Internet J Intern Med 2009;8(2):1–10.
14. Budhiraja R, Budhiraja P, Quan SF. Sleep-disordered breathing and cardiovascular disorders. Respir Care 2010;55(10):1322–32.
15. Peker Y, Hedner J, Kraiczi H, et al. Respiratory disturbance index: an independent predictor of mortality in coronary artery disease. Am J Respir Crit Care Med 2000;162(1):81–6.
16. Vgontzas AN, Bixler EO, Chrousos GP. Sleep apnea is a manifestation of the metabolic syndrome. Sleep Med Rev 2005;9(3):211–24.
17. Hudgel DW. Neuropsychiatric manifestations of obstructive sleep apnea: a review. Int J Psychiatry Med 1989;19(1):11–22.
18. Allen RP, Picchietti D, Hening WA, et al. Restless legs syndrome: diagnostic criteria, special considerations, and epidemiology: a report from the Restless Legs Syndrome Diagnosis and Epidemiology Workshop at the National Institutes of Health. Sleep Med 2003;4:101–19.
19. Garnaldo CE, Benbrook AR, Allen RP, et al. Childhood and adult factors associated with restless legs syndrome (RLS) diagnosis. Sleep Med 2007;8(7–8):716–22.
20. Hening W, Walters AS, Allen AP, et al. Impact, diagnosis, and treatment of restless legs syndrome (RLS) in a primary care population: the REST (RLS epidemiology, symptoms, and treatment) primary care study. Sleep Med 2004;5:3–237.

21. Yeh P, Walters A, Tsuang JW. Restless legs syndrome: a comprehensive review on its epidemiology, risk factors, and treatment. Sleep Breath 2012;16: 987–1007.

22. Yules RB, Lippman ME, Freedman DX. Alcohol administration prior to sleep: the effect on EEG sleep stages. Arch Gen Psychiatry 1967;16(1):94–7.

23. Irish LA, Kline CE, Gunn HE, et al. The role of sleep hygiene in promoting public health: a review of the empirical evidence. Sleep Med Rev 2015;22:23–36.

24. Vitiello MV, Prinz PN, Personius JP, et al. History of chronic alcohol abuse is associated with increased nighttime hypoxemia in older men. Alcohol Clin Exp Res 1987;11(4):368–71.

25. Vitiello MV, Prinz PN, Personius JP, et al. Nighttime hypoxemia is increased in abstaining chronic alcoholic men. Alcohol Clin Exp Res 1990;14(1):38–41.

26. McKinnon A, Terpening Z, Hickie IB, et al. Prevalence and predictors of poor sleep quality in mild cognitive impairment. J Geriatr Psychiatry Neurol 2014; 27(3):204–11.

27. Yang PY, Ho K-H, Chen H-C, et al. Exercise training improves sleep quality in middle-aged and older adults with sleep problems: a systematic review. J Physiother 2012;58:157–63.

28. Edinger JD, Morey MC, Sullivan RJ, et al. Aerobic fitness, acute exercise and sleep in older men. Sleep 1993;16(4):351–9.

29. Leblanc MF, Desjardins S, Desgagné A. The relationship between sleep habits, anxiety, and depression in the elderly. Nat Sci Sleep 2015;7:33–42.

30. Werth E, Dijk D-J, Achermann P, et al. Dynamics of the sleep EEG after an early evening nap: experimental data and simulations. Am J Physiol 1996;271: R501–10.

31. Campbell SS, Sanchina MD, Schlang JR, et al. Effects of a month-long napping regimen in older individuals. J Am Geriatr Soc 2011;59(2):224–32.

32. Dhand R, Sohal H. Good sleep, bad sleep! The role of daytime naps in healthy adults. Curr Opin Pulm Med 2006;12(6):379–82.

33. Stang A, Dragano N, Moebus S, et al. Midday naps and the risk of coronary artery disease: results of the Heinz Nixdorf Recall Study. Sleep 2012;35(12): 1705–12.

34. Massey LK. Caffeine and the elderly. Drugs Aging 1998;13(1):43–50.

35. Wolkove N, Elkholy O, Baltzan M, et al. Sleep and aging: 1. Sleep disorders commonly found in older people. CMAJ 2007;176(9):1299–304.

36. Robillard R, Bouchard M, Cartier A, et al. Sleep is more sensitive to high doses of caffeine in the middle years of life. J Psychopharmacol 2015;29(6):688–97.

37. Aurora RN, Crainicenau C, Caffo B, et al. Sleep-disordered breathing and caffeine consumption: results of a community-based study. Chest 2012; 142(3):631–8.

38. Kromhout MA, Jongerling J, Achterberg WP. Relation between caffeine and behavioral symptoms in elderly patients with dementia: an observational study. J Nutr Health Aging 2014;18(4):407–10.

39. Krause KH, Dressel SH, Krause J, et al. Stimulant-like action of nicotine on striatal dopamine transporter in the brain of adults with attention deficit hyperactivity disorder. Int J Neuropsychopharmacol 2002;5(2):111–3.

40. Cohrs S, Rodenbeck A, Riemann D, et al. Impaired sleep quality and sleep duration in smokers—results from the German Multicenter Study on Nicotine Dependence. Addict Biol 2014;19(3):286–96.

41. Zhang L, Samet J, Caffo B, et al. Cigarette smoking and nocturnal sleep architecture. Am J Epidemiol 2006;164(6):529–37.

42. Ohayon MM. Interactions between sleep normative data and sociocultural characteristics in the elderly. J Psychosom Res 2004;56(5):479–86.
43. Lin YN, Li QY, Zhang XJ. Interaction between smoking and obstructive sleep apnea: not just participants. Chin Med J (Engl) 2012;125(17):3150–6.
44. Gourlay SG, Benowitz NL. The benefits of stopping smoking and the role of nicotine replacement therapy in older patients. Drugs Aging 1996;9(1):8–23.
45. Smith TM, Winters FD. Smoking cessation: a clinical study of the transdermal nicotine patch. J Am Osteopath Assoc 1995;95(11):655–6, 661-2.
46. Steffens DC, Fisher GG, Langa KM, et al. Prevalence of depression among older Americans: the Aging, Demographics, and Memory Study. Int Psychogeriatr 2009;21(5):879–88.
47. Cole MG, Dendukuri N. Risk factors for depression among elderly community subjects: a systematic review and meta-analysis. Am J Psychiatry 2003;16(6): 1147–56.
48. Buysse DJ. Insomnia, depression, and aging. Assessing sleep and mood interactions in older adults. Geriatrics 2004;59(2):47–51.
49. Aziz R, Steffens DC. What are the causes of late-life depression? Psychiatr Clin North Am 2013;36:497–516.
50. Monk TH, Germain A, Reynolds CF. Sleep disturbance in bereavement. Psychiatr Ann 2008;38(10):671–5.
51. Spira AP, Friedman L, Flint A, et al. Interaction of sleep disturbances and anxiety in later life: perspectives and recommendations for future research. J Geriatr Psychiatry Neurol 2005;18:109–15.
52. Schaub RT, Linden M. Anxiety and anxiety disorders in the old and very old—results from the Berlin Aging Study (BASE). Compr Psychiatry 2000;41(2 Suppl 1):48–54.
53. Magee JC, Carmin CN. The relationship between sleep and anxiety in older adults. Curr Psychiatry Rep 2010;12:13–9.
54. Potvin O, Lorrain D, Belleville G, et al. Subjective sleep characteristics associated with anxiety and depression in older adults: a population-based study. Int J Geriatr Psychiatry 2014;29(12):1262–70.
55. Wetherell JL, Le Roux H, Gatz M. DSM-IV criteria for generalized anxiety disorder in older adults: distinguishing the worried from the well. Psychol Aging 2003; 18:622–7.
56. Marcks BA, Weisberg RB, Edelen MO, et al. The relationship between sleep disturbance and the course of anxiety disorders in primary care patients. Psychiatry Res 2010;178(3):487–92.
57. Takaesu Y, Inoue Y, Komada Y, et al. Effects of nasal continuous positive airway pressure on panic disorder comorbid with obstructive sleep apnea syndrome. Sleep Med 2012;13(2):156–60.
58. Edmonds JC, Yang H, King TS, et al. Claustrophobic tendencies and continuous positive airway pressure therapy non-adherence in adults with obstructive sleep apnea. Heart Lung 2015;44(2):100–6.
59. Peskind ER, Bonner LT, Hoff DJ, et al. Prazosin reduces trauma-related nightmares in older men with chronic post-traumatic stress disorder. J Geriatr Psychiatry Neurol 2003;16(3):165–71.
60. Cook JM, Dinnen S, O'Donnell C. Older women survivors of physical and sexual violence: a systematic review of the quantitative literature. J Womens Health (Larchmt) 2011;20(7):1075–81.
61. Krakow B, Germain A, Tandberg D, et al. Sleep breathing and sleep movement disorders masquerading as insomnia in sexual-assault survivors. Compr Psychiatry 2000;41:49–56.

62. Bottche M, Kuwert P, Knaevelsrud C. Posttraumatic stress disorder in older adults: an overview of characteristics and treatment approaches. Int J Geriatr Psychiatry 2012;27(3):230–9.
63. Lapp LK, Agbokou C, Ferreri F. PTSD in the elderly: the interaction between trauma and aging. Int Psychogeriatr 2011;23(6):858–68.
64. Hiskey S, Luckie M, Davies S, et al. The emergence of posttraumatic distress in later life: a review. J Geriatr Psychiatry Neurol 2008;21(4):232–41.
65. Sadavoy J. Survivors: a review of late-life effects of prior psychological trauma. Am J Geriatr Psychiatry 1997;5:287–301.
66. Yaffe K, Falvey CM, Hoang T. Connections between sleep and cognition in older adults. Lancet Neurol 2014;13(10):1017–28.
67. Blackwell T, Yaffe K, Laffan A, et al. Associations between sleep-disordered breathing, nocturnal hypoxemia, and subsequent cognitive decline in older community-dwelling men: the osteoporotic fractures in men sleep study. J Am Geriatr Soc 2015;63(3):453–61.
68. Dlugaj M, Weinreich G, Weimar C, et al. Sleep-disordered breathing, sleep quality, and mild cognitive impairment in the general population. J Alzheimers Dis 2014;41(2):479–97.
69. Musiek ES, Xiong DD, Holtzman DM. Sleep, circadian rhythms, and the pathogenesis of Alzheimer's disease. Exp Mol Med 2015;47:e148.
70. Vitiello MV, Prinz PN. Sleep/wake patterns and sleep disorders in Alzheimer's disease. In: Thorpy MJ, editor. Handbook of sleep disorders. New York: Marcel Dekker; 1990. p. 703–18.
71. Hatfield CF, Herbert J, van Someren EJ, et al. Disrupted daily activity/rest cycles in relation to daily cortisol rhythms of home-dwelling patients with early Alzheimer's dementia. Brain 2004;127:1061–74.
72. Carvalho-Bos SS, Riemersma-van der Lek RF, Waterhouse J, et al. Strong association of the rest-activity rhythm with well-being in demented elderly women. Am J Geriatr Psychiatry 2007;15:92–100.
73. Scarmeas N, Brandt J, Blacker D, et al. Disruptive behavior as a predictor in Alzheimer disease. Arch Neurol 2007;64:1755–61.
74. Pollak CP, Perlick D. Sleep problems and institutionalization of the elderly. J Geriatr Psychiatry Neurol 1991;4:204–10.
75. Gallagher-Thompson D, Brooks JO III, Bliwise D, et al. The relations among caregiver stress, "sundowning" symptoms, and cognitive decline in Alzheimer's disease. J Am Geriatr Soc 1992;40:807–10.
76. Klaffke S, Staedt J. Sundowning and circadian rhythm disorders in dementia. Acta Neurol Belg 2006;106(4):168–75.
77. De Jonghe A, Korevaar JC, van Munster BC, et al. Effectiveness of melatonin treatment on circadian rhythm disturbances in dementia. Are there implications for delirium? A systematic review. Int J Geriatr Psychiatry 2010;25(12): 1201–8.
78. McKeith IG, Dickson DW, Lowe J, et al, Consortium on DLB. Diagnosis and management of dementia with Lewy bodies: third report of the DLB Consortium. Neurology 2005;65(12):1863–72.
79. Karantzoulis S, Galvin JE. Update on dementia with Lewy bodies. Curr Transl Geriatr Exp Gerontol Rep 2013;2(3):196–204.
80. Boeve BF, Dickson DW, Olson EJ, et al. Insights into REM sleep behavioral disorder pathophysiology in brainstem-predominant Lewy body disease. Sleep Med 2007;8(1):60–4.
81. Molano JRV. Dementia with Lewy bodies. Semin Neurol 2013;33:330–5.

82. Bozek K, Relogio A, Kielbasa SM, et al. Regulation of clock-controlled genes in mammals. PLoS One 2009;4(3):e4882.
83. Meagher DJ, Moran M, Raju ZB, et al. Phenomenology of delirium Assessment of 100 adult cases using standardized measures. Br J Psychiatry 2007;190:135–41.
84. Fitzgerald JM, Adamis D, Trzepacz PT, et al. Delirium: a disturbance of circadian integrity? Med Hypotheses 2013;81(4):568–76.
85. Verceles AC, Silhan L, Terrin M, et al. Circadian rhythm disruption in severe sepsis: the effect of ambient light on urinary 6-sulfatoxymelatonin secretion. Intensive Care Med 2012;38(5):804–10.
86. Van Rompaey B, Elseviers MM, Schuurmans MJ, et al. Risk factors for delirium in intensive care patients: a prospective cohort study. Crit Care 2009;13(3):R77.
87. Gabor JY, Cooper AB, Crombach SA, et al. Contribution of the intensive care unit environment to sleep disruption in mechanically ventilated patients and healthy subjects. Am J Respir Crit Care Med 2003;167(5):708–15.
88. Freedman NS, Kotzer N, Schwab RJ. Patient perception of sleep quality and etiology of sleep disruption in the intensive care unit. Am J Respir Crit Care Med 1999;159(4 Pt 1):1155–62.
89. Wilson LM. Intensive care delirium. The effect of outside deprivation in a windowless unit. Arch Intern Med 1972;130(2):225–6.
90. Keep P, James J, Inman M. Windows in the intensive therapy unit. Anaesthesia 1980;35(3):257–62.
91. Beauchemin KM, Hays P. Dying in the dark: sunshine, gender and outcomes in myocardial infarction. J R Soc Med 1998;91(7):352–4.
92. Videnovic A, Golombek D. Circadian and sleep disorders in Parkinson's disease. Exp Neurol 2013;243:45–56.
93. Schrempf W, Brandt MD, Storch A, et al. Sleep disorders in Parkinson's disease. J Parkinsons Dis 2014;4(2):211–21.
94. Suzuki K, Miyamoto M, Miyamoto T, et al. Parkinson's disease and sleep/wake disturbances. Curr Neurol Neurosci Rep 2015;15:8.
95. Stocchi F, Abbruzzese G, Ceravolo R, et al. Prevalence of fatigue in Parkinson disease and its clinical correlates. Neurology 2014;83(3):215–20.
96. Mahale R, Yadav R, Pal PK. Quality of sleep in young onset Parkinson's disease: any difference from older onset Parkinson's disease. Parkinsonism Relat Disord 2015;21(5):461–4.
97. Van Doorn B, Bosch JL. Nocturia in older men. Maturitas 2012;71(1):8–12.
98. Bosch JL, Weiss JP. The prevalence and causes of nocturia. J Urol 2013;189(1 Suppl):S86–92.
99. Doo SW, Lee HJ, Ahn J, et al. Strong impact of nocturia on sleep quality in patients with lower urinary tract symptoms. World J Mens Health 2012;30(2):123–30.
100. Cakir OO, McVary KT. LUTS and sleep disorders: emerging risk factor. Curr Urol Rep 2012;13:407–12.
101. American Geriatrics Society 2012 Beers Criteria Expert Panel. American Geriatrics Society updated Beers criteria for potentially inappropriate medication use in older adults. J Am Geriatr Soc 2012;60:616–31.
102. Mannino DM, Buist AS. Global burden of COPD: risk factors, prevalence, and future trends. Lancet 2007;370:765–73.
103. McNicholas WT. Impact of sleep in COPD. Chest 2000;117(Suppl 2):48S–53S.
104. Soler X, Gaio E, Powell FL, et al. High prevalence of obstructive sleep apnea in patients with moderate to severe COPD. Ann Am Thorac Soc 2015. [Epub ahead of print].

105. Klink M, Quan SF. Prevalence of reported sleep disturbances in a general adult population and their relationship to obstructive airways diseases. Chest 1987; 91:540–6.
106. Roth T. Hypnotic use for insomnia management in chronic obstructive pulmonary disease. Sleep Med 2009;10:19–25.
107. Kryger M, Roth T, Wang-Weigand S, et al. The effects of ramelteon on respiration during sleep in subjects with moderate to severe chronic obstructive pulmonary disease. Sleep Breath 2009;13:79–84.
108. Kapella MC, Herdegen JJ, Perlis ML, et al. Cognitive behavioral therapy for insomnia comorbid with COPD is feasible with preliminary evidence of positive sleep and fatigue effects. Int J Chron Obstruct Pulmon Dis 2011;6:625–35.
109. Lloyd-Owen SJ, Donaldson GG, Ambrosino N, et al. Patterns of home mechanical ventilation use in Europe: results from the Eurovent survey. Eur Respir J 2005;25:1025–31.
110. AGS Panel on Persistent Pain in Older Persons. The management of persistent pain in older persons. A GS panel on persistent pain in older persons. J Am Geriatr Soc 2002;50(6 Suppl):S205–24.
111. Pilowsky I, Crettenden I, Townley M. Sleep disturbance in pain clinic patients. Pain 1985;23(1):27–33.
112. Morin CM, Gibson D, Wade J. Self-reported sleep and mood disturbance in chronic pain patients. Clin J Pain 1998;14(4):311–4.
113. Benca RM, Ancoli-Israel S, Moldofsky H. Special considerations in insomnia diagnosis and management: depressed, elderly, and chronic pain populations. J Clin Psychiatry 2004;65(Suppl 8):26–35.
114. Schredl M, Weber B, Braus D, et al. The effect of rivastigmine on sleep in elderly healthy subjects. Exp Gerontol 2000;35(2):243–9.
115. Schredl M, Weber B, Leins ML, et al. Donepezil-induced REM sleep augmentation enhances memory performance in elderly, healthy persons. Exp Gerontol 2001;36(2):353–61.
116. Riemann D, Gann H, Dressing H, et al. Influence of the cholinesterase inhibitor galanthamine hydrobromide on normal sleep. Psychiatry Res 1993;51(3): 253–67.
117. Kanbayashi T, Sugiyama T, Aizawa R, et al. Effects of donepezil (Aricept) on the rapid eye movement sleep of normal subjects. Psychiatry Clin Neurosci 2002; 56(3):307–8.
118. Markowitz JS, Gutterman EM, Lilienfeld S, et al. Sleep-related outcomes in persons with mild to moderate Alzheimer disease in a placebo-controlled trial of galantamine. Sleep 2003;26(5):602–6.
119. Stoschitzky K, Sakotnik A, Lercher P, et al. Influence of beta-blockers on melatonin release. Eur J Clin Pharmacol 1999;55:111–5.
120. Van Den Heuvel CJ, Reid KJ, Dawson D. Effect of atenolol on nocturnal sleep and temperature in young men: reversal by pharmacological doses of melatonin. Physiol Behav 1997;61:795–802.
121. Prenner B, Anolik R, Danzig M, et al. Efficacy and safety of fixed-dose loratadine/montelukast in seasonal allergic rhinitis: effects on nasal congestion. Allergy Asthma Proc 2009;30(3):263–9.
122. Wolkowitz OM, Rubinow D, Doran AR, et al. Prednisone effects on neurochemistry and behavior. Arch Gen Psychiatry 1990;47:963–8.
123. Kenna HA, Poon AW, de los Angeles CP, et al. Psychiatric complications of treatment with corticosteroids: review with case report. Psychiatry Clin Neurosci 2011;65(6):549–60.

124. Wichniak A, Wierzbicka A, Jernajczyk W. Sleep and antidepressant treatment. Curr Pharm Des 2012;18(36):5802–17.
125. Jensen E, Dehlin O, Hagberg B, et al. Insomnia in an 80-year-old population: relationship to medical, psychological, and social factors. J Sleep Res 1998; 7(3):183–9.
126. Morin CM. Dysfunctional beliefs and attitudes about sleep among older adults with and without insomnia complaints. Psychol Aging 1993;8(3):463–7.
127. Montgomery P, Dennis J. Cognitive behavioural interventions for sleep problems in adults aged 60+. Cochrane Database Syst Rev 2003;(1):CD003161.
128. Bootzin RR, Epstein D, Wood JM. Stimulus control instructions. In: Hauri P, editor. Case studies in insomnia. New York: Plenum Medical; 1991. p. 19–23.
129. Spielman AJ, Saskin P, Thorpy MJ. Treatment of chronic insomnia by restriction of time in bed. Sleep 1987;10:45–56.
130. Wurtman RJ, Zhdanova I. Improvement of sleep quality by melatonin. Lancet 1995;346(8988):1491.
131. Trotti LM. REM sleep behavior disorder in older individuals: epidemiology, pathophysiology, and management. Drugs Aging 2010;27(6):457–70.
132. Vural EM, van Munster BC, de Rooij SE. Optimal dosages for melatonin supplementation therapy in older adults: a systematic review of current literature. Drugs Aging 2014;31(6):441–51.
133. James SP, Mendelson WB. The use of trazodone as a hypnotic: a critical review. J Clin Psychiatry 2004;65(6):752–5.
134. Mendelson WB. A review of the evidence for the efficacy and safety of trazodone in insomnia. J Clin Psychiatry 2005;66(4):469–76.
135. Haria M, Fitton A, McTavish D. Trazodone. A review of its pharmacology, therapeutic use in depression and therapeutic potential in other disorders. Drugs Aging 1994;4(4):331–55.
136. Salzman C. Pharmacologic treatment of disturbed sleep in the elderly. Harv Rev Psychiatry 2008;16:271–8.
137. De Gage SB, Moride Y, Ducruet T, et al. Benzodiazepine use and risk of Alzheimer's disease: case-control study. BMJ 2014;349:g5205.
138. Huang AR, Mallet L, Rochefort CM, et al. Medication-related falls in the elderly: causative factors and preventive strategies. Drugs Aging 2012; 29(5):359–76.
139. Salzman C, Fisher J, Nobel K, et al. Cognitive improvement following benzodiazepine discontinuation in elderly nursing home residents. Int J Geriatr Psychiatry 1992;7:89–93.
140. Krystal AD. A compendium of placebo-controlled trials of the risks/benefits of pharmacological treatments for insomnia: the empirical basis for U.S. clinical practice. Sleep Med Rev 2009;13(4):265–74.
141. Dolder C, Nelson M, McKinsey J. Use of non-benzodiazepine hypnotics in the elderly: are all agents the same? CNS Drugs 2007;21(5):389–405.
142. McCall WV, Fleischer AB Jr, Feldman SR. Diagnostic codes associated with hypnotic medications during outpatient physician-patient encounters in the United States from 1990-1998. Sleep 2002;25:221–3.
143. Silber MH. Clinical practice. Chronic insomnia. N Engl J Med 2005;353:803–10.
144. Winokur A, Sateia MJ, Hayes JB, et al. Acute effects of mirtazapine on sleep continuity and sleep architecture in depressed patients: a pilot study. Biol Psychiatry 2000;48:75–8.
145. Wiegand MH. Antidepressants for the treatment of insomnia: a suitable approach? Drugs 2008;68(17):2411–7.

146. Kang JE, Lim MM, Bateman RJ, et al. Amyloid-beta dynamics are regulated by orexin and the sleep-wake cycle. Science 2009;326:1005–7.

147. Huang Y, Potter R, Sigurdson W, et al. Effects of age and amyloid deposition on Abeta dynamics in the human central nervous system. Arch Neurol 2012;69: 51–8.

148. Lucey BP, Bateman RJ. Amyloid-beta diurnal pattern: possible role of sleep in Alzheimer's disease pathogenesis. Neurobiol Aging 2014;35(Suppl 2):S29–34.

149. Ju YE, Lucey BP, Holtzman DM. Sleep and Alzheimer disease pathology—a bidirectional relationship. Nat Rev Neurol 2014;10(2):115–9.

150. Sultan SS. Assessment of role of perioperative melatonin in prevention and treatment of postoperative delirium after hip arthroplasty under spinal anesthesia in the elderly. Saudi J Anaesth 2010;4(3):169–73.

151. Al-Aama T, Brymer C, Gutmanis I, et al. Melatonin decreases delirium in elderly patients: a randomized, placebo-controlled trial. Int J Geriatr Psychiatry 2011; 26(7):687–94.

152. Hatta K, Kishi Y, Wada K, et al. Preventive effects of ramelteon on delirium: a randomized placebo-controlled trial. JAMA Psychiatry 2014;71(4):397–403.

153. De Jonghe A, van Munster BC, Goslings JC, et al. Effect of melatonin on incidence of delirium among patients with hip fracture: a multicenter, double-blind randomized controlled trial. CMAJ 2014;186(14):E547–56.

Sleep Disturbances in Mood Disorders

Meredith E. Rumble, PhD*, Kaitlin Hanley White, PhD, Ruth M. Benca, MD, PhD

KEYWORDS

- Depression • Sleep • Insomnia • Hypersomnia • Polysomnography
- Circadian rhythm • Actigraphy • Therapeutics

KEY POINTS

- Self-reported and objective sleep disturbances are common in people with depressive, bipolar, and other mood disorders.
- Sleep disturbance alone is a risk factor for future onset of depressive disorders and dys-regulated rest-activity patterns are a risk factor for onset of affective episodes in people with bipolar disorders.
- Residual sleep disturbance is common in people with remitted mood disorders and can lead to higher risk of relapse.
- Other sleep disorders are more prevalent in people with mood disorders and should be considered, and medications potentially helpful for mood disorders may be disruptive to sleep.
- Effective treatments are available for sleep disturbances comorbid with mood disorders and show promise for improving not only sleep but also mood more broadly.

MOOD DISORDERS OVERVIEW

Mood disorders are among the most prevalent and debilitating psychiatric conditions affecting the population worldwide. They make up the second most common category of psychiatric illness following anxiety disorders, and estimates suggest that approximately 12% of individuals meet criteria for a mood disorder during their lifetimes.[1] Mood disorders are associated with increased morbidity and mortality from other illnesses and, in 6% to 15% of those affected, can result in eventual suicide.[2] The societal burden of mood disorders is enormous, with a projected cost of $14.1 billion for bipolar disorders and $36.6 billion for major depressive disorder in terms of annual

Disclosures: Dr M.E. Rumble reports grant support from Merck; Dr K.H. White has no disclosures to report; Dr R.M. Benca has served as a consultant to Jazz and Merck, Inc, and receives grant support from Merck.
Department of Psychiatry, University of Wisconsin, 6001 Research Park Boulevard, Madison, WI 53719, USA
* Corresponding author.
E-mail address: rumble@wisc.edu

Psychiatr Clin N Am 38 (2015) 743–759
http://dx.doi.org/10.1016/j.psc.2015.07.006
0193-953X/15/$ – see front matter © 2015 Elsevier Inc. All rights reserved.

Abbreviations	
AOR	Adjusted odds ratio
CBT	Cognitive behavior therapy
CRH	Corticotropin-releasing hormone
DSM-5	Diagnostic and Statistical Manual, Fifth edition
EEG	Electroencephalogram
IPSRT	Interpersonal and social rhythm therapy
MAOI	Monoamine oxidase inhibitor
MDD	Major depressive disorder
NREM	Non–rapid eye movement
OSA	Obstructive sleep apnea
PSG	Polysomnography
REM	Rapid eye movement
SCN	Suprachiasmatic nucleus
SNRI	Serotonin and norepinephrine reuptake inhibitor
SRM-II-5	Social Rhythm Metric II, 5-Item Version
SRT	Social rhythm therapy
SSRI	Selective serotonin reuptake inhibitor
STAR*D trial	Sequenced Treatment Alternatives to Relieve Depression trial
SWS	Slow wave sleep
TCA	Tricyclic antidepressant

human capital loss in the United States, where bipolar disorder is associated with 65.5 and unipolar depression with 27.2 annual lost work days per ill worker.[3] A strong association between sleep disturbances and mood disorders has long been acknowledged, and the Diagnostic and Statistical Manual of Mental Disorders, fifth edition (DSM-5), diagnostic criteria reflect their central role in the diagnosis of mood disorders.[4]

DSM-5 differentiates what have historically been categorized as mood disorders into bipolar and related disorders and depressive disorders. Mood disorders are distinguished by the presence of mood episodes, which may be mania, hypomania, or depression. The most common depressive disorder is major depressive disorder (MDD). MDD is associated with at least 1 episode of major depression. Up to 85% of people having 1 episode of major depression later develop another episode (ie, recurrent subtype).[5] In the United States, lifetime prevalence of MDD with a seasonal pattern is estimated at 0.4%, with typical onset in the fall or winter.[6] Persistent depressive disorder, previously dysthymia, is distinguished by the experience of depressed mood and at least 2 other symptoms of depression on more days than not for at least 2 years, not meeting criteria for a full major depressive episode.

Bipolar I disorder is characterized by lifetime presence of at least 1 manic episode, whereas bipolar II disorder is characterized by at least 1 hypomanic episode and at least 1 major depressive episode. Cyclothymia refers to the presence of numerous hypomanic symptoms that do not meet full criteria for a hypomanic episode and depressive symptoms that do not meet criteria for a major depressive episode, occurring for at least half the time for 2 years with no more than 2 months of remission of symptoms.

Other bipolar and depressive disorders include substance-induced/medication-induced and medically induced disorders, which refer to the symptoms previously described that are related specifically to substance-related, medication-related, or medical-related conditions. In addition, specified and unspecified bipolar and depressive disorders refer to other conditions resembling these disorders that do not meet full criteria for those previously described.

COMMON SLEEP DISTURBANCES IN MOOD DISORDERS

Box 1 presents an overview of common sleep disturbances in mood disorders as measured by self-report, polysomnography, and actigraphy.

Self-reported Sleep, Fatigue, and Sleepiness in Mood Disorders

Individuals with mood disorders describe a range of difficulties with sleep continuity and quality as well as related daytime difficulties. Estimates suggest that up to 90% of individuals in a depressive episode report sleep quality complaints.[7] About two-thirds of these complaints can be classified as insomnia, whereas about 15% indicate hypersomnia.[8,9] Specifically, MDD is related to more frequent reports of difficulty falling asleep, difficulty staying asleep, and waking up too early in the morning, as well as nonrestorative sleep, significantly increased or decreased total sleep time (ie, dependent on insomnia or hypersomnia as the primary concern), lower sleep efficiency, and more frequent disturbing dreams.[10] In addition, individuals with MDD report greater daytime sleepiness,[11-13] and continued fatigue has been noted as the second most common residual symptom in depression.[14]

A central distinguishing symptom of manic episodes is the perception of a decreased need for sleep.[4] Sleep disturbances continue between mood episodes for bipolar spectrum disorders, including continued difficulty falling and staying asleep, longer time spent in bed, and lower sleep efficiency than in controls.[15] Furthermore, interepisode bipolar disorders are associated with significant intraindividual variability in terms of sleep continuity (ie, total sleep time, time to fall asleep, wake time after sleep onset, and sleep efficiency). Bipolar individuals also report greater daytime fatigue and sleepiness. Compared with individuals with primary insomnia, those with interepisode bipolar spectrum disorders tend to show better sleep continuity but report similar levels of daytime sleepiness.[16]

Beyond information gathered in a clinical interview, questionnaires and daily sleep logs are often helpful in further assessing sleep disturbances so that treatment can be appropriately tailored to the sleep concern. The following are several instruments that can be used easily within clinical practice: the Insomnia Severity Index to assess insomnia,[17] the Consensus Sleep Diary to assess daily sleep-wake patterns,[18] and the Epworth Sleepiness Scale to assess level of sleepiness.[19]

Polysomnography Findings in Mood Disorders

Many psychiatric disorders are associated with impacts on sleep architecture as assessed by polysomnography (PSG).[20] MDD has received by far the most attention in terms of PSG and related approaches. Disturbances of sleep continuity that are frequently found, based on PSG assessments, include a longer time to fall asleep, increased wake time after falling asleep, and more awakenings early in the morning, leading to lower overall sleep time and sleep efficiency.[20,21] Furthermore, patients in a depressive episode show a decreased amount and percentage of stage 3 sleep, with slow wave sleep (SWS) loss most evident during the first non–rapid eye movement (NREM) period but also reduced delta power and slow wave counts throughout the night.[21] The distribution of SWS during the night differs among depressed patients, with a lower amount of SWS in the first NREM period versus the second.[22] Decreased rapid eye movement (REM) latency is the most robust finding in depression,[20] but other REM abnormalities include a prolonged first REM sleep period and increased REM density. REM sleep has been shown to be important for affect regulation.[23-25] These findings have largely been replicated in persistent depressive disorder (previously dysthymia), but not with the same severity.[26,27]

Box 1
Common sleep disturbances in mood disorders

Self-reported sleep symptoms

- Insomnia, including difficulty initiating sleep, difficulty maintaining sleep, and/or early morning awakenings
- Nonrestorative sleep/poor sleep quality
- Hypersomnia
- Disturbing dreams/nightmares
- Decreased need for sleep[a]
- Fatigue
- Excessive sleepiness

Polysomnographic sleep disturbances

Decreased sleep continuity

- Longer sleep onset latency
- Greater wake time after sleep onset
- More early morning awakenings
- Decreased total sleep time
- Decreased sleep efficiency (percentage of time spent in sleeping during sleep period)

Differences in sleep architecture

- Increased percentage of stage 1 sleep
- Decreased percentage of stage 3 sleep
- Decreased slow wave sleep
- Decreased rapid eye movement (REM) latency
- Increased first REM sleep period
- Increased REM density

Rest-activity disturbances

Activity counts/self-reported daily rhythms

- Lower actigraphic activity counts
- Less rhythmic self-reported daily routines[a]

Differences in actigraphic sleep continuity

- Increased sleep onset latency[a]
- Increased total sleep time[a]
- Increased wake time after sleep onset[a]
- Increased variability of total sleep time[a]
- Increased variability of sleep onset latency[a]
- Increased variability of wake time after sleep onset[a]

[a] Bipolar and related disorders only.

The findings discussed earlier have been further supported by advanced sleep analysis using electroencephalogram (EEG) methods, including power spectral analysis and high-density EEG.[28–30] Automated analysis of SWS indicates a lower ratio of delta sleep (ie, deep sleep) in the first NREM period compared with the second NREM period for depressed patients.[28] This association may be informative regarding prediction of treatment response, because depressed patients with higher delta sleep ratios have been reported to respond better to treatment and those with lower delta sleep ratios were more likely to have recurrent episodes.[31,32] Studies have also suggested that SWS abnormalities may be affected by the sex, with men tending to show lower slow wave power and slower dissipation of slow wave activity during the night.[33,34] Studies using high-density EEG during sleep have identified that depressed women showed increased slow wave activity in prefrontal regions.[35]

Notably, REM sleep differences may precede the development of a depressive episode and are often found in first-degree relatives of those who have depression, suggesting a potential biological marker of the disorder.[36] Furthermore, REM sleep and SWS abnormalities can persist during remission from a depressive episode and predict relapse and poor treatment outcome.

Although not as extensively studied, PSG findings in manic episodes seem to be similar to those of a major depressive episode and include severe sleep continuity disturbances, reduced stage 3 sleep, short latency to REM sleep, and increased numbers of rapid eye movements.[37] Interepisode bipolar spectrum disorders have been associated with a significantly higher percentage of stage 1 sleep than healthy controls, but no other differences in terms of sleep continuity, SWS, non-REM sleep, or REM sleep.[15] A study of children with bipolar disorder found lower sleep efficiency, total sleep time, percentage of sleep spent in REM sleep, and percentage of stage 3 sleep compared with healthy controls.[38] Thus, even between episodes of mania and depression, adults and children with bipolar spectrum disorders continue to show some distinctions in PSG-measured sleep compared with healthy controls. Although sleep studies are not diagnostic of mood disorders, the presence of sleep abnormalities such as short REM sleep latency or early morning awakening should trigger consideration for possible mood disorder. In contrast, further sleep evaluation in patients with significant sleep complaints that persist despite remission of their mood episodes should be considered.

Rest-Activity Disturbances in Mood Disorders

A host of biological processes occur within living organisms in circadian cycles over an approximately 24-hour period. Circadian rhythms are orchestrated endogenously by the central clock in the suprachiasmatic nucleus (SCN) within the hypothalamus and are also behaviorally based in that they are sensitive to external input such as light exposure, which sends signals directly from the eyes to the SCN.[39] Mood-disordered patients show evidence of circadian rhythm disruption, including patterns of abnormal melatonin secretion in both depressed[40] and bipolar patients.[41]

An alternative marker of circadian rhythm dysregulation is the diurnal pattern of rest and activity as measured by wrist-worn actigraphy, which uses a highly sensitive accelerometer to objectively quantify activity. Several measures can be derived from raw activity data, including measures more directly related to activity (eg, average activity counts, variability in rest-activity patterns) as well as average sleep statistics derived from algorithms of rest and activity patterns to approximate sleep and wake. Thus, application of this measure to mood disorder populations may be clinically useful given that activity and sleep dysregulation are often a crucial part of mood disorders.

In depression, one systematic review identified 19 articles using actigraphy in depressive samples.[42] The main findings of this review were that (1) affected patients had significantly lower mean daytime activity counts than controls; (2) daytime activity counts significantly increased with depression treatment; and (3) nighttime activity significantly decreased with depression treatment. Few studies reported actigraphic sleep statistics or variability in rest-activity patterns, so no conclusive statements could be made on these measures.

In bipolar disorder, a recent systematic review of 9 studies and another of 21 studies of patients with remitted bipolar disorder showed that affected patients had significantly longer sleep onset latencies, longer sleep durations, and greater wake time after sleep onset than controls.[15,43] One review found affected patients to have less efficient sleep than controls,[43] whereas the other did not.[15] Ng and colleagues[15] found that affected patients had significantly greater variability in total sleep time, sleep onset latency, and wake time after sleep onset (across 3 studies), and lower activity counts (across 4 studies) than controls.

Similarly, there has been a body of work examining social zeitgebers (ie, social cues within the environment related to rest-activity rhythms) through the use of the Social Rhythm Metric.[44] A shortened version, the Social Rhythm Metric II, 5-Item Version (SRM-II-5[45]), monitors the timing of 5 daily activities strongly related to outcome in previous studies (ie, out of bed, first contact with another person, start of work/volunteering/school, dinner, and to bed). Studies examining rest-activity rhythmicity in patients with rapid cycling bipolar disorder as well as those with remitted bipolar disorder found that affected patients have significantly fewer rhythmic daily routines than healthy controls.[46,47] In addition, one study found that a collection of morning activities were more phase delayed in affected patients than in controls and more likely to occur within affected patients during depressive than hypomanic or euthymic episodes.[46]

Collectively, these findings underscore the importance of assessing rest-activity patterns when treating individuals with mood disorders. Moreover, although collection of biomarkers and actigraphy are not currently practical in most clinical settings, an understanding of rest-activity patterns can be gathered through the patient and family interviewing process or through sleep logs or assessments such as the SRM-II-5 so that treatment targets can be better defined.

SLEEP DISTURBANCE AS A RISK FACTOR AND INTEREPISODE PERSISTENCE OF SLEEP DISTURBANCE

Historically within psychiatry, sleep-wake disturbances, including insomnia, hypersomnia, and rest-activity dysregulation, have been considered secondary to the mood disorder. That is, as the mood disorder improved, sleep disturbances would improve and, if depression worsened, sleep disturbance would do so as well. However, there is a large body of epidemiologic data that instead supports the contention that sleep disturbance can be independent of, and have a bidirectional relationship with, psychiatric concerns (eg, the comorbid model of insomnia). More specifically, one meta-analysis of 18 epidemiologic studies found that patients with insomnia symptoms and without depression at baseline were 2.6 more times likely to develop future depression than those without insomnia symptoms at baseline.[48] In addition to self-report data, there is also evidence that objective abnormalities in sleep latency, continuity, and duration, as assessed by polysomnography, also predicted future depression onset.[49]

Hypersomnia has been less studied as a risk factor for future depression. A 4-year prospective, longitudinal study within older adults found excessive daytime sleepiness to be an independent risk factor for subsequent depressive symptoms,[50] whereas another prospective, longitudinal study following participants from ages 20 to 40 years found that excessive daytime sleepiness did not predict future depression.[51] However, in the latter study, sleepiness correlated with insomnia symptoms, which were predictive of depression.[51] Importantly, a recent meta-analysis showed that patients who are depressed with sleep disturbance were 3.1 times more likely to have suicidal behaviors than those who are depressed without sleep disturbance.[52] Thus, not only is insomnia a risk factor for onset of depression, and hypersomnia potentially a similar risk factor in some populations, sleep disturbance is also linked with increased likelihood of suicidality.

Rest-activity patterns have also been investigated as a risk factor for future onset of affective episodes in patients with bipolar disorder. One prospective longitudinal study found that less social rhythm regularity predicted onset of both depressive and hypomanic/manic episodes in those with cyclothymia and bipolar II disorder.[53] Thus, sleep-wake disturbance in a variety of forms may precede the onset of mood disturbance and could potentially contribute to the onset of a first lifetime mood disturbance. This finding points to the importance of treating sleep issues in individuals with no history of mood disorder because continued sleep disturbance may contribute to future onset of mood disorder.

Furthermore, in individuals with sleep disturbance in the context of a mood disorder, sleep disturbance can often persist even when the mood disorder is considered remitted. For example, one study from the Sequenced Treatment Alternatives to Relieve Depression (STAR*D) trial showed that sleep disturbance occurred as the most common residual symptom with approximately 72% of remitted patients treated with citalopram complaining of sleep issues.[54] Similarly, a 3-year prospective study of 267 depressed primary care patients found that sleep problems were present for 85% to 94% of the time during a depressive episode but also persisted for 39% to 44% of the time when depression was in remission.[55] In addition, many studies examining subjects with remitted bipolar disorder find that sleep and rest-activity disturbance continues and actigraphic measures of sleep and rest-activity patterns as well as self-reported sleep quality, insomnia severity, and daytime sleepiness differentiate affected patients from controls.[15] Thus, in psychiatric practice, these findings underscore that treating both sleep and mood issues as residual sleep disturbance can lead to relapse of the mood disorder.

MECHANISMS FOR SLEEP CHANGES IN MOOD DISORDERS

Several potential mechanisms have been proposed to explain the association of sleep disturbances with mood disorders. Early theories primarily attempted to account for the REM sleep abnormalities that seemed to be most characteristic of depression.

One of the first theories was related to the neurotransmitter imbalance hypothesis for depression, initially proposed by Janowsky and colleagues[56] in 1972. They suggested that depression was related to a relative increase in cholinergic activity and decrease in monoaminergic activity in the brain. At about the same time, Hobson and colleagues[57] proposed the reciprocal interaction model of NREM/REM sleep cycling; increased brainstem cholinergic activity was associated with turning on REM sleep episodes, whereas increased brainstem monoaminergic activity suppressed the pontine REM-on neurons. The REM sleep abnormalities often seen in depressed patients, including reduced REM latency and increased REM density and REM sleep amounts, could therefore be explained by increased cholinergic activity and/or decreased monoaminergic activity. Increased cholinergic activity could also account for suppression of slow wave activity.[58] Most, but not all, antidepressants tend to increase monoaminergic activity and suppress REM sleep, and studies have shown that the ability of a medication to suppress REM sleep may be associated with eventual antidepressant effect.[59]

Alternatively, Papousek's[60] description of the early appearance of REM sleep in depressives was related to a phase advance of the circadian rhythm. REM sleep propensity is tightly linked to the circadian rhythm, and thus a phase advance of the endogenous circadian rhythm could account for reduced latency to REM sleep as well as early morning awakening. However, studies have suggested that mood-disordered patients, including those with major depression as well as bipolar disorder, may show delayed as well as advanced circadian rhythms and even disruptions of circadian rhythms can exacerbate depression. More recent work has shown association of circadian clock gene variants and mood disorders in some but not all studies, but the circadian system could affect mood regulation indirectly through effects on neurotransmitter and neuroendocrine systems[61] (additional coverage of this topic is provided elsewhere in this issue). Furthermore, treatments designed to entrain circadian rhythms, such as light therapy and interpersonal social rhythm therapy, have been effective in treating mood disorders.

Borbély[62] described the 2-process model of sleep regulation in 1982, which remains widely accepted today. Sleep depends on the homeostatic sleep drive (process S) that builds up during wakefulness and the circadian sleep propensity (process C). He then suggested that, in depression, there is a deficiency in process S that explains not only the earlier appearance of REM sleep but also the deficiencies in SWS and total sleep amounts that are often present in depression.[27] Although SWS deficits now seem to be less consistent in depression, there is still some evidence for abnormalities in the homeostatic function of sleep.[29,63]

Depression is also associated with overactivity of the hypothalamic-pituitary-adrenal axis, which may account for depressive symptoms as well as sleep disturbance.[64] Increases in both corticotropin-releasing hormone (CRH) level and glucocorticoid levels can lead to decreased slow wave activity, reduced REM sleep latency and increased REM density.[59] CRH antagonists have been shown to increase SWS and decrease REM density, and CRH antagonists are being developed as potential treatments for a variety of mood-related and anxiety-related disorders.[65]

More recent studies have focused on the role of sleep-related neuroplasticity in depression. Genes related to plasticity show increased expression during waking, and those related to synaptic downscaling are preferentially expressed during sleep, particularly during SWS[66]; the renormalization of synaptic strength and restoration of cellular homeostasis during sleep are necessary for optimal brain function (discussed elsewhere in this issue). Mechanisms involved in brain plasticity are similar to those thought to mediate most of the core features in mood disorders.[67] Antidepressants seem to exert their clinical effects in part by inducing neuroplastic changes, which generally take several weeks to occur.[68] More rapidly acting treatments for depression, including sleep deprivation and ketamine, likely act by increasing synaptic strength and synaptic plasticity more immediately,[69] and the increase in slow wave activity following ketamine infusion or sleep deprivation have been correlated with an antidepressant response.[63,70,71]

SLEEP DISORDERS IN PATIENTS WITH MOOD DISORDERS

Patients with mood disorders may also have increased rates of other primary sleep disorders and vice versa, so it should not be assumed that all sleep complaints in psychiatric patients are related to psychiatric illness. Patients with depression have an increased prevalence of obstructive sleep apnea (OSA), and individuals with apnea have higher rates of depression.[72] Moreover, OSA is a risk factor for developing depression, and in those with apnea, depression contributes to the severity of daytime fatigue. In contrast, treatment of OSA may lead to improvement in depression.[73] There is significant overlap of symptoms between depression and apnea, particularly in the vegetative symptoms of fatigue, cognitive complaints, and lack of motivation, which can make diagnosis of these comorbid conditions challenging.

Epidemiologic studies have found an increased rate of depression in patients with restless legs syndrome.[74] Although some antidepressant medications can exacerbate restless legs, the diagnosis of restless legs often precedes the diagnosis of the psychiatric disorder, suggesting that the association is not primarily mediated by antidepressant therapy.

As described previously, circadian rhythm disturbances of sleep and waking are also more prevalent in patients with mood disorders. Delayed sleep phase has been reported in unipolar and particularly bipolar depression,[75,76] most prominently in adolescents and young adults. Treatments designed to correct circadian misalignment have been shown to improve the course of bipolar disorder[77] (discussed elsewhere in this issue).

Narcoleptics have significantly increased rates of major depression (adjusted odds ratio [AOR] = 2.67) and bipolar disorder (AOR = 4.56),[78] and increased depressive symptoms have been reported in idiopathic hypersomnia.[79] Although a significant minority of patients with depression report hypersomnia, and narcolepsy is a rare disorder, depressed patients with pathologic sleepiness should be screened for central nervous system hypersomnia disorders such as narcolepsy.

Confusional arousal, a parasomnia that involves confusional behavior following an awakening, often accompanied by at least partial amnesia, were found to be associated with a variety of psychiatric disorders, but particularly mood and anxiety disorders, as well as use of antidepressant medications.[80] However, other SWS parasomnias, such as sleepwalking, are not necessarily associated with increased rates of psychiatric disorders. A broader review of primary sleep disorders in psychiatric populations is provided elsewhere in this issue.

EFFECTS OF PSYCHIATRIC DRUGS ON SLEEP

Most medications used in the treatment of depression can have effects on sleep (reviewed in Ref.[81]). Sedating antidepressants, including trazodone, mirtazapine, and tricyclic antidepressants (TCAs) such as amitriptyline are frequently used as sleep-promoting agents in doses that are subtherapeutic for depression. Only doxepin has been approved by the US Food and Drug Administration as a hypnotic, also in a dose that is considerably less than is needed for an antidepressant effect. Mood stabilizers such as lithium carbonate and anticonvulsants, as well as antipsychotic agents used in treating bipolar disorder or in treatment-resistant depression, can also cause sedation. In patients with mood disorders and significant insomnia, these agents may be useful to manage both sleep and mood symptoms.

Many of the newer antidepressants, including selective serotonin reuptake inhibitors (SSRIs), and serotonin-norepinephrine reuptake inhibitors (SNRIs), as well as the older monoamine oxidase inhibitors (MAOIs), tend to cause insomnia. Although their activating effects may be helpful in depressed patients with fatigue or hypersomnia, their use in patients with depression and insomnia may worsen sleep disturbance, leading to the need for addition of hypnotics or sedating antidepressants specifically for sleep.

Antidepressants and mood stabilizers can also lead to changes in sleep architecture. Many antidepressants lead to REM sleep suppression, including TCAs, SSRIs, SNRIs, and MAOIs; they can produce REM sleep rebound and insomnia if discontinued abruptly. In contrast, bupropion does not typically suppress REM sleep and may even lead to increases in REM sleep amounts.[82] Increases in SWS have been reported with trazodone, lithium carbonate, and some antipsychotic drugs.

Primary sleep disorders can also be precipitated or exacerbated by psychiatric medications. Drugs that increase arousal threshold or produce weight gain, as do many antidepressants, antipsychotics, and mood stabilizers, can exacerbate the tendency for OSA. Sleep-related movement disorders such as restless legs and periodic limb movements have been associated with most antidepressants (eg, SSRIs, SNRIs, TCAs, mirtazapine) as well as antipsychotics.[83,84] REM sleep behavior disorder, as well as increased REM sleep without atonia, has also been reported in patients using REM sleep–suppressing antidepressants.[85] SSRIs have also been shown to lead to increased eye movements during NREM sleep, sometime referred to as Prozac eyes; this effect can persist even after discontinuation of medication.[86]

Effects of Treating Sleep on Mood Disorders

Insomnia may be treated with medication and/or cognitive behavior therapy (CBT) for insomnia. CBT is an evidence-based treatment of insomnia[87] that has been shown to be effective in those with insomnia and comorbid psychiatric disorders.[88] CBT for insomnia typically consists of a multicomponent approach including stimulus control, sleep restriction therapy, sleep hygiene practices, and cognitive therapy (for further details see Ref.[89]). Two smaller randomized controlled trials have examined the concurrent treatment of insomnia (ie, randomization to CBT for insomnia or a behavioral control group) and depression (ie, all participants receiving standard antidepressant medication). Both of these studies showed not only greater improvement in insomnia for the group receiving CBT for insomnia but also improvement in depressive symptoms compared with those receiving only antidepressant treatment with a behavioral control group.[90,91] In addition, in an uncontrolled clinical sample of veterans with insomnia receiving CBT for insomnia, results showed that improvement in insomnia was related to a significant decrease in suicidal ideation, even when controlling for change in depressive symptom severity more broadly over the course of treatment.[92]

Several studies examining insomnia treatment with medications such as eszopiclone, zolpidem, and lorazepam all found a reduction in insomnia symptoms.[93–95] Furthermore, the study using eszopiclone in combination with antidepressant treatment showed additional benefit in depressive symptoms compared with subjects receiving antidepressant treatment and a sleep placebo.[93] Thus, specific insomnia treatment is beneficial for insomnia in the context of depression. Moreover, CBT for insomnia seems to be a promising adjunctive therapy in patients with unipolar depression to further depressive treatment response.

Related to the association of mood disorders with circadian rhythm abnormalities, behavioral chronotherapeutic interventions have also been shown to help improve both sleep and the underlying mood disorder; these therapies include sleep deprivation therapy, bright light therapy, and social rhythm therapy. A variety of sleep manipulations, including total and partial sleep deprivation, have been shown to have rapid-onset antidepressant effects, with response rates similar to those seen with antidepressant drug therapy (ie, average response rate of about 60% across diagnostic subgroups; for further details see Ref.[96]). Several patient characteristics have been identified as predictive of better response, including a more pronounced diurnal pattern of mood[97,98] and bipolar disorder.[99]

Although effective initially, one drawback of sleep deprivation therapies is that the initial gains are typically quickly lost after an episode of recovery sleep. However, studies have shown a better ability to sustain the initial mood improvements when combining sleep deprivation therapy with other forms of treatment, including medication and light therapy.[100] However, sleep deprivation therapies have not come into widespread clinical use, likely because of the difficulty in administering them. Furthermore, these findings should not lead clinicians to conclude that the insufficient sleep is generally helpful for patients with depression. Sleep deprivation or restriction therapies should be used with caution in patients with bipolar disorder because they can trigger mania. In patients with severe or treatment-nonresponsive depression, sleep deprivation or the sleep restriction therapy component of CBT for insomnia may be helpful for both sleep and mood.

More common in clinical practice is the use of bright light therapy. Light therapy entails administration of full-spectrum white light at 5000 to 10,000 lux in the morning on awakening. A meta-analysis of randomized controlled trials examining light therapy in the treatment of mood disorders showed that bright light treatment (minimum of 3000 lux daily) led to a significant reduction in depressive symptoms in both individuals with seasonal affective disorder (effect size = 0.85) and nonseasonal depression (effect size = 0.53).[101] More recently the retinal melanopsin receptor has been identified as the mediator of the circadian, alerting, and mood effects of light, with greatest sensitivity to light with a wavelength of 460 to 480 nm (blue light).[102] As a result, new light therapy devices often enrich for light in this wavelength.

Social rhythm therapy (SRT) has shown strong efficacy in patients with bipolar disorder when combined with Klerman and colleagues'[103] interpersonal psychotherapy to form interpersonal and social rhythm therapy (IPSRT).[104] The SRT component of this treatment entails helping individuals to develop more structured schedules across the day, often with key targets, including regular times each day for getting out of bed; having first contact with another person; starting work, school, or volunteer work; having dinner; and going to bed. A 2-year outcome study from a large randomized controlled trial in bipolar patients showed that participants assigned to IPSRT (vs intensive clinical management) had higher regularity of social rhythms by the end of acute treatment and then were recurrence free for longer during the maintenance period.[105] Similarly, a recent randomized controlled study incorporated SRT into CBT for insomnia for patients with interepisode bipolar I disorder and insomnia. Patients randomized to CBT for insomnia/SRT had improved insomnia compared with those randomized to psychoeducation. Moreover, in the 6-month follow-up period, subjects in the active sleep treatment condition had fewer days in an affective episode and lower hypomania/mania recurrence rates compared with the psychoeducation group.[106]

Thus, a variety of sleep therapeutic options have shown efficacy in treating sleep issues in the context of mood disorders. The findings that many of these therapies lead not only to improvement in sleep and rhythmicity but also to improvement in mood underscores the need to consider adding specific sleep-related treatment when approaching treatment of patients with mood disorders.

SUMMARY

Both self-reported and objective sleep disturbances, including insomnia, hypersomnia, changes in sleep architecture, and rest-activity dysregulation, are common in people with mood disorders. In addition, this population often is at greater risk for other primary sleep disorders, such as OSA, restless legs syndrome, and circadian rhythm disorders, and although some psychiatric medications may be beneficial for sleep, others may disrupt sleep. Attending to sleep disturbances in this population is of utmost importance given that sleep disturbances are a risk factor for onset of mood disorders, they often continue as a residual symptom in patients with remitted mood disorders, and they can lead to exacerbation (including greater risk of suicidality) and relapse of mood disorders. However, several effective treatments are available for sleep disturbances comorbid with mood disorders and show promise for treating not only sleep but also improving mood outcomes.

REFERENCES

1. Kessler RC, Aguilar-Gaxiola S, Alonso J, et al. The global burden of mental disorders: an update from the WHO World Mental Health (WMH) surveys. Epidemiol Psichiatr Soc 2009;18(1):23–33.
2. World Health Organization. Preventing suicide: a resource for general physicians. Geneva (Switzerland): World Health Organization; 2000.
3. Kessler RC, Akiskal HS, Ames M, et al. Prevalence and effects of mood disorders on work performance in a nationally representative sample of U.S. workers. Am J Psychiatry 2006;163(9):1561–8.
4. American Psychiatric Association. Diagnostic and statistical manual of mental disorders. 5th edition. Washington, DC: American Psychiatric Association; 2013.
5. Mueller TI, Leon AC, Keller MB, et al. Recurrence after recovery from major depressive disorder during 15 years of observational follow-up. Am J Psychiatry 1999;156(7):1000–6.
6. Blazer DG, Kessler RC, Swartz MS. Epidemiology of recurrent major and minor depression with a seasonal pattern. The National Comorbidity Survey. Br J Psychiatry 1998;172:164–7.
7. Tsuno N, Besset A, Ritchie K. Sleep and depression. J Clin Psychiatry 2005; 66(10):1254–69.
8. Perlis ML, Giles DE, Buysse DJ, et al. Which depressive symptoms are related to which sleep electroencephalographic variables? Biol Psychiatry 1997;42(10): 904–13.
9. Hamilton M. Frequency of symptoms in melancholia (depressive illness). Br J Psychiatry 1989;154:201–6.
10. Yates WR, Mitchell J, Rush AJ, et al. Clinical features of depressed outpatients with and without co-occurring general medical conditions in STAR*D. Gen Hosp Psychiatry 2004;26(6):421–9.
11. Fava M. Daytime sleepiness and insomnia as correlates of depression. J Clin Psychiatry 2004;65(Suppl 16):27–32.
12. Breslau N, Roth T, Rosenthal L, et al. Sleep disturbance and psychiatric disorders: a longitudinal epidemiological study of young adults. Biol Psychiatry 1996;39(6):411–8.
13. Hublin C, Kaprio J, Partinen M, et al. Daytime sleepiness in an adult, Finnish population. J Intern Med 1996;239(5):417–23.
14. Nierenberg AA, Keefe BR, Leslie VC, et al. Residual symptoms in depressed patients who respond acutely to fluoxetine. J Clin Psychiatry 1999;60(4):221–5.
15. Ng TH, Chung KF, Ho FY, et al. Sleep-wake disturbance in interepisode bipolar disorder and high-risk individuals: a systematic review and meta-analysis. Sleep Med Rev 2015;20:46–58.

16. St-Amand J, Provencher MD, Bélanger L, et al. Sleep disturbances in bipolar disorder during remission. J Affect Disord 2013;146(1):1.12–9.
17. Bastien CH, Vallières A, Morin CM. Validation of the Insomnia Severity Index as an outcome measure for insomnia research. Sleep Med 2001;2(4):297–307.
18. Carney CE, Buysse DJ, Ancoli-Israel S, et al. The consensus sleep diary: standardizing prospective sleep self-monitoring. Sleep 2012;35(2):287–302.
19. Johns MW. A new method for measuring daytime sleepiness: the Epworth sleepiness scale. Sleep 1991;14(6):540–5.
20. Benca RM, Obermeyer WH, Thisted RA, et al. Sleep and psychiatric disorders. A meta-analysis. Arch Gen Psychiatry 1992;49(8):651–68 [discussion: 669–70].
21. Borbély AA, Tobler I, Loepfe M, et al. All-night spectral analysis of the sleep EEG in untreated depressives and normal controls. Psychiatry Res 1984;12(1):27–33.
22. Kupfer DJ, Jarrett DB, Frank E. Relationship among selected neuroendocrine and sleep measures in patients with recurrent depression. Biol Psychiatry 1984;19(11):1525–36.
23. Kramer M, Roth T. The mood regulatory function of sleep. In: Koella W, Levin P, editors. Sleep, physiology, biochemistry, psychology, pharmacology. New York: S Karger; 1972. p. 562–71.
24. Cartwright R, Luten A, Young M, et al. Role of REM sleep and dream affect in overnight mood regulation: a study of normal volunteers. Psychiatry Res 1998; 81(1):1–8.
25. Cartright R, Baehr E, Kirkby J, et al. REM sleep reduction, mood regulation and remission in untreated depression. Psychiatry Res 2003;121(2):159–67.
26. Akiskal HS, Judd LL, Gillin JC, et al. Subthreshold depressions: clinical and polysomnographic validation of dysthymic, residual and masked forms. J Affect Disord 1997;45(1–2):53–63.
27. Borbély AA. The S-deficiency hypothesis of depression and the two-process model of sleep regulation. Pharmacopsychiatry 1987;20(1):23–9.
28. Kupfer DJ. Sleep research in depressive illness: clinical implications–a tasting menu. Biol Psychiatry 1995;38(6):391–403.
29. Plante DT, Goldstein MR, Landsness EC, et al. Altered overnight modulation of spontaneous waking EEG reflects altered sleep homeostasis in major depressive disorder: a high-density EEG investigation. J Affect Disord 2013;150(3): 1167–73.
30. Plante DT, Goldstein MR, Landsness EC, et al. Topographic and sex-related differences in sleep spindles in major depressive disorder: a high-density EEG investigation. J Affect Disord 2013;146(1):120–5.
31. Jindal RD, Thase ME, Fasiczka AL, et al. Electroencephalographic sleep profiles in single-episode and recurrent unipolar forms of major depression: II. Comparison during remission. Biol Psychiatry 2002;51(3):230–6.
32. Nissen C, Feige B, König A, et al. Delta sleep ratio as a predictor of sleep deprivation response in major depression. J Psychiatr Res 2001;35(3):155–63.
33. Armitage R, Hoffmann R, Fitch T, et al. Temporal characteristics of delta activity during NREM sleep in depressed outpatients and healthy adults: group and sex effects. Sleep 2000;23(5):607–17.
34. Lopez J, Hoffmann R, Emslie G, et al. Sex differences in slow-wave electroencephalographic activity (SWA) in adolescent depression. Ment Illn 2012; 4(1):e4.
35. Plante DT, Landsness EC, Peterson MJ, et al. Sex-related differences in sleep slow wave activity in major depressive disorder: a high-density EEG investigation. BMC Psychiatry 2012;12:146.

36. Palagini L, Baglioni C, Ciapparelli A, et al. REM sleep dysregulation in depression: state of the art. Sleep Med Rev 2013;17(5):377–90.
37. Hudson JI, Lipinski JF, Keck PE, et al. Polysomnographic characteristics of young manic patients. Comparison with unipolar depressed patients and normal control subjects. Arch Gen Psychiatry 1992;49(5):378–83.
38. Mehl RC, O'Brien LM, Jones JH, et al. Correlates of sleep and pediatric bipolar disorder. Sleep 2006;29(2):193–7.
39. Mohawk JA, Green CB, Takahashi JS. Central and peripheral circadian clocks in mammals. Annu Rev Neurosci 2012;35:445–62.
40. Crasson M, Kjiri S, Colin A, et al. Serum melatonin and urinary 6-sulfatoxymelatonin in major depression. Psychoneuroendocrinology 2004;29(1):1–12.
41. Kennedy SH, Kutcher SP, Ralevski E, et al. Nocturnal melatonin and 24-hour 6-sulphatoxymelatonin levels in various phases of bipolar affective disorder. Psychiatry Res 1996;63(2–3):219–22.
42. Burton C, McKinstry B, Szentagotai Tătar A, et al. Activity monitoring in patients with depression: a systematic review. J Affect Disord 2013;145(1):21–8.
43. Geoffroy PA, Scott J, Boudebesse C, et al. Sleep in patients with remitted bipolar disorders: a meta-analysis of actigraphy studies. Acta Psychiatr Scand 2015; 131(2):89–99.
44. Monk TH, Kupfer DJ, Frank E, et al. The Social Rhythm Metric (SRM): measuring daily social rhythms over 12 weeks. Psychiatry Res 1991;36(2):195–207.
45. Monk TH, Frank E, Potts JM, et al. A simple way to measure daily lifestyle regularity. J Sleep Res 2002;11(3):183–90.
46. Ashman SB, Monk TH, Kupfer DJ, et al. Relationship between social rhythms and mood in patients with rapid cycling bipolar disorder. Psychiatry Res 1999;86(1):1–8.
47. Rosa AR, Comes M, Torrent C, et al. Biological rhythm disturbance in remitted bipolar patients. Int J Bipolar Disord 2013;1:6.
48. Baglioni C, Battagliese G, Feige B, et al. Insomnia as a predictor of depression: a meta-analytic evaluation of longitudinal epidemiological studies. J Affect Disord 2011;135(1–3):10–9.
49. Szklo-Coxe M, Young T, Peppard PE, et al. Prospective associations of insomnia markers and symptoms with depression. Am J Epidemiol 2010; 171(6):709–20.
50. Jaussent I, Bouyer J, Ancelin ML, et al. Insomnia and daytime sleepiness are risk factors for depressive symptoms in the elderly. Sleep 2011;34(8):1103–10.
51. Hasler G, Buysse DJ, Gamma A, et al. Excessive daytime sleepiness in young adults: a 20-year prospective community study. J Clin Psychiatry 2005;66(4): 521–9.
52. Malik S, Kanwar A, Sim LA, et al. The association between sleep disturbances and suicidal behaviors in patients with psychiatric diagnoses: a systematic review and meta-analysis. Syst Rev 2014;3:18.
53. Shen GH, Alloy LB, Abramson LY, et al. Social rhythm regularity and the onset of affective episodes in bipolar spectrum individuals. Bipolar Disord 2008; 10(4):520–9.
54. Nierenberg AA, Husain MM, Trivedi MH, et al. Residual symptoms after remission of major depressive disorder with citalopram and risk of relapse: a STAR*D report. Psychol Med 2010;40(1):41–50.
55. Conradi HJ, Ormel J, de Jonge P. Presence of individual (residual) symptoms during depressive episodes and periods of remission: a 3-year prospective study. Psychol Med 2011;41(6):1165–74.

56. Janowsky DS, el-Yousef MK, Davis JM, et al. A cholinergic-adrenergic hypothesis of mania and depression. Lancet 1972;2(7778):632–5.
57. Hobson JA, McCarley RW, Wyzinski PW. Sleep cycle oscillation: reciprocal discharge by two brainstem neuronal groups. Science 1975;189(4196):55–8.
58. Steriade M, Dossi RC, Nuñez A. Network modulation of a slow intrinsic oscillation of cat thalamocortical neurons implicated in sleep delta waves: cortically induced synchronization and brainstem cholinergic suppression. J Neurosci 1991;11(10):3200–17.
59. Steiger A. Neurochemical regulation of sleep. J Psychiatr Res 2007;41(7): 537–52.
60. Papousek M. Chronobiological aspects of cyclothymia (author's transl). Fortschr Neurol Psychiatr Grenzgeb 1975;43(8):381–440 [in German].
61. McClung CA. How might circadian rhythms control mood? Let me count the ways. Biol Psychiatry 2013;74(4):242–9.
62. Borbély AA. A two process model of sleep regulation. Hum Neurobiol 1982;1(3): 195–204.
63. Landsness EC, Goldstein MR, Peterson MJ, et al. Antidepressant effects of selective slow wave sleep deprivation in major depression: a high-density EEG investigation. J Psychiatr Res 2011;45(8):1019–26.
64. Gold PW. The organization of the stress system and its dysregulation in depressive illness. Mol Psychiatry 2015;20(1):32–47.
65. Zorrilla EP, Logrip ML, Koob GF. Corticotropin releasing factor: a key role in the neurobiology of addiction. Front Neuroendocrinol 2014;35(2):234–44.
66. Tononi G, Cirelli C. Sleep and the price of plasticity: from synaptic and cellular homeostasis to memory consolidation and integration. Neuron 2014;81(1): 12–34.
67. Pittenger C. Disorders of memory and plasticity in psychiatric disease. Dialogues Clin Neurosci 2013;15(4):455–63.
68. Krishnan V, Nestler EJ. The molecular neurobiology of depression. Nature 2008; 455(7215):894–902.
69. Zarate CA, Mathews DC, Furey ML. Human biomarkers of rapid antidepressant effects. Biol Psychiatry 2013;73(12):1142–55.
70. Duncan WC, Zarate CA. Ketamine, sleep, and depression: current status and new questions. Curr Psychiatry Rep 2013;15(9):394.
71. Duncan WC, Gillin JC, Post RM, et al. Relationship between EEG sleep patterns and clinical improvement in depressed patients treated with sleep deprivation. Biol Psychiatry 1980;15(6):879–89.
72. Peppard PE, Szklo-Coxe M, Hla KM, et al. Longitudinal association of sleep-related breathing disorder and depression. Arch Intern Med 2006;166(16): 1709–15.
73. Povitz M, Bolo CE, Heitman SJ, et al. Effect of treatment of obstructive sleep apnea on depressive symptoms: systematic review and meta-analysis. PLoS Med 2014;11(11):e1001762.
74. Becker PM, Sharon D. Mood disorders in restless legs syndrome (Willis-Ekbom disease). J Clin Psychiatry 2014;75(7):e679–94.
75. Robillard R, Naismith SL, Rogers NL, et al. Delayed sleep phase in young people with unipolar or bipolar affective disorders. J Affect Disord 2013; 145(2):260–3.
76. Robillard R, Naismith SL, Smith KL, et al. Sleep-wake cycle in young and older persons with a lifetime history of mood disorders. PLoS One 2014; 9(2):e87763.

77. Frank E. Interpersonal and social rhythm therapy: a means of improving depression and preventing relapse in bipolar disorder. J Clin Psychol 2007;63(5):463–73.
78. Ohayon MM. Narcolepsy is complicated by high medical and psychiatric comorbidities: a comparison with the general population. Sleep Med 2013; 14(6):488–92.
79. Dauvilliers Y, Lopez R, Ohayon M, et al. Hypersomnia and depressive symptoms: methodological and clinical aspects. BMC Med 2013;11:78.
80. Ohayon MM, Mahowald MW, Leger D. Are confusional arousals pathological? Neurology 2014;83(9):834–41.
81. DeMartinis NA, Winokur A. Effects of psychiatric medications on sleep and sleep disorders. CNS Neurol Disord Drug Targets 2007;6(1):17–29.
82. Nofzinger EA, Reynolds CF, Thase ME, et al. REM sleep enhancement by bupropion in depressed men. Am J Psychiatry 1995;152(2):274–6.
83. Hoque R, Chesson AL. Pharmacologically induced/exacerbated restless legs syndrome, periodic limb movements of sleep, and REM behavior disorder/REM sleep without atonia: literature review, qualitative scoring, and comparative analysis. J Clin Sleep Med 2010;6(1):79–83.
84. Fulda S, Kloiber S, Dose T, et al. Mirtazapine provokes periodic leg movements during sleep in young healthy men. Sleep 2013;36(5):661–9.
85. McCarter SJ, St Louis EK, Sandness DJ, et al. Antidepressants increase REM sleep muscle tone in patients with and without REM sleep behavior disorder. Sleep 2015;38(6):907–17.
86. Geyer JD, Carney PR, Dillard SC, et al. Antidepressant medications, neuroleptics, and prominent eye movements during NREM sleep. J Clin Neurophysiol 2009;26(1):39–44.
87. Smith MT, Perlis ML, Park A, et al. Comparative meta-analysis of pharmacotherapy and behavior therapy for persistent insomnia. Am J Psychiatry 2002; 159(1):5–11.
88. Taylor DJ, Pruiksma KE. Cognitive and behavioural therapy for insomnia (CBT-I) in psychiatric populations: a systematic review. Int Rev Psychiatry 2014;26(2): 205–13.
89. Edinger JD, Means MK. Cognitive-behavioral therapy for primary insomnia. Clin Psychol Rev 2005;25(5):539–58.
90. Manber R, Edinger JD, Gress JL, et al. Cognitive behavioral therapy for insomnia enhances depression outcome in patients with comorbid major depressive disorder and insomnia. Sleep 2008;31(4):489–95.
91. Ashworth DK, Sletten TL, Junge M, et al. A randomized controlled trial of cognitive behavioral therapy for insomnia: an effective treatment for comorbid insomnia and depression. J Couns Psychol 2015;62(2):115–23.
92. Trockel M, Karlin BE, Taylor CB, et al. Effects of cognitive behavioral therapy for insomnia on suicidal ideation in veterans. Sleep 2015;38(2):259–65.
93. Krystal A, Fava M, Rubens R, et al. Evaluation of eszopiclone discontinuation after cotherapy with fluoxetine for insomnia with coexisting depression. J Clin Sleep Med 2007;3(1):48–55.
94. Fava M, Shelton RC, Zajecka JM. Evidence for the use of l-methylfolate combined with antidepressants in MDD. J Clin Psychiatry 2011;72(8):e25.
95. Buysse DJ, Reynolds CF, Houck PR, et al. Does lorazepam impair the antidepressant response to nortriptyline and psychotherapy? J Clin Psychiatry 1997; 58(10):426–32.
96. Dallaspezia S, Benedetti F. Sleep deprivation therapy for depression. Curr Top Behav Neurosci 2015;25:483–502.

97. Martiny K, Refsgaard E, Lund V, et al. The day-to-day acute effect of wake therapy in patients with major depression using the HAM-D6 as primary outcome measure: results from a randomised controlled trial. PLoS One 2013; 8(6):e67264.
98. Reinink E, Bouhuys N, Wirz-Justice A, et al. Prediction of the antidepressant response to total sleep deprivation by diurnal variation of mood. Psychiatry Res 1990;32(2):113–24.
99. Barbini B, Colombo C, Benedetti F, et al. The unipolar-bipolar dichotomy and the response to sleep deprivation. Psychiatry Res 1998;79(1):43–50.
100. Colombo C, Lucca A, Benedetti F, et al. Total sleep deprivation combined with lithium and light therapy in the treatment of bipolar depression: replication of main effects and interaction. Psychiatry Res 2000;95(1):43–53.
101. Golden RN, Gaynes BN, Ekstrom RD, et al. The efficacy of light therapy in the treatment of mood disorders: a review and meta-analysis of the evidence. Am J Psychiatry 2005;162(4):656–62.
102. Hughes S, Hankins MW, Foster RG, et al. Melanopsin phototransduction: slowly emerging from the dark. Prog Brain Res 2012;199:19–40.
103. Klerman G, Weissman M, Rounsaville B, et al. Interpersonal psychotherapy of depression. New York: Basic Books; 1998.
104. Frank E, Swartz HA, Boland E. Interpersonal and social rhythm therapy: an intervention addressing rhythm dysregulation in bipolar disorder. Dialogues Clin Neurosci 2007;9(3):325–32.
105. Frank E, Kupfer DJ, Thase ME, et al. Two-year outcomes for interpersonal and social rhythm therapy in individuals with bipolar I disorder. Arch Gen Psychiatry 2005;62(9):996–1004.
106. Harvey AG, Soehner AM, Kaplan KA, et al. Treating insomnia improves mood state, sleep, and functioning in bipolar disorder: a pilot randomized controlled trial. J Consult Clin Psychol 2015;83(3):564–77.

Recent Advances in the Study of Sleep in the Anxiety Disorders, Obsessive-Compulsive Disorder, and Posttraumatic Stress Disorder

CrossMark

Elaine M. Boland, PhD[a,b,*], Richard J. Ross, MD, PhD[b,c]

KEYWORDS

- Sleep • Anxiety • Generalized anxiety disorder • Obsessive-compulsive disorder
- Posttraumatic stress disorder • Circadian rhythms

KEY POINTS

The information provided in this review is designed to help mental health professionals and researchers understand the following:

- The prevalence of sleep disturbance in anxiety disorders, obsessive-compulsive disorder (OCD), and posttraumatic stress disorder (PTSD).
- Advances in identifying the mechanisms of sleep disturbance in anxiety disorders, OCD, and PTSD.
- The burgeoning research in circadian rhythms in anxiety disorders, OCD, and PTSD and its potential role in treatment advancement.
- The importance of dimensional measurement of cognitive processes related to sleep disturbance across diagnostic boundaries.
- Recent advances in psychotherapeutic and pharmacologic treatments for sleep disturbance in anxiety disorders, OCD, and PTSD.

Funding Sources: Dr E.M. Boland: Office of Academic Affiliations, Advanced Fellowship Program in Mental Illness Research and Treatment, Department of Veterans Affairs. Dr R.J. Ross: Department of Defense.

Conflict of Interest: None.

[a] Behavioral Health, Mental Illness Research Education and Clinical Center, Corporal Michael J. Crescenz Veterans Affairs Medical Center, 3900 Woodland Avenue, Philadelphia, PA 19104, USA; [b] Department of Psychiatry, Perelman School of Medicine, University of Pennsylvania, 423 Guardian Drive, Philadelphia, PA 19104, USA; [c] Corporal Michael J. Crescenz Veterans Affairs Medical Center, 3900 Woodland Avenue, Philadelphia, PA 19104, USA
* Corresponding author. Corporal Michael J. Crescenz Veterans Affairs Medical Center, Mental Illness Research Education and Clinical Center, 3900 Woodland Avenue, Philadelphia, PA 19104.
E-mail addresses: elaine.boland@va.gov; bolande@mail.med.upenn.edu

Psychiatr Clin N Am 38 (2015) 761–776
http://dx.doi.org/10.1016/j.psc.2015.07.005
0193-953X/15/$ – see front matter Published by Elsevier Inc.

psych.theclinics.com

Abbreviations	
CAPS	Clinician Administered PTSD Scale
CBT	Cognitive behavioral therapy
CBT-I	Cognitive behavioral therapy for insomnia
CPT	Cognitive processing therapy
DSM-IV/5	*Diagnostic and Statistical Manual of Mental Disorders, Fourth/Fifth Edition*
ERP	Exposure and response prevention therapy
fMRI	Functional MRI
GAD	Generalized anxiety disorder
IR	Imagery rehearsal
MAOI	Monoamine oxidase inhibitors
N2	Stage 2 sleep
NP	Nocturnal panic
OCD	Obsessive-compulsive disorder
OSA	Obstructive sleep apnea
PD	Panic disorder
PE	Prolonged exposure
PLM	Periodic limb movements
PSG	Polysomnography
PTSD	Posttraumatic stress disorder
P-wave	Pontine wave
RBD	REM behavior disorder
RCT	Randomized controlled trial
REMS	Rapid eye movement sleep
SNP	Single nucleotide polymorphism
SNRI	Serotonin and norepinephrine reuptake inhibitor
SSRI	Selective serotonin reuptake inhibitor
SWS	Slow wave sleep
TCA	Tricyclic antidepressants

Anxiety disorders are highly comorbid with sleep disorders. In fact, for disorders such as generalized anxiety disorder (GAD), the core diagnostic criteria may include sleep disturbance. High rates of co-occurrence and diagnostic overlap are suggestive of common diatheses among anxiety and sleep disorders. There is a considerable literature documenting sleep disturbances in anxiety disorders (see Refs.[1,2] for comprehensive reviews). However, important advances at the interface of sleep and anxiety disorders research have occurred in the past decade, yielding new insights into the etiology and treatment of sleep disturbances in the anxiety disorders. Here, we review and discuss these advances to bring attention to the development of new themes in sleep research in the context of anxiety.

A major advance in psychiatric research is the advent of the Research Domain Criteria,[3] which encourage the dimensional examination of behavior to better inform the diagnosis and treatment of mental disorders. In this review, we pay specific attention to ways in which several biological and psychological processes that are not unique to anxiety disorders may be implicated in the relationship between anxiety and sleep disturbance. As an example, we review the burgeoning literature on circadian rhythm disturbances in these disorders and discuss the implications of new findings for the development of novel treatments.

Another significant advance is the recategorization of mental disorders in the fifth edition of the *Diagnostic and Statistical Manual of Mental Disorders* (DSM-5).[4] Obsessive-compulsive disorder (OCD) and posttraumatic stress disorder (PTSD) are no longer included among the anxiety disorders, but rather are categories of obsessive-compulsive and related disorders and trauma-related and stressor-related disorders, respectively. For the purpose of highlighting commonalities in the sleep disturbances of the anxiety disorders as defined by the DSM-IV, including OCD and PTSD, and for maintaining continuity with previous reviews, we include a discussion of the latter 2 disorders here.

GENERALIZED ANXIETY DISORDER

GAD, characterized by excessive, persistent, and unrealistic worry, affects approximately 3.1% of adults in the United States.[5] Fifty percent to 70% of patients with GAD report insomnia, which can manifest as initial-onset insomnia, sleep continuity disturbance, or early morning awakening. Sleep disturbances in GAD have been shown to persist despite remission of waking anxiety symptoms.[6] This is consistent with a view of insomnia as an independent disorder that can be comorbid with other mental disorders.[7]

Sleep Architecture in Generalized Anxiety Disorder

Polysomnographic (PSG) studies of GAD have been well reviewed elsewhere.[1,2] These typically demonstrate significantly longer sleep onset latency, decreased sleep time, and reduced stage 2 sleep (N2) in patients with GAD compared with healthy individuals. A longer rapid eye movement sleep (REMS) latency recently has been observed in nonmedicated, nondepressed children diagnosed with GAD relative to age- and gender-matched children free of psychiatric or sleep disorders.[8] To date, there are no PSG studies comparing patients with GAD and patients with insomnia disorder, although, given the overlap of symptoms, this may be an important direction for future research.

Dimensions of Psychological Contributions to Sleep Disturbance in Generalized Anxiety Disorder

The cardinal feature of GAD is excessive cognitive activity, predominantly future-oriented worry and the tendency to think repetitively about causes, contexts, and consequences of negative experiences, referred to as rumination.[9] These forms of cognition also have been shown to be relevant to the sleep disturbances in other disorders, including depression, and to sleep difficulties among individuals without mental health diagnoses. An examination of these processes as they pertain to sleep disturbance broadly may aid in the development of more targeted interventions for the sleep disturbance in GAD. For example, in a sample of individuals without a GAD diagnosis, those who were characterized as "worriers" evidenced increased sleep disturbance compared with nonworriers.[10] Similarly, "worry about the future" was a significant contributor to sleep disturbance among college students who were not diagnosed with GAD.[11] Rumination also has been associated with sleep disturbance. A longitudinal study of a nonclinical sample found that rumination at baseline predicted a reduction in sleep quality at follow-up, and rumination, specifically, was associated with poorer sleep quality among individuals who expressed high levels of worry.[12] Future research on the sleep disturbance in GAD may benefit from a focus on the distinct effects of rumination and worry.

There is some evidence that emotional dysregulation, also referred to as mood lability or difficulty modulating emotional responses, may play an important role in the relationship between sleep disturbance and anxiety in GAD. One study demonstrated that, relative to healthy controls, individuals with GAD experienced greater sleep discontinuity, daytime sleepiness, difficulty waking in the morning, daytime dysfunction, and nightmare frequency; and that poor emotion regulation fully mediated the relationship between GAD diagnosis and most of these parameters, most notably daytime dysfunction.[13]

Circadian Rhythms in Generalized Anxiety Disorder

Circadian rhythm abnormalities have long been identified as key mechanisms in mood disorders, with important treatment implications.[14] Similarly, examination of the role of circadian rhythms in GAD may provide new avenues for treating the sleep disturbance in GAD. Sipilä and colleagues[15] examined 12 circadian clock-related genes in individuals with anxiety disorders compared with healthy controls and found evidence of an association of two single nucleotide polymorphisms (SNP) with GAD specifically; two additional SNP were associated with a group of anxiety disorders that included GAD. This finding suggests that there is a genetic predisposition to GAD that implicates circadian processes. Consistent with this view, GAD also has been associated with a diminished circadian rhythm of blood pressure among patients with hypertension.[16] The hypothesis that individuals with GAD have a genetic predisposition to circadian rhythm abnormalities and may be more susceptible to sleep disturbance, including the development of comorbid insomnia disorder, warrants empirical validation. Future research on the role of circadian rhythm disruption in GAD may be important to advancing treatment for disturbed sleep in GAD.

Treatment of Generalized Anxiety Disorder Sleep Disturbances: Psychotherapy

There is some evidence that the treatment of GAD can ameliorate insomnia in affected individuals. Individual and group cognitive behavioral therapy (CBT) for GAD, not specifically targeting sleep disturbance, has been shown to significantly reduce insomnia symptoms.[17,18]

To the best of our knowledge, CBT for insomnia (CBT-I) has not been studied in patients with GAD, although some studies of the efficacy of CBT-I have included in their samples a small proportion of participants with concomitant psychiatric diagnoses including GAD.[19] It has been suggested that sleep restriction, a core component of CBT-I, would be poorly tolerated by highly anxious patients, as it might increase anxiety about not getting enough sleep, which could further reduce sleep time.[20] Similarly, although some stimulus control strategies promoted by CBT-I may be beneficial for patients with GAD (eg, scheduling a worry time, getting out of bed when unable to control anxious thoughts), others may lead to worry about adhering to a strict sleep/wake schedule.[20] Future research could identify predictors of positive response to CBT-I among individuals with GAD. Additionally, the development of a treatment protocol that incorporates elements of CBT-I into the concurrent treatment of anxiety symptoms could be highly beneficial in GAD with a significant insomnia component.

Treatment of Generalized Anxiety Disorder Sleep Disturbances: Pharmacotherapy

Several medications have been shown to be effective in treating the sleep disturbance characteristic of GAD. The addition of eszopiclone, a nonbenzodiazepine drug that acts as an agonist at the benzodiazepine receptor, to the selective serotonin reuptake inhibitor (SSRI) escitalopram significantly improved sleep and daytime function, and decreased anxiety, in a placebo-controlled study in patients with GAD.[21] Treatment with pregabalin, approved as an anticonvulsant and for neuropathic pain, was well tolerated and associated with significant reductions in insomnia and daytime anxiety among individuals with GAD.[22] The melatonin receptor agonist ramelteon was associated with reduced sleep-onset latency and increased sleep time, as well as improvement in other, non–sleep-related GAD symptoms, in a community sample of adults with GAD.[23] Agomelatine, a melatonin agonist and serotonergic antagonist, was effective in reducing insomnia and daytime symptoms in individuals with GAD.[24] Given the importance of melatonin in circadian rhythm regulation, this finding provides additional evidence that a disruption of the sleep/wake cycle may be central to the pathogenesis of GAD.

PANIC DISORDER

Panic disorder (PD), characterized by sudden, recurrent panic attacks, occurs in approximately 5% of the US population.[5] Sleep architecture in PD has been reviewed elsewhere,[1,2] with mixed findings that range from a minimal reduction in sleep time and slow wave sleep (SWS) to a substantial increase in sleep-onset latency. The core feature of sleep disturbance in PD, however, is nocturnal panic attacks (NP). These occur in 44% to 71% of individuals with PD[25]; they have been found to emerge from the transition between N2 and SWS.[26] NP, abrupt awakenings from sleep in a state of panic, usually accompanied by subjective fear and discomfort and physiologic symptoms, including racing heart, shortness of breath, and chest tightness, are a major cause of insomnia in PD. This sleep disruption can result from the attacks themselves, from cognitive distortions about sleep, or from a conditioned fear of sleeping.

Correlates of Sleep Disturbance in Panic Disorder

Recent studies have uncovered other factors associated with sleep disturbance in PD in addition to NP. In one study, anxiety sensitivity, defined as the belief that anxiety-related sensations are harmful and cause for fear, was associated with increased sleep latency in patients with PD.[27] Such sensitivity may relate to difficulties with cognitive inhibition, that is, the ability to "tune out" irrelevant stimuli, and there is some evidence that poor cognitive inhibition may lead to sleep disturbances in PD. A recent study in patients with PD measured cognitive inhibition using the inhibition condition of the Stroop task. In this task, color names are printed in differently colored ink (eg, the word "blue" printed in red ink), and participants are required to say the name of the ink color, inhibiting the natural response, which is to read the color word. In this study, difficulties with cognitive inhibition were associated with increased sleep latency and reduced sleep quality.[28] Impaired cognitive inhibition may be related to the inability of patients with PD to ignore the internal physiologic sensations from which panic attacks evolve.

Treatment of Panic Disorder Sleep Disturbances

An adaptation of CBT designed for NP was found to be more effective than a waitlist control, with efficacy persisting over a 9-month follow-up period.[29] However, a more recent study comparing this adapted CBT protocol with traditional CBT for PD found that both were associated with significant reductions in NP that lasted through a 1-year follow-up period.[30] Generalizability of these findings is limited by small sample sizes and lack of randomization. Randomized controlled trials (RCT) comparing CBT adapted for NP and standard CBT for PD are warranted. Given research demonstrating an association between increased anxiety sensitivity and increased sleep-onset latency, pharmacotherapy addressing anxiety sensitivity may be helpful in individuals with PD and insomnia, sleep-onset insomnia in particular. For example, paroxetine and clonazepam have been shown to decrease anxiety sensitivity in patients with PD and could, via this mechanism, improve insomnia symptoms.[31]

OBSESSIVE-COMPULSIVE DISORDER

OCD is characterized by intrusive, unwanted, repeated, and uncontrollable thoughts, feelings, impulses, or images, and repetitive behaviors that are aimed at reducing the associated anxiety. Sleep disturbance in OCD is often characterized by increased sleep-onset latency, reduced overall sleep duration, and reduced sleep efficiency.[32] Greater severity of OCD symptoms has been associated with more severe sleep disturbance.[32]

The Specific Effect of Obsessional Thinking on Sleep

Recent research suggests that obsessions, rather than compulsions, may play a larger role in generating the insomnia often observed in OCD. For example, Timpano and colleagues[33] found that insomnia was significantly associated with obsessions but not with compulsions; depression, which frequently is comorbid with OCD, did not explain the relationship between OCD and disturbed sleep. This finding is particularly compelling in the context of the previously reviewed research on worry and rumination in GAD, both of which have been associated with increased sleep disturbance (see Dimensions of Psychological Contributions to Sleep Disturbance in Generalized Anxiety Disorder, earlier in this article). Taken together, there is evidence of an association between sleep disturbance and aspects of what could be termed "cognitive interference." Future research on this dimension of cognition across psychiatric disorders could be highly useful for treatment development.

Circadian Rhythms in Obsessive-Compulsive Disorder

There is evidence that circadian rhythms influence vulnerability to, and presentation of, OCD. For example, a growing literature supports the importance of delayed sleep phase in OCD.[32] One study of inpatients with OCD revealed that 17.6% met criteria for delayed sleep phase,[34] compared with a rate of 0.17% to 8.9% (depending on the exact definition) in the general population.[35] A recent meta-analysis of sleep and circadian rhythms in OCD reported a higher overall prevalence of delayed sleep phase in patients with OCD than in controls, a finding that was not affected by the exclusion of individuals with comorbid depression.[36] Therefore, circadian rhythm disruption appears to be a salient feature of OCD that cannot be explained completely by comorbid depression, in which circadian dysregulation is well documented.

Sleep Architecture in Obsessive-Compulsive Disorder

Sleep architecture in OCD has been thoroughly reviewed elsewhere,[1,2] with variable results. Some studies reveal increased sleep discontinuity and reduced REMS latency, whereas others report little abnormality. Thus far, PSG studies have been unable to parse the differential effects on sleep of OCD and comorbid depression. In one study, nondepressed patients with OCD, relative to healthy controls, demonstrated a moderate disturbance in sleep continuity but no abnormalities of SWS or REMS timing or amount, which have been described in depression.[37] However, another controlled study of a similar sample reported only a reduction in stage 4 sleep, which is often seen in depression.[38] Given these conflicting results and the relatively small number of studies of sleep architecture in OCD, future research is needed to understand the sleep disturbances that are intrinsic to OCD and to distinguish these from others associated with comorbid depression.

Treatment of Sleep Disturbances in Obsessive-Compulsive Disorder

SSRIs and serotonin and norepinephrine reuptake inhibitors (SNRI) are frequently prescribed for the treatment of OCD; however, many of these drugs may have deleterious effects on sleep.[39] Given the relationship between obsessional thinking and sleep quality, CBT for OCD may have positive effects on sleep as well as waking symptoms. Exposure and response prevention therapy (ERP) is an empirically supported treatment for OCD.[40] Future studies should address whether targeting obsessional thinking via ERP improves sleep in individuals with OCD.

POSTTRAUMATIC STRESS DISORDER

The vast majority of individuals with PTSD report the two sleep disturbances included in the DSM-5 classification of the disorder: recurrent nightmares as a form of reexperiencing the traumatic event and insomnia. Insomnia is a symptom of many mental disorders, but recurrent nightmares of a traumatic experience are quite specific to PTSD, perhaps pathognomonic.[41] We review here recent developments in our understanding of the phenomenology and pathophysiology of PTSD sleep disturbances and current strategies to treat these frequently disabling sleep problems.

An increased prevalence of obstructive sleep apnea (OSA) in PTSD was not confirmed in one controlled study; however, there was evidence that OSA could increase PTSD severity.[42] The investigators recommended further research on the implications of these findings for treating PTSD comorbid with OSA. This topic will not be discussed further here.

Tonic Rapid Eye Movement Sleep Alterations in Posttraumatic Stress Disorder: the Importance of Time Posttrauma

There is considerable evidence for fundamental REMS alterations in PTSD. In one study, REMS fragmentation in the early aftermath of trauma predicted the development of PTSD.[43] Fragmented, preserved, and enhanced REMS continuity following trauma all have been described.[44,45] Mellman and colleagues[45] have helped to reconcile these seemingly discrepant observations by noting the importance of the time elapsed posttrauma as a moderating variable. In a nonclinical community sample of young adults, they found that both REMS percentage (REMS time/total sleep time) and REMS segment length increased with PTSD duration, as assessed retrospectively. They suggested that increases in REMS amount and REMS continuity over time could reflect successful adaptation to a stressor, a hypothesis that they viewed as broadly consistent with a current view that REMS is essential to the successful processing of emotional memories.[46] An equally compelling hypothesis is that the reconstituted REMS observed long after a traumatic experience may be the outcome of maladjustment to a stressor and the neurobiological substrate of the recurrent nightmares that severely disrupt sleep in PTSD.[44]

Phasic Rapid Eye Movement Sleep Alterations in Posttraumatic Stress Disorder: Basic and Clinical Studies

A comprehensive description of REMS architecture in PTSD should include phasic as well as tonic REMS measures, the latter indicating REMS amount and REMS continuity versus fragmentation.[44] Phasic REMS processes are transient brain macropotentials and peripheral physiologic events, with rapid eye movements the best studied phasic event in humans. In their meta-analysis of 20 PSG studies of PTSD, Kobayashi and colleagues[47] found an increased REM density (number of rapid eye movements/REMS time). The significance of this finding may best be understood in the context of the animal literature on the role of REMS phasic mechanisms in the processing of fearful stimuli.

In the rat, the pontine wave (P-wave), recorded in the pons, is the prototypical REMS phasic event. Datta[48] observed that P-wave density increased following 2-way active avoidance training in rats and hypothesized that P-wave generation is essential for effective REMS-dependent memory processing. Ross[44] suggested that severe psychological stress initiates a phasic REMS response that either facilitates successful emotional adaptation or, alternatively, lays the groundwork for the development of PTSD. Based on a study of fear conditioning in two rat strains with different levels of stress sensitivity, DaSilva et al[49] proposed that the inability to mount a strong phasic REMS response following exposure to a severe stressor could lead eventually to the increase in phasic activity that characterizes sleep in chronic PTSD.

The behavioral response threshold in healthy individuals has been reported to be elevated during phasic compared with tonic REMS.[50] Elevated REMS phasic activity in PTSD could explain the increased arousal threshold during REMS that has been observed in patients compared with controls.[51]

Neurocircuitry of Rapid Eye Movement Sleep Alterations in Posttraumatic Stress Disorder

Although the neurocircuitry responsible for REMS changes in PTSD remains to be fully elucidated, there is much evidence for the involvement of the limbic system, and more specifically, the amygdala. This structure plays an essential role in emotion and in the regulation of arousal states.[52] Amygdalar activation during REMS has been observed in healthy humans.[52]

Schwartz and Maquet[53] proposed that, using functional neuroimaging (fMRI) techniques, there could be demonstrated a relationship of "common fear experience in dreams to the activation of the limbic system, in particular the amygdala." As a disorder characterized by recurrent nightmares, PTSD deserves to be studied with complementary fMRI and dream content analysis methods. Increased activation of the amygdala has been demonstrated during waking in some studies of PTSD.[54] It can be predicted that the investigation of amygdalar function across the sleep-wake cycle will provide important insights into the brain mechanisms of the PTSD sleep disturbance. As an example, using [18-F]-flurodeoxyglucose PET neuroimaging, Germain and colleagues[55] observed hypermetabolism in "brain regions involved in arousal regulation, fear responses, and reward processing" during REMS as well as waking in Operations Enduring Freedom and Iraqi Freedom veterans with PTSD compared with controls.

Circadian Rhythm Abnormalities in Posttraumatic Stress Disorder

Hasler and colleagues[56] observed that self-reported evening chronotype (referring to the propensity for an individual to sleep later in the 24-hour period) in combat-exposed military veterans with a varying level of posttraumatic stress symptoms was associated with greater sleep disturbance and lifetime posttraumatic stress severity. Nielsen[57] reviewed the evidence that PTSD is characterized by "an apparent phase advance in dreaming such that vivid nightmares, which usually occur in late REM sleep, occur in PTSD patients also early in the sleep episode...." This raises the question of whether individuals with PTSD may purposefully delay their sleep onset to avoid sleeping when nightmares are most distressing. However, van Liempt and colleagues[42] measured mean melatonin onset time and found no evidence of a phase advance in small samples of subjects with PTSD compared with controls.

Sleep Movement Disturbances in Posttraumatic Stress Disorder

Individuals with PTSD frequently describe excessive movement during sleep, reports that often are corroborated by bed partners. These movements could be a result of the prominent muscle activation that occurs during spontaneous awakenings from sleep.[58] An early PSG study in "trauma survivors" noted extreme motor activity, sometimes violent, during REMS.[59] This suggests that the pathophysiology of PTSD could involve neural circuitry that also is disrupted in REM behavior disorder (RBD). Although RBD typically is not associated with psychopathology,[60] Husain and colleagues[61] reported that 56% of a sample of patients with RBD had comorbid PTSD. Complicating the consideration of any association between PTSD and RBD is the well-known relationship between antidepressant medications used to treat PTSD (see Treatment of Posttraumatic Stress Disorder Sleep Disturbances: Pharmacotherapy for Posttraumatic Stress Disorder, later in this article) and the occurrence of RBD symptoms.[62]

Compared with healthy controls, combat veterans with PTSD may show phasic motor dysregulation during non-REMS, in the form of periodic limb movements (PLM).[63] Cantor and Ross[63] suggested a potential link between the neural mechanisms of PLM and those of PTSD. This is based on the observation that a group of individuals with PLM had an abnormal blink reflex, one component of the startle reflex that is characteristically exaggerated during wakefulness in PTSD.[63] Another potential link between the pathophysiology of PLM and that of PTSD is provided by the evidence that sympathetic nervous system activity, which is elevated in PTSD,[64] has an essential role in producing PLM.[65] PLM can be associated with partial arousal or awakening,[66] and might thereby contribute to insomnia in PTSD. The antidepressant medications used to treat PTSD (see Treatment of Posttraumatic Stress Disorder Sleep Disturbances: Pharmacotherapy for Posttraumatic Stress Disorder, later in this article) can increase PLM, thereby promoting arousal and exacerbating insomnia.[66]

Apparently paradoxically, Woodward and colleagues[67] observed that, compared with healthy controls, a group of combat veterans with PTSD showed a reduction in sleep movement time. Noting the uncertain relationship between movement time and brief body movements, they saw no incompatibility between their finding and reports of elevated phasic motor activity in PTSD.

Treatment of Posttraumatic Stress Disorder Sleep Disturbances: Psychotherapy for Posttraumatic Stress Disorder

Existing meta-analyses of the effectiveness of psychotherapies for PTSD have paid little attention to sleep outcomes.[68] The VA/DoD 2010 Clinical Practice Guideline[69] supports the use of exposure-based therapies, prolonged exposure (PE) in particular, and cognitive processing therapy (CPT). Galovski and colleagues[70] found that both PE and CPT were somewhat effective in reducing global sleep disturbance in adult, female rape survivors; however, sleep impairment remained clinically significant despite an overall improvement in PTSD symptoms. Examining long-term changes in sleep symptoms after CPT and PE, Gutner and colleagues[71] found no improvement in sleep disturbance, again in the context of a remission of the waking symptoms of PTSD.

Treatment of Posttraumatic Stress Disorder Sleep Disturbances: Psychotherapy for Insomnia

There is some evidence that CBT-I is effective for insomnia related to PTSD.[68] Talbot and colleagues[72] conducted an RCT of CBT-I in a community sample with PTSD. Compared with waitlist controls, the CBT-I group had a superior response on sleep diary measures, on Pittsburgh Sleep Quality Index (PSQI) scores, and on PSG-derived total sleep time, effects that remained significant at 6-month follow-up. However, both the CBT-I and waitlist control groups had reductions in PTSD symptom severity and posttraumatic nightmares, indicating that trials with an active treatment control group will be essential to demonstrating the efficacy of CBT-I specifically.

Treatment of Posttraumatic Stress Disorder Sleep Disturbances: Psychotherapy for Recurrent Nightmares

Imagery rehearsal (IR),[73,74] the best studied psychotherapeutic intervention for recurrent nightmares, may promote increased mastery of nightmare content.[75] A variety of protocols exist, all having these essential components: choosing a recurrent nightmare, rescripting it during waking, and rehearsing the new dream script imaginally at bedtime. Most forms of IR include additional potentially active treatment elements, such as CBT-I techniques. Only one RCT of IR has included a potentially active psychotherapy control.[76] In a study of Vietnam War veterans with chronic, severe PTSD and recurrent nightmares, there was no significant difference in reducing nightmare frequency and PTSD severity and improving sleep quality between IR and a comparison treatment that included components of CBT-I.[76] Harb and colleagues[74] emphasized the limitations of the extant IR literature and identified strategies to advance the field. Exposure, relaxation, and rescripting therapy is a variant of IR that has shown promise for reducing nightmares and insomnia in predominantly civilian samples with posttraumatic symptoms.[77]

Treatment of Posttraumatic Stress Disorder Sleep Disturbances: Pharmacotherapy for Posttraumatic Stress Disorder

The SSRIs have the strongest evidence base among pharmacotherapies for PTSD[69]; however, there is remarkably little evidence that insomnia and recurrent nightmares in PTSD respond to these drugs.[68] To the best of our knowledge, only a small open-label trial of fluvoxamine in Vietnam War combat veterans demonstrated an improvement in subjective sleep quality and a decrease in dreams related to combat trauma.[78]

The use of selective SNRI, in particular venlafaxine, is supported by clinical guidelines for treating PTSD.[69] However, in a pooled analysis of two controlled trials, there was no advantage of venlafaxine ER in reducing distressing dreams as assessed with the CAPS-SX17 (Clinician Administered PTSD Scale).[79] Accordingly, the "Best Practice Guide for the Treatment of Nightmare Disorder in Adults" does not recommend venlafaxine for treating PTSD-associated nightmares.[73]

The tricyclic antidepressants (TCA) and monoamine oxidase inhibitors (MAOI) have not been studied in large clinical trials in PTSD.[79] Currently there is only weak support for the usefulness of the TCA and the MAOI in controlling recurrent nightmares.[73] This is particularly interesting in light of the prominent REMS suppressant effect of the MAOI, given that most nightmares emerge from REMS.[73]

The atypical antipsychotic drugs have been investigated as a treatment for PTSD. One controlled trial of olanzapine monotherapy found a greater reduction in the total CAPS score with the medication, but only the decrease in the avoidance and numbing subscore achieved significance.[80] A small placebo-controlled trial of adjunctive olanzapine for combat-related PTSD unresponsive to SSRI treatment showed a greater improvement in sleep, as measured by the PSQI, in the olanzapine group.[81] The largest study of an atypical antipsychotic drug in PTSD showed no significant effect of risperidone in veterans.[82] No completed RCTs of quetiapine, ziprasidone, or aripiprazole have been carried out in PTSD populations.

Treatment of Posttraumatic Stress Disorder Sleep Disturbances: Pharmacotherapy for Insomnia

Few studies have examined the benefits of pharmacotherapy for insomnia in individuals with PTSD. There was no significant advantage of the benzodiazepine clonazepam in a small, single-blind, placebo-controlled trial.[83] However, clonazepam, the mainstay of pharmacologic treatment for RBD, could have a place in the treatment of excessive movement during sleep in PTSD, a topic for future research. In an RCT, Pollack and colleagues[84] found that a 3-week treatment with eszopiclone, a nonbenzodiazepine that acts at the benzodiazepine receptor, led to greater improvements in PTSD symptoms, including sleep disturbance.

There is some evidence that the 5-HT$_2$ antagonist/SSRI trazodone, an antidepressant drug with prominent sedative properties, may be useful in treating insomnia and recurrent nightmares in individuals with PTSD.[85] Nefazodone, an antidepressant with a similar pharmacologic mechanism, showed some utility in open-label trials,[78] but concerns about hepatotoxicity have limited further investigation with this medication.

Treatment of Posttraumatic Stress Disorder Sleep Disturbances: Pharmacotherapy for Recurrent Nightmares

There is low-level evidence for the usefulness of topiramate, low-dose cortisol, and gabapentin in treating recurrent nightmares. There are conflicting data on the benefit of the antihistamine cyproheptadine.[73] The introduction of the alpha-1 adrenoceptor antagonist prazosin is arguably the most important advance in the pharmacotherapy of the nightmare disturbance in PTSD.

Two placebo-controlled trials of prazosin in US military veterans reported a decrease in nightmares.[65] A placebo-controlled trial in civilians with PTSD also showed an advantage of prazosin in reducing trauma nightmares.[65] Additionally, Raskind and colleagues[86] reported a decrease in combat-related nightmares in active duty US service members treated with prazosin compared with placebo; sleep quality and overall PTSD symptoms were improved as well. Notably, prazosin has also been found to reduce non-nightmare distressed awakenings, that is, those awakenings from sleep accompanied by extreme psychological distress without any recall of dream mentation.[87] Other drugs that reduce central noradrenergic activity could also be expected to ameliorate the nightmare disturbance in PTSD. There are positive case reports for clonidine, an alpha-2 adrenoceptor agonist that inhibits the firing of noradrenergic locus coeruleus neurons,[88] but no clinical trial of this drug has been conducted.

SUMMARY: DIRECTIONS FOR FUTURE RESEARCH

The past decade has seen numerous advances in our understanding of both the mechanisms of sleep disturbance in anxiety disorders, OCD, and PTSD, and in their treatment. Research in GAD, PD, and OCD has uncovered common dimensional processes at the interface of sleep disturbance and anxiety disorders. Many of these processes cluster around difficulties with cognitive control (eg, worry, rumination, anxiety sensitivity, obsessional thinking, impaired cognitive inhibition). Together, this research suggests that treatments for sleep disturbance in these disorders may benefit from the utilization of cognitive strategies aimed at reducing mental activity before sleep onset and during midsleep waking periods. Cognitive restructuring of negative beliefs about sleep is already an important component of CBT-I. Individuals with GAD, PD, and OCD may benefit from the addition to CBT-I of anxiety-specific cognitive strategies.

The brain mechanisms underlying the sleep disturbance in PTSD are increasingly understood. These advances have depended in part on the translation from basic research in animals. Although non-REMS can be affected in PTSD, for example, in the form of PLM, attention has focused on REMS processes. Abnormalities of REMS control may evolve with the passage of time posttrauma. Neuroimaging during sleep will likely provide important insights into the underlying neural circuitry. The alpha-1 adrenoceptor antagonist prazosin has assumed an important role in the treatment of recurrent nightmares in PTSD. Identifying effective psychotherapies for the sleep disturbance in PTSD is a field poised for further investigation.

Circadian rhythm disturbances have been observed in GAD and OCD, and there is reason to suspect the presence of circadian abnormalities in PTSD. Although research in this area is still in its early stages, identifying the ways in which circadian rhythm abnormalities contribute to sleep disturbances in anxiety disorders, PTSD, and OCD could lead to important developments in both pharmacotherapy and psychotherapy. An example is the reported benefit of agomelatine in treating GAD and associated insomnia.

Finally, although the DSM-5 no longer considers GAD, PD, OCD, and PTSD under the umbrella of "anxiety disorders," this review has highlighted areas of overlap in the pathophysiology and treatment of the sleep disturbances in these disorders. Dimensional approaches to the study of sleep across psychiatric disorders is likely to be key in introducing new treatments and improving the quality of life for affected individuals.

REFERENCES

1. Mellman TA. Sleep and anxiety disorders. Psychiatr Clin North Am 2006;29:1047–58.
2. Uhde TW, Cortese BM. Anxiety and sleep problems: emerging concepts and theoretical treatment implications. Curr Psychiatry Rep 2009;11:269–76.
3. Insel T, Cuthbert B, Gravey M, et al. Research Domain Criteria (RDoC): toward a new classification framework for research on mental disorders. Am J Psychiatry 2010;167(7):748–51.
4. American Psychiatric Association. Diagnostic and statistical manual of mental disorders. 5th edition. Washington, DC: American Psychiatric Association; 2013.
5. Kessler RC, Chiu WT, Demier O, et al. Prevalence, severity, and comorbidity of 12-month DSM-IV disorders in the National Comorbidity Survey Replication. Arch Gen Psychiatry 2005;62(6):617.
6. Belleville G, Cousineau H, Levrier K, et al. The impact of cognitive-behavior therapy for anxiety disorders on concomitant sleep disturbances: a meta-analysis. J Anxiety Disord 2010;24:379–86.
7. Lichstein KL. Secondary insomnia: a myth dismissed. Sleep Med Rev 2006;10(1):3–5.
8. Alfano C, Reynolds K, Nikia S, et al. Polysomnographic sleep patterns of non-depressed, non-medicated children with generalized anxiety disorder. J Affect Disord 2013;147:379–84.
9. Nolen-Hoeksema S. The role of rumination in depressive disorders and mixed anxiety/depressive symptoms. J Abnorm Psychol 2000;109:504–11.
10. Kertz SJ, Woodruff-Borden J. Human and economic burden of GAD, subthreshold GAD and worry in a primary care sample. J Clin Psychol Med Settings 2011;18:281–90.
11. Lund HG, Reider BD, Whiting AB, et al. Sleep patterns and predictors of disturbed sleep in a large population of college students. J Adolesc Health 2010;46:124–32.

12. Takano K, Iijima Y, Tanno Y. Repetitive thought and self-reported sleep disturbance. Behav Ther 2012;43(4):779–89.

13. Tsypes A, Aldao A, Mennin DS. Emotion dysregulation and sleep difficulties in generalized anxiety disorder. J Anxiety Disord 2013;27(2):197–203.

14. Wirz-Justice A. Biological rhythm disturbances in mood disorders. Int Clin Psychopharmacol 2006;21:S11–5.

15. Sipilä T, Kananen L, Greco D, et al. An association analysis of circadian genes in anxiety disorders. Biol Psychiatry 2010;67(12):1163–70.

16. Ma LL, Kong DG, Qi XW, et al. Generalized anxiety disorder and the circadian rhythm of blood pressure in patients with hypertension. Int J Psychiatry Clin Pract 2008;12:292–5.

17. Bush AL, Armento MEA, Weiss BJ, et al. The Pittsburgh Sleep Quality Index in older primary care patients with generalized anxiety disorder: psychometrics and outcomes following cognitive behavioral therapy. Psychiatry Res 2012;199:24–30.

18. Belanger L, Morin CM, Langlous F, et al. Insomnia and generalized anxiety disorder: effects of cognitive behavior therapy for GAD on insomnia symptoms. J Anxiety Disord 2004;18:561–71.

19. Harvey AG, Sharpley AL, Ree MJ, et al. An open trial of cognitive therapy for chronic insomnia. Behav Res Ther 2007;45(10):2491–501.

20. Smith MT, Huang MI, Manber R. Cognitive behavior therapy for chronic insomnia occurring within the context of medical and psychiatric disorders. Clin Psychol Rev 2005;25(5):559–92.

21. Pollack M, Kinrys G, Krystal A, et al. Eszopiclone coadministered with escitalopram in patients with insomnia and comorbid generalized anxiety disorder. Arch Gen Psychiatry 2008;65(5):551–62.

22. Holsboer-Trachsler E, Prieto R. Effects of pregabalin on sleep in generalized anxiety disorder. Int J Neuropsychopharmacol 2013;16:925–36.

23. Gross PK, Nourse R, Wasser TE. Ramelton for insomnia symptoms in a community sample of adults with generalized anxiety disorder: an open label study. J Clin Sleep Med 2009;5(1):28–33.

24. Stein DJ, Ahokas AA, de Bodinat C. Efficacy of agomelatine in generalized anxiety disorder: a randomized, double-blind, placebo-controlled study. J Clin Psychopharmacol 2008;28:561–6.

25. Craske MG, Tsao JCI. Assessment and treatment of nocturnal panic attacks. Sleep Med Rev 2005;9(3):173–84.

26. Mellman TA, Uhde TW. Electroencephalographic sleep in panic disorder. A focus on sleep-related panic attacks. Arch Gen Psychiatry 1989;46:178–84.

27. Hoge EA, Marques L, Wechsler RS, et al. The role of anxiety sensitivity in sleep disturbance in panic disorder. J Anxiety Disord 2011;25(4):536–8.

28. Hovland A, Pallesen A, Hammar A, et al. Subjective sleep quality in relation to inhibition and heart rate variability in patients with panic disorder. J Affect Disord 2013;150(1):152–5.

29. Craske MG. Cognitive behavioral therapy for nocturnal panic. Behav Ther 2005; 36(1):43–54.

30. Marchand L, Marchand A, Landry P, et al. Efficacy of two cognitive-behavioral treatment modalities for panic disorder with nocturnal panic attacks. Behav Modif 2013;37(5):680–704.

31. Simon NM, Otto MW, Smits JAJ, et al. Changes in anxiety sensitivity with pharmacotherapy for panic disorder. J Psychiatr Res 2004;38:491–5.

32. Paterson JL, Reynolds AC, Ferguson SA, et al. Sleep and obsessive-compulsive disorder (OCD). Sleep Med Rev 2013;17:465–74.

33. Timpano KR, Carbonella JY, Bernert RA, et al. Obsessive compulsive symptoms and sleep difficulties: exploring the unique relationship between insomnia and obsessions. J Psychiatr Res 2014;57:101–7.
34. Mukhopadhyay S, Fineberg NA, Drummond LM, et al. Delayed sleep phase in severe obsessive-compulsive disorder: a systematic case-report survey. CNS Spectr 2008;13:406–13.
35. Nesbit AD, Dijk DJ. Out of synch with society: an update on delayed sleep phase disorder. Curr Opin Pulm Med 2014;20(6):581–7.
36. Nota JA, Sharkey KM, Coles ME. Sleep, arousal, and circadian rhythms in adults with obsessive-compulsive disorder: a meta-analysis. Neurosci Biobehav Rev 2015;51:100–7.
37. Voderholzer U, Riemann D, Huwig-Poppe C, et al. Sleep in obsessive compulsive disorder: polysomnographic studies under baseline conditions and after experimentally induced serotonin deficiency. Eur Arch Psychiatry Clin Neurosci 2007; 257:173–82.
38. Kluge M, Schussler P, Dresler M, et al. Sleep onset REM periods in obsessive compulsive disorder. Psychiatry Res 2007;152:29–35.
39. Ferguson JM. SSRI antidepressant medications: adverse effects and tolerability. Prim Care Companion J Clin Psychiatry 2001;3(1):22–7.
40. Freeston MH, Ladouceur R, Gagnon F, et al. Cognitive behavioral treatment of obsessive thoughts: a controlled study. J Consult Clin Psychol 1997;65(3):405–13.
41. Ross RJ, Ball WA, Sullivan KA, et al. Sleep disturbance as the hallmark of posttraumatic stress disorder. Am J Psychiatry 1989;146:697–707.
42. Van Liempt S, Arends J, Cluitmans PJM, et al. Sympathetic activity and hypothalamo-pituitary-adrenal axis activity during sleep in post-traumatic stress disorder: a study assessing polysomnography with simultaneous blood sampling. Psychoneuroendocrinology 2013;38(1):155–65.
43. Mellman T, Bustamante V, Fins A, et al. REM sleep and the early development of posttraumatic stress disorder. Am J Psychiatry 2002;159:1696–701.
44. Ross RJ. The changing REM sleep signature of posttraumatic stress disorder. Sleep 2014;37:1281–2.
45. Mellman TA, Kobayashi I, Lavela J, et al. A relationship between REM sleep measures and the duration of posttraumatic stress disorder in a young adult urban minority population. Sleep 2014;37(8):1321–6.
46. Goldstein AN, Walker MP. The role of sleep in emotional brain function. Annu Rev Clin Psychol 2014;10:679–708.
47. Kobayashi I, Boarts JM, Delahanty DL. Polysomnographically measured sleep abnormalities in PTSD: a meta-analytic review. Psychophysiology 2007;44(4): 660–9.
48. Datta S. Avoidance task training potentiates phasic pontine-wave density in the rat: a mechanism for sleep-dependent plasticity. J Neurosci 2000;20(22):8607–13.
49. DaSilva JK, Lei Y, Madan V, et al. Fear conditioning fragments REM sleep in stress-sensitive Wistar-Kyoto, but not Wistar, rats. Prog Neuropsychopharmacol Biol Psychiatry 2011;35(1):67–73.
50. Price LJ, Kremen I. Variations in behavioral response threshold within the REM period of human sleep. Psychophysiology 1980;17(2):133–40.
51. Lavie P, Katz N, Pillar G, et al. Elevated awaking thresholds during sleep: characteristics of chronic war-related posttraumatic stress disorder patients. Biol Psychiatry 1998;44:1060–5.
52. Sanford L, Ross R. Amygdalar regulation of REM sleep. In: Mallick B, Pandi-Perumal S, McCarley R, et al, editors. Rapid eye movement sleep. Regulation

and function. Cambridge (United Kingdom): Cambridge University Press; 2011. p. 110–20.

53. Schwartz S, Maquet P. Sleep imaging and the neuropsychological assessment of dreams. Trends Cogn Sci 2002;6(1):23–30.

54. Liberzon I, Garfinkel S. Functional neuroimaging in post-traumatic stress disorder. In: Shiromani P, Keane T, LeDoux J, editors. Post-traumatic stress disorder. Basic science and clinical practice. New York: Humana Press; 2009. p. 297–317.

55. Germain A, James J, Insana S, et al. A window in the invisible wound of war: functional neuroimaging of REM sleep in returning combat veterans with PTSD. Psychiatry Res 2013;211:176–9.

56. Hasler BP, Insana SP, James JA, et al. Evening-type military veterans report worse lifetime posttraumatic stress symptoms and greater brainstem activity across wakefulness and REM sleep. Biol Psychol 2013;94(2):255–62.

57. Nielsen TA. Chronobiology of dreaming. In: Kryger MH, Roth T, Dement WC, editors. Principles and practice of sleep medicine. Philadelphia: WB Saunders; 2005. p. 535–50.

58. Horner RRL. Arousal from sleep—perspectives relating to autonomic function. Sleep 2003;26(6):644–5.

59. Hefez A, Metz L, Lavie P. Long-term effects of extreme situational stress on sleep and dreaming. Am J Psychiatry 1987;144:344–7.

60. Schenck CH, Bundlie SR, Ettinger MG, et al. Chronic behavioral disorders of human REM sleep: a new category of parasomnia. Sleep 1986;9(2):293–308.

61. Husain AM, Miller PP, Carwile ST. REM sleep behavior disorder: potential relationship to post-traumatic stress disorder. J Clin Neurophysiol 2001;18(2):148–57.

62. Schenck CH, Mahowald MW, Kim SW, et al. Prominent eye movements during NREM sleep and REM sleep behavior disorder associated with fluoxetine treatment of depression and obsessive-compulsive disorder. Sleep 1992;15:226–35.

63. Cantor C, Ross R. Psychiatric aspects of movement during sleep. In: Chokroverty S, Allen R, Walters A, et al, editors. Sleep and movement disorders. Oxford (United Kingdom): Oxford University Press; 2013. p. 722–44.

64. Raskind M. Pharmacologic treatment of PTSD. In: Shiromani P, Keane T, LeDoux J, editors. Post-traumatic stress disorder. Basic science and clinical practice. New York: Humana Press; 2009. p. 337–61.

65. Guggisberg AG, Hess CW, Mathis J. The significance of the sympathetic nervous system in the pathophysiology of periodic leg movements in sleep. Sleep 2007; 30:755–66.

66. Desautels A, Michaud M, Lanfranchi P, et al. Periodic limb movements in sleep. In: Chokroverty S, Allen R, Walters A, et al, editors. Sleep and movement disorders. Oxford (United Kingdom): Oxford University Press; 2013. p. 650–63.

67. Woodward SH, Leskin GA, Sheikh JL. Movement during sleep: associations with posttraumatic stress disorder, nightmares and comorbid panic disorder. Sleep 2002;25(6):669–76.

68. Brownlow JA, Harb GC, Ross RJ. Treatment of sleep disturbances in post-traumatic stress disorder: a review of the literature. Curr Psychiatry Rep 2015;17(6):41.

69. The Management of Post-Traumatic Stress Working Group. VA/DoD clinical practice guideline for management of post-traumatic stress. Version 2.0. Department of Veterans Affairs. Department of Defense; 2010.

70. Galovski TE, Monson C, Bruce SE, et al. Does cognitive-behavioral therapy for PTSD improve perceived health and sleep impairment? J Trauma Stress 2009; 22(3):197–204.

71. Gutner CA, Casement MD, Stavitsky GK, et al. Change in sleep symptoms across cognitive processing therapy and prolonged exposure: a longitudinal perspective. Behav Res Ther 2013;51(2):817–22.
72. Talbot LS, Maguen S, Metzler TJ, et al. Cognitive behavioral therapy for insomnia in posttraumatic stress disorder: a randomized controlled trial. Sleep 2014;37(2): 327–41.
73. Aurora RN, Zak RS, Auerbach SH, et al. Best practice guide for the treatment of nightmare disorder in adults. J Clin Sleep Med 2010;6(4):389–401.
74. Harb GC, Phelps AJ, Forbes D, et al. A critical review of the evidence base of imagery rehearsal for posttraumatic nightmares: pointing the way for future research. J Trauma Stress 2013;26(5):570–9.
75. Germain A, Krakow B, Faucher B, et al. Increased mastery elements associated with imagery rehearsal treatment for nightmares in sexual assault survivors with PTSD. Dreaming 2004;14:195–206.
76. Cook JM, Harb GC, Gehrman PR, et al. Imagery rehearsal for posttraumatic nightmares: a randomized controlled trial. J Trauma Stress 2010;23(5):553–63.
77. Davis JL, Wright DC. Exposure, relaxation and rescripting treatment for trauma-related nightmares. J Trauma Dissociation 2006;7(1):5–18.
78. Neylan TC, Metzler TJ, Schoenfeld FB, et al. Fluvoxamine and sleep disturbances in posttraumatic stress disorder. J Trauma Stress 2001;14:461–7.
79. Ravindran LN, Stein MB. Pharmacotherapy of PTSD: premises, principles, and priorities. Brain Res 2009;1293:24–39.
80. Carey P, Suliman S, Ganesan K, et al. Olanzapine monotherapy in posttraumatic stress disorder: efficacy in a randomized, double-blind, placebo-controlled study. Hum Psychopharmacol 2012;27(4):386–91.
81. Stein MB, Kline NA, Matloff JL. Adjunctive olanzapine for SSRI-resistant combat-related PTSD: a double-blind, placebo-controlled study. Am J Psychiatry 2002; 159(10):1777–9.
82. Krystal JH, Rosenheck RA, Cramer JA, et al. Adjunctive risperidone treatment for antidepressant-resistant symptoms of chronic military service-related PTSD: a randomized trial. JAMA 2011;306(5):493–502.
83. Cates ME, Bishop MH, Davis LL, et al. Clonazepam for treatment of sleep disturbances associated with combat-related posttraumatic stress disorder. Ann Pharmacother 2004;38(9):1395–9.
84. Pollack MH, Hoge EA, Worthington JJ, et al. Eszopiclone for the treatment of posttraumatic stress disorder and associated insomnia: a randomized, double-blind, placebo-controlled trial. J Clin Psychiatry 2011;72(7):892–7.
85. Warner MD, Dorn MR, Peabody CA. Survey of the usefulness of trazodone in patients with PTSD with insomnia or nightmares. Pharmacopsychiatry 2001;34: 128–31.
86. Raskind MA, Peterson K, Williams T, et al. A trial of prazosin for combat trauma PTSD with nightmares in active-duty soldiers returned from Iraq and Afghanistan. Am J Psychiatry 2013;170(9):1003–10.
87. Thompson CE, Taylor FB, McFall ME, et al. Nonnightmare distressed awakenings in veterans with posttraumatic stress disorder: response to prazosin. J Trauma Stress 2008;21(4):417–20.
88. Alao A, Selvarajah J, Razi S. The use of clonidine in the treatment of nightmares among patients with co-morbid PTSD and traumatic brain injury. Int J Psychiatry Med 2012;44(2):165–9.

Sleep Disturbances in Schizophrenia

Jayesh Kamath, MD, PhD*, Sundeep Virdi, MD, JD, Andrew Winokur, MD, PhD

KEYWORDS

- Sleep disturbances • Schizophrenia • Polysomnography • Clinical correlates
- Neurotransmitter • Clock genes • Antipsychotic medication

KEY POINTS

- Sleep disturbances play an important role in the symptomatology and pathophysiology of schizophrenia.
- Slow wave sleep deficits, shortened rapid eye movement latency, and unchanged rapid eye movement sleep are primary polysomnography (PSG) findings.
- Correlations have been established between certain critical clinical aspects of schizophrenia and the PSG findings.
- Dysregulation of specific neurotransmitter systems and clock genes may play a role in the pathophysiology of schizophrenia and schizophrenia-related sleep disturbances.
- Antipsychotic medications can impact sleep structure but also play a role in the treatment of sleep disturbances.

OVERVIEW

Although rarely the primary complaint, insomnia and other sleep related abnormalities are a common symptom in schizophrenia, reported in 30% to 80% of schizophrenic patients.[1,2] The wide prevalence range is related to variation in several factors such as acuity of illness, specifically severity of psychotic symptomatology, age, gender, and medication status.[2] A difference in the prevalence of sleep disorders between patients with "acute schizophrenia" and "chronic psychosis" has been demonstrated, with 1 study reporting that 83% of patients with 'acute schizophrenia' experienced sleep difficulties compared with 47% of those with "chronic psychosis."[2] In the Clinical Antipsychotic Trials of Intervention Effectiveness (CATIE) study, 16% to 30% of patients across treatment arms reported insomnia and 24% to 31% of patients reported hypersomnia.[3]

Disclosure: The authors have nothing to disclose.
Department of Psychiatry, University of Connecticut School of Medicine, 263 Farmington Avenue, Farmington, CT 06030-6415, USA
* Corresponding author.
E-mail address: jkamath@uchc.edu

Psychiatr Clin N Am 38 (2015) 777–792
http://dx.doi.org/10.1016/j.psc.2015.07.007
0193-953X/15/$ – see front matter © 2015 Elsevier Inc. All rights reserved.

Abbreviations	
5-HT	Serotonin/Serotonergic
CATIE	Clinical antipsychotic trials of intervention effectiveness
DA	Dopamine
GABA	Gamma-aminobutyric acid
OSA	Obstructive sleep apnea
PLMS	Periodic limb movements syndrome
PSG	Polysomnography/Polysomnographic
REM	Rapid eye movement
REM-L	Rapid eye movement latency
SE	Sleep efficiency
SOL	Sleep onset latency
SWS	Slow wave sleep
TST	Total sleep time
WASO	Wake time after sleep onset

Sleep difficulties must occur for at least 1 month and be associated with daytime fatigue or impaired daytime functioning to be considered related to schizophrenia.[4] Subjective impairment of sleep quality in patients with schizophrenia is similar to the impairment seen in individuals suffering from primary insomnia or major depression.[2] These impairments include difficulty with sleep initiation and maintenance, as well as early morning awakening.[2] Prolonged sleep onset latency (SOL) and problems with sleep maintenance are among the most often reported difficulties.[5] Other symptoms reported by schizophrenic patients include restlessness, agitation, hypnagogic hallucinations, nightmares, and sleep reversal, that is, the major sleep period occurring during the day with wakefulness at night.[5] Sleep disturbances are often part of the prodromal phase before the development of manifest psychotic symptomatology and are involved in the pathophysiology of various aspects of the illness in these patients.[2] Abrupt and pronounced deterioration in the sleep–wake cycle of a patient with schizophrenia often serves as an early warning sign of an impending psychotic decompensation.[6] Acute exacerbations of psychosis are associated with restless and agitated sleep.[1] Even after resolution of psychotic agitation, patients continue to report prolonged SOL, reduced total sleep time (TST), and fragmented sleep.[7] Medicated and stable patients with schizophrenia commonly report early and middle insomnia and sleep reversal.[8,9] Comorbid alcohol use and use of other substances, frequently seen in these patients, can negatively impact sleep quality and lead to relapse.[7] Poor sleep quality in these patients has been associated with reduced quality of life and poor coping skills.[10] Schizophrenic patients with insomnia reported lower mean scores on all quality of life domains that were independent of depression, distress, and side effects related to their antipsychotic medications.[10]

OBJECTIVE ASSESSMENTS

Several studies have evaluated objective measures of sleep abnormalities in patients with schizophrenia by means of polysomnographic (PSG) techniques.[5] These studies have validated many of the subjective findings of sleep cycle disturbances in these patients.[5] However, the findings are not consistent across studies.[11,12] The discrepancies are owing to factors such as inclusion of diverse phenotypes, differences in study design, differences in quantification of sleep variables, differences in control groups and sample sizes, and differences in inclusion/exclusion criteria, for example, differences in demographic and clinical characteristics, medication status, and chronicity of illness.[13] Despite these methodologic confounds, some consistent findings have emerged across studies.[7] The most consistent findings include prolonged SOL and increased wake time after sleep onset (WASO).[7] These studies also documented poor sleep efficiency (SE) with reduction in TST owing to initial, middle, and late insomnia.[1] Evidence from PSG studies suggests that sleep-onset insomnia as well as difficulty reaching a state of persistent sleep is highly characteristic of the sleep of schizophrenic patients.[1,11,12]

Many PSG studies conducted in patients with schizophrenia have quantified the latency of onset of the first period of rapid eye movement (REM) sleep. Some of these studies have found that subgroups of patients with schizophrenia have an abnormal shortening of the interval between sleep onset and the first REM episode.[7] About one-half of the studies have reported diminished slow wave sleep (SWS) time in patients with schizophrenia compared with healthy controls.[14] SWS deficits have been correlated with several factors, including age, severity of negative symptoms, and duration of illness.[15] It has been suggested that the SWS deficits indicate impaired homeostatic drive in these patients[7] and might be the consequence of defective synaptic pruning during the second decade of life.[16] Benson[1] suggests that the shortened REM latency (REM-L) might be owing to the reduction in SWS. Ordinarily, the presence of SWS exerts an inhibitory effect on the initiation of a REM episode. Benson[1] proposed that a diminution of the SWS episode would permit the passive advance of the first REM period, leading to shortened REM-L. Findings across several studies have indicated that REM sleep remains unchanged in patients with schizophrenia.[7]

Some of the variability of the findings concerning SWS and REM sleep parameters in schizophrenia might be related to the clinical diversity of patients studied.[2] Evidence suggests that lower REM-L may be related to higher genetic loading, that is, a family history of affective disorders.[15]

Polysomnography Findings According to the Phase of Clinical Course

Studies conducted in patients experiencing their first psychotic episode or an acute exacerbation of schizophrenia have documented a reduction in TST and an increase in N2 sleep latency. Patients experiencing their first psychotic episode demonstrated a shortening of REM-L.[16] Chouinard and colleagues[12] found increased total awake time and decreased percentage of stage 2 sleep in antipsychotic-naïve schizophrenic patients. Studies conducted in patients during the chronic phase of their illness have also reported reduced TST and increased N2 sleep latency.[13] Many of these studies also documented shortening of REM-L and unchanged REM.[13] Monti and associates[16] summarized their analyses across evaluable studies and concluded that the findings of sleep onset prolongation and impairment of sleep maintenance were observed in studies involving patients with schizophrenia irrespective of their medication status and irrespective of the phase of clinical course, that is, first episode, acute exacerbation, or chronic stage of illness. They also concluded that shortening of REM-L, SWS reduction, and unchanged REM are other consistent findings across several studies.[16]

Studies have quantified sleep-related brain wave activity in patients with schizophrenia. These include slow wave activity in the delta band, sleep-spindle events, and high-frequency activity in the beta and gamma ranges.[7] These studies reported decreases in slow wave activity in patients with schizophrenia in comparison with health controls[7]; high-frequency activity in the beta and gamma ranges were found to be greater in unmedicated patients with schizophrenia relative to healthy controls and correlated with psychotic symptoms.[7] In medicated patients with schizophrenia, the number and amplitude of non-REM sleep spindles was found to be less, suggesting abnormality in thalamic–reticular and thalamocortical circuitry.[7]

CLINICAL CORRELATES

Schizophrenia is a complex illness with a broad range of symptomatic disturbances that include positive symptoms, such as delusions and hallucinations, and negative symptoms, such as flattened affect, social withdrawal, lack of interest and motivation, neurocognitive impairment, and suicidality. Correlations have been found between PSG findings and symptom domains in patients with schizophrenia.[7]

Positive Symptoms

Positive symptoms have been associated with poor SE, longer SOL, increased REM and increased high-frequency activity in the electroencephalogram.[17,18] The degree of positive symptoms has been found to correlate with REM density in medicated and unmedicated patients.[19,20] REM-L was found to correlate inversely with the severity of positive symptoms in unmedicated and medication-naïve patients.[21,22]

Negative Symptoms

Negative symptoms have been correlated with shorter REM-L, SWS deficits and reduced delta-band slow wave activity. An increase in negative symptoms have been correlated with a reduction in SWS duration, SWS percentage, and stage 4 sleep after accounting for confounders such as age and depression.[23–25] Keshavan and colleagues[25] found that negative symptoms correlated with a reduction in SWS as well as decreases in brain anabolic processes. Similar to positive symptoms, negative symptoms were found to correlate inversely with REM density and REM-L, independent of depression.[21,24,26]

Suicide Risk

The mortality rate of schizophrenics owing to suicide is high relative to other psychiatric illnesses.[5] Studies have shown an apparent relationship between suicidality in schizophrenic patients and REM sleep variables.[2,27] Severe sleep disruption may contribute to suicidal behavior in these patients.[4] Schizophrenic patients with suicidal behavior have demonstrated increased whole night REM sleep time and REM activity compared with nonsuicidal patients.[28]

Neurocognitive Impairment

The symptom of schizophrenia that is often considered most essential is cognitive impairment.[7] Thus, it is important to recognize that there is an association between sleep structure and cognitive impairment in schizophrenic patients.[2] Several studies have shown sleep-related cognitive impairment in schizophrenics compared with healthy controls.[1] A normal rest–activity cycle may be essential for sufficient cognitive functioning in individuals who suffer from schizophrenia.[29] Several cognitive domains may demonstrate impairment in patients with decreased SWS, including difficulties in abstract, stereotyped thinking, cognitive disorganization, poor insight and judgment, tension, mannerisms, posturing, and deficiencies in attention.[20] One study showed failure of sleep-dependent consolidation of procedural learning in chronic, medicated schizophrenic patients when compared with healthy controls.[30] Visuospatial memory is another dimension of neurocognitive performance that has demonstrated a correlation with a reduction in SWS and SE.[31] Although some have attributed this correlation to a functional interrelationship between regulation of SWS and performance in visuospatial memory in schizophrenia, others have hypothesized that both SWS and cognitive impairment have the same morphologic base contributing to the correlation.[32] Attention is another neurocognitive parameter of importance. Forest and colleagues[33] found a negative correlation between reaction time on a selective attention task and sleep spindle density and also a negative correlation between reaction time and the duration of stage 4 sleep in both selective and the sustained attention tasks.

Severity of Illness

The association between objective sleep variables and the severity of illness and outcomes in patients with schizophrenia has been studied by several investigators. Objective sleep variables are measured using PSG and severity of illness is usually determined via the Brief Psychiatric Rating Scale or the Positive and Negative Syndrome Scale.[2] Studies have demonstrated a significant association between the severity of illness and selected REM sleep parameters.[14,20] Studies have reported that total scores on the Brief Psychiatric Rating Scale correlated positively with the percentage of REM sleep and negatively with REM-L and REM density.[14,21,34]

Outcomes

Patients with schizophrenia often suffer from a poorer quality of life than those with other psychiatric disorders, because most battle lifelong mental disability and the accompanying social and economic problems.[7] They tend to marry less, are institutionalized more often, and have more difficulty in the work setting.[7] There is a significant association between the poor subjective sleep quality of schizophrenic patients and a decreased quality of life.[2,13] This correlation exists even after correcting for depression and adverse drug effects.[2] Continued sleep difficulties may also adversely affect a patient's clinical outcome.[7] Additionally, poor sleep quality is correlated with maladaptive coping styles, which include a reduced preference for positive reappraisal.[2] SWS deficits and short REM-L have been found to be associated with poorer outcomes from 4 weeks to 2 years after initial PSG assessments. The percentage of delta sleep at baseline predicted outcomes at 1 and 2 years.[25] Studies found that the short REM-L was associated with poorer outcomes, including severe symptomatology, lack of employment, decreased social activity, and impaired global functioning.[34,35]

Evidence accumulated from PSG studies and their clinical correlates suggests that sleep structure abnormalities can serve as potential therapeutic targets or biomarkers in future investigations (**Fig. 1**). Such investigations can include subjective and objective assessments of sleep structure when novel pharmacologic and nonpharmacologic interventions are evaluated targeting schizophrenia and schizophrenia-related sleep disturbances.

UNDERLYING MECHANISMS AND PATHOPHYSIOLOGY

Dopamine (DA) dysfunction plays a critical role in the pathophysiology of schizophrenia. Evidence suggests that an increase in the synthesis and release of DA in the striatum is associated with the positive symptoms of schizophrenia, whereas negative symptoms and cognitive deficits have been associated with deficit of a DA in the dorsolateral prefrontal cortex.[36,37] Disruption of other neurotransmitter circuits, including glutamate and gamma-aminobutyric acid (GABA) have been implicated in the pathophysiology of schizophrenia.[38,39]

It has been proposed that overactivity of DA may play a role in the pathophysiology of sleep disturbances in schizophrenia. Indirect evidence derived from DA receptor

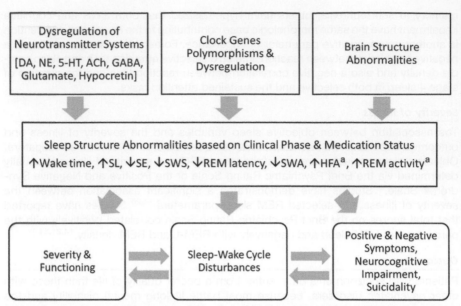

Fig. 1. Underlying mechanism and pathophysiology of schizophrenia and schizophrenia-related sleep-wake cycle disturbances. 5-HT, serotonin; ACh, acetylcholine/cholinergic; DA, dopamine; GABA, γ-aminobutyric acid; HFA, high-frequency activity; NE, norepinephrine; REM, rapid eye movement; SE, sleep efficiency; SL, sleep onset latency; SWA, slow wave activity; SWS, slow wave sleep; WAKE, wake after sleep onset; ↓, decreased; ↑, increased.
[a] During positive symptoms.

agonist/antagonist studies supports this hypothesis. DA D2 receptor agonists such as bromocriptine, pergolide, and apomorphine have been shown to enhance wakefulness and reduce sleep, whereas selective DA D2 receptor blocking agents have been shown to enhance light sleep in animal models.[40,41] Disruption of GABA and glutamate systems may also play a role in the pathophysiology of sleep disturbances in schizophrenia.[42,43] However, currently there is no evidence to support these hypotheses.

SWS deficits, a major sleep architecture abnormality seen in patients with schizophrenia, have been associated with impaired serotonergic (5-HT) mechanisms.[44] In unmedicated patients with schizophrenia, a positive correlation was found between SWS time and cerebrospinal fluid levels of the 5-HT metabolite, 5-hydroxyindole acetic acid.[44] Increased cerebrospinal fluid levels of norepinephrine and its metabolite, 3-methoxy 4-hydroxyphenylgycol, have been found in patients with insomnia during psychotic decompensation.[45] Hypocretin (orexin), located in the lateral hypothalamus, is a wake-promoting neurotransmitter and is known to play a major role in the normal sleep–wake cycle.[46] In unmedicated patients with schizophrenia, hypocretin levels in the cerebrospinal fluid were found to correlate positively with sleep latency, suggesting a potential role for hypocretin in hyperarousal in patients with schizophrenia.[47] Under normal conditions, REM sleep is facilitated by cholinergic and inhibited by 5-HT and noradrenergic neurons located in the brainstem.[48] It has been proposed that shortened REM-L may be related to enhanced cholinergic or diminished 5-HT and noradrenergic neurotransmission (cholinergic–aminergic imbalance hypothesis).[49] Shortened REM-L may be partially related to such an imbalance in neurotransmission, but evidence to support this notion is lacking. Future studies are needed to investigate the multiple neurotransmitter systems involved in the disruption of sleep architecture in patients with schizophrenia.[16]

Abnormalities in brain structure in schizophrenics have been discovered in post-mortem studies and in living subjects via computed tomography and MRI.[7] These abnormalities include enlarged lateral and third ventricles, loss of total gray matter tissue, frontal and temporal lobe volume, and a reduction in total brain size.[7] A relationship between sleep and brain structural abnormalities has been shown to exist in patients with schizophrenia.[2] Specifically, an enlarged ventricular brain ratio has been shown to be associated with various sleep parameters, including decreased stage 4 sleep and longer SOL.[23,50] In addition, sleep continuity and time spent asleep has shown a negative correlation with third ventricle width.[2] There are other important associations of brain structure and sleep disturbances in schizophrenic patients to note. Global cortical and prefrontal atrophy demonstrated a negative correlation with number awakenings, whereas ventricular brain ratio, caudate ratios, and anterior horn ratios showed a negative correlation with SE and a positive correlation with REM-L.[51]

Circadian rhythms are driven by the self-regulatory interaction between of a set of clock genes and their protein products.[52,53] The mammalian circadian timing apparatus includes oscillators that are found universally at a cellular level and a central pacemaker generator located in the hypothalamic suprachiasmatic nuclei.[54] Preliminary evidence links polymorphisms of certain clock genes with schizophrenia and sleep–wake patterns in schizophrenia.[55,56] It is interesting to note that dopaminergic signaling through DA D2 receptors has been associated with circadian regulation by certain clock gene protein products.[57] It has been suggested that clock gene polymorphisms leading to aberrant dopaminergic transmission may be involved in the pathophysiology of schizophrenia and sleep–wake cycle disturbances in schizophrenia.[55]

EFFECTS OF ANTIPSYCHOTIC MEDICATIONS ON SLEEP

Several review articles provide extensive information and commentary on this topic, which we can only summarize briefly in this article.[2,4,58,59] Drugs used in the treatment of schizophrenia, including typical antipsychotic drugs such as chlorpromazine and haloperidol, and atypical antipsychotic drugs, such as clozapine, risperidol, olanzapine, and others, are known to produce a broad array of pharmacologic effects.[60,61] The hallmark pharmacologic effect of all marketed antipsychotic drugs involves inhibition of DA D2 receptors, and to date, no drug has been shown to be effective in the treatment of symptoms of schizophrenia that lacks DA D2 receptor inhibitory effects. However, additional pharmacologic effects have been demonstrated across the full range of antipsychotic drugs. In the case of the atypical antipsychotic drugs, a defining pharmacologic profile has been proposed to include potent inhibition of 5-HT-2 receptors in conjunction with DA D2 receptor blockade.[62] Inhibition of 5-HT-2 receptors by atypical antipsychotic drugs is of plausible relevance to their effects on sleep physiology in light of the fact that data from a number of studies implicate blockade of this 5-HT receptor subtype with enhancement of SWS activity.[58,63–67] To different extents, antipsychotic drugs produce pharmacologic effects on numerous other neuroreceptor targets, many of which exert significant modulatory effects on sleep–wake function, as described in Chapter 2. In particular, inhibitory effects on muscarinic acetylcholine receptors, norepinephrine-1 receptors, and histamine H-1 receptors have all been documented in studies using in vitro brain homogenate techniques to examine effects produced by various antipsychotic agents.[68]

Clinical studies examining effects of antipsychotic drugs on parameters of sleep continuity and sleep architecture by means of PSG assessments in schizophrenic patients have been reported for some, but not all, of the commonly used antipsychotic drugs (Table 1). Thus, the available evidence base to guide clinical practice is somewhat limited. This situation is further complicated by the fact that significant methodologic limitations are associated with the majority of published reports in this area, a topic that has been discussed in detail in other reviews.[4,16] In a previous review, we identified cogent results from 7 studies describing effects of selected typical antipsychotic drugs on sleep parameters in schizophrenic patients.[59] We summarized the methodologic details and specific main findings from each of these 7 reports. Herein, we provide a general summary of the major findings for the effects of typical antipsychotic drugs on sleep parameters in schizophrenic patients: increases in TST and SE, along with decreases in SOL and wake time after sleep onset, findings indicative of an improvement in sleep continuity in patients with schizophrenia (see Table 1). In general, SWS was not altered by the typical antipsychotic drugs tested, whereas in some studies REM-L was increased.

Studies examining effects of several of the atypical antipsychotic drugs on sleep physiology have been published, including studies with clozapine, risperidone, olanzapine, quetiapine, ziprasidone, and paliperidone. However, studies involving assessment of effects of atypical antipsychotic drugs on sleep parameters in schizophrenic patients have only been reported for clozapine, risperidone, olanzapine, and paliperidone.[59] Of the limited studies involving assessment of effects of atypical antipsychotic drugs on sleep in schizophrenic patients, a report examining the effects of paliperidone is noteworthy because of the large sample size of schizophrenic patients enrolled and because of the rigor of the methodologic design involved.[68] There are also PSG studies describing effects of quetiapine and ziprasidone on sleep parameters in healthy volunteer subjects, but not in patients with schizophrenia.[69,70] Among the remaining atypical antipsychotic drugs that are currently approved and marketed in the United States, namely, aripiprazole, iloperidone, asenapine, and lurasidone, no studies have been published to date involving PSG assessments of the effects of these drugs on sleep physiology in either normal subjects or in patients with schizophrenia. In general, the effects of the atypical antipsychotic drugs clozapine,

Table 1
Effects of antipsychotic medications on polysomnography sleep variables

Antipsychotic	Increased	Decreased
Clozapine	TST, SE, stage N2	WASO, SOL, SWS[a]
Olanzapine	TST, SE, stage N2, SWS, REM-D	WASO, SOL, stage N1
Paliperidone	TST, SE, stage N2, REM sleep time	SOL, stage N1, # AW, Time awake
Quetiapine[b]	TST, SE, stage N2	SOL, WASO, REM sleep time
Ziprasidone[b]	TST, SE, stage N2, SWS, REM-L	WASO, #AW, stage N1, REM-D, REM%
Risperidone	Sleep maintenance, SWS[a]	—
Haloperidol	TST, stage N1, REM-L	SOL, stage N2, WASO
Chlorpromazine	TST, SWS, REM-L	SOL, WASO

Abbreviations: #AW, number of awakenings; REM, rapid eye movement; REM%, percentage of REM; REM-D, REM-density; REM-L, REM latency; SE, sleep efficiency; stage N1, stage 1 sleep; stage N2 sleep, stage 1 sleep; SOL, sleep-onset latency; SWS, slow wave sleep; TST, total sleep time; WASO, wake after sleep onset.
[a] In some studies.
[b] Studies conducted in normal subjects.

risperidone, olanzapine, and paliperidone on sleep are characterized by producing improvement in sleep continuity measures, including increases in TST and SE, along with decreases in in SOL and wake time after sleep onset (see **Table 1**). Similar findings have been reported in PSG studies conducted in normal subjects receiving administration of quetiapine or ziprasidone, with the exception that ziprasidone administration did not produce a decrease in SOL (see **Table 1**).

Sedation is an effect that has long been associated with both the typical and atypical antipsychotic drugs.[71] Within both categories of antipsychotic drugs, the potency of sedation produced ranges from mild to marked. For example, within the typical antipsychotic drug class, haloperidol is viewed as being minimally sedating, whereas the sedation associated with chlorpromazine administration is of moderate to marked severity. Among the atypical antipsychotic drugs, clozapine is associated with marked sedation, and quetiapine and olanzapine are also considered to exert prominent sedating effects. In contrast, risperidone, ziprasidone, and aripiprazole, among others, are generally thought to be only mildly sedating atypical antipsychotic agents. From a clinical perspective, drugs that produce more prominent sedating effects are frequently chosen to help address insomnia symptoms along with psychotic symptoms in patients with schizophrenia, even though no antipsychotic drug has been officially approved for the treatment of insomnia. This approach represents an analogous strategy to the common "off-label" use of trazodone to manage insomnia symptoms in depressed patients. A cautionary note about the use of sedating agents to treat insomnia symptoms in schizophrenic patients relates to the fact that producing a state of sedation is not equivalent to improving the quality of sleep in an individual with a sleep disturbance. Additionally, in some cases, the use of prominently sedating antipsychotic drugs may produce an undesirable adverse effect of excessive daytime somnolence, which may interfere with efforts to obtain improvement in functional recovery after acute treatment of psychotic symptoms in schizophrenic patients. Antipsychotic medications, especially atypical antipsychotic medications (eg, olanzapine), have been associated with serious cardiometabolic risk. Use of these medications just to treat insomnia should be avoided as much as possible.

SLEEP-DISORDERED BREATHING AND SLEEP-RELATED MOVEMENT DISORDERS

Two sleep disorders unrelated to disruption of sleep architecture, sleep-disordered breathing and sleep-related movement disorders, have been associated with schizophrenia. Both conditions have been partially linked (directly or indirectly) to antipsychotic medications used to treat schizophrenia.[7]

Sleep-Disordered Breathing

Sleep-disordered breathing, specifically obstructive sleep apnea (OSA), can cause somnolence and fatigue in patients with schizophrenia.[7] Some studies have found a greater prevalence of OSA in patients with schizophrenia compared with the general population,[72,73] whereas others report no difference in prevalence.[74] This discrepancy can be partially explained by obesity and differences in body mass index. A Japanese study reporting a lower prevalence of OSA also reported normal body mass index in their study participants.[74] Obesity is the best predictor of OSA.[75] Obesity in patients with schizophrenia has been linked to genetic factors, lifestyle factors, and antipsychotic medications used in the treatment of schizophrenia.[76] Use of antipsychotic medications in these patients, especially second-generation antipsychotic medications, has been linked to weight gain, high body mass index, and cardiometabolic issues.[76] OSA should be diagnosed and treated aggressively in these patients because obesity and OSA have serious medical consequences, including cardiometabolic and respiratory disorders, as noted in Chapter 11.[75]

Sleep-related Movement Disorders

Restless legs syndrome and periodic limb movements syndrome (PLMS) have been associated with schizophrenia and may contribute to sleep-onset insomnia. DA deficiency plays a critical role in the pathophysiology of sleep-related movement disorders.[77] The use of antipsychotic medications, via their effects on the DA system, has been associated with sleep-related movement disorders in patients with schizophrenia.[1] Studies investigating the prevalence of restless legs syndrome and PLMS are limited in patients with schizophrenia and the results from these studies are contradictory.[7,78] The prevalence of restless legs syndrome and PLMS in antipsychotic-free patients remains unknown.

MANAGEMENT

Sleep disturbances are prevalent in patients with schizophrenia, are associated with significant negative functional impact, and may herald the onset of an acute psychotic episode.[2,6,79] There are no established guidelines and few published reports providing guidance about the management of sleep disorders in schizophrenic patients. Herein, we offer some suggestions regarding the management of sleep disturbances in schizophrenic patients.

Evaluation and Management of Primary Sleep Disorders

Carefully evaluate the presence of symptoms of sleep disturbance in all schizophrenic patients, including symptoms of insomnia, complaints or manifestations of excessive daytime somnolence, and symptoms suggestive of OSA or PLMS, as well as evidence of altered circadian rhythm sleep–wake schedule. In addition to obtaining information from patients, it is often important to obtain collateral information from relatives or health care providers. In cases where evidence of a primary sleep disorder is obtained, it is important to initiate an appropriate treatment for the disorder, such as setting up arrangements for a schizophrenic patient with OSA to be treated with continuous positive airway pressure therapy, in light of the serious medical morbidity associated with untreated OSA. It is to be noted that schizophrenic patients have increased risk factors for the development of OSA.

Application of Behavioral and Sleep Hygiene Approaches to Manage Sleep Disturbances in Schizophrenic Patients

Patients with schizophrenia may be at risk for the development of sleep disturbances related to the neurobiology of their primary psychiatric disorder, but there are a number of environmental factors that impact adversely on sleep quality in this population, including markedly altered sleep–wake schedules, which may be associated with disruptions of circadian rhythms, poor diet, lack of exercise, and extensive use of caffeine, nicotine, alcohol, and drugs of abuse. The importance of using sleep hygiene approaches coupled with positive health-promoting lifestyle changes has been emphasized in recent guidelines with regard to the management of insomnia in general, and such approaches should be emphasized in patients with schizophrenia who manifest sleep disturbances characterized by insomnia and/or circadian rhythm sleep–wake alterations. It must be acknowledged that there is a lack of experimental evidence demonstrating the efficacy of these approaches in this patient population. Additionally, it is recognized that patients with schizophrenia may be difficult to engage in self-directed, health-promoting behavioral changes. These limitations not withstanding, we still strongly advocate the clinical wisdom of pursuing such approaches to the extent possible.

Pharmacologic Approaches for the Management of Insomnia and Other Sleep Disturbances in Schizophrenic Patients

There is a lack of published evidence with regard to the pharmacologic management of sleep disturbances in patients with schizophrenic patients, yet clinicians are confronted with the manifestations of sleep disorders in schizophrenic patients on a regular basis. The first suggestion in this regard is to evaluate the exact nature of the sleep disturbance(s), as noted. Many patients with schizophrenia demonstrate prominent alterations in circadian rhythm sleep–wake schedules.[16] A few studies have reported favorable responses to the administration of melatonin in schizophrenic patients who manifest circadian rhythm sleep schedule abnormalities.[80–82] The use of sedating antipsychotic medications, such as quetiapine, either as monotherapy or to supplement treatment with a minimally sedating antipsychotic drug in the treatment of schizophrenic patients with sleep disturbances, has clearly become a favored strategy for many psychiatrists.[83] Many of the prominently sedating antipsychotic agents, including quetiapine, olanzapine, and clozapine, are associated with a significant risk for producing symptoms associated with the metabolic syndrome. Additionally, the potential for such agents to produce significant daytime somnolence, and thus bring about negative consequences with regard to functional improvement must be carefully considered. Limited data are available to judge the efficacy and adverse effects of approved sleep medications such as zolpidem, eszopiclone, and zaleplon in this population, so the use of these agents becomes a matter of clinical judgment, not guided by an evidence-base. Additionally, the use of a low-dose sedating antidepressant drug, such as trazodone or doxepin, represents another plausible, although unproven strategy in this population, as does the potential use of the melatonin agonist ramelteon. Finally, as noted in Chapter 14, suvorexant is a recently approved treatment for insomnia that has a novel mechanism of action. It remains to be determined whether this new pharmacologic option may be of value in patients with schizophrenia who manifest prominent symptoms of insomnia.

SUMMARY

Sleep disturbance is a critical aspect of the symptomatology and pathophysiology of schizophrenia regardless of the medication status or clinical phase of the illness. Substantial evidence indicates reduced sleep quality with decreased TST and SE in patients with schizophrenia. Consistent findings from PSG studies conducted in schizophrenic patients include SWS deficits, shortened REM-L, and unchanged REM duration. Several clinical aspects, including positive, negative, and neurocognitive symptoms, suicidality, severity of illness, and outcomes have been associated with sleep architecture abnormalities. Preliminary evidence suggests that dysregulation of selected neurotransmitters and pathways related to the clock genes may play a role in the pathophysiology of sleep–wake cycle disturbances in patients with schizophrenia. Antipsychotic medications usually have a positive impact on sleep quality owing to their sedative effects. Their impact on sleep structure varies depending on their pharmacology and specifically related to their effects on different neurotransmitters systems. Nonpharmacologic and pharmacologic treatments play a role in the management of schizophrenia-sleep disturbances. Accumulated evidence suggests that sleep structure abnormalities identified in schizophrenia can serve as potential therapeutic targets or biomarkers in future investigations.

REFERENCES

1. Benson KL. Sleep in schizophrenia: impairments, correlates, and treatment. Psychiatr Clin North Am 2006;29(4):1033–45.
2. Cohrs S. Sleep disturbances in patients with schizophrenia: impact and effect of antipsychotics. CNS Drugs 2008;22(11):939–62.
3. Lieberman JA, Stroup TS, McEvoy JP, et al. Effectiveness of antipsychotic drugs in patients with chronic schizophrenia. N Engl J Med 2005;353(12):1209–53.
4. Monti JM, Monti D. Sleep in schizophrenia patients and the effects of antipsychotic drugs. Sleep Med Rev 2004;8(2):133–48.
5. Benson KL, Feinberg I. Schizophrenia. In: Kryger MH, Roth T, Dement WC, editors. Principles and practice of sleep medicine. 5th edition. Philadelphia: Elsevier Saunders; 2010. p. 1501–11.
6. Chemerinski E, Beng-Choon H, Flaum M, et al. Insomnia as a predictor for symptom worsening following antipsychotic withdrawal in schizophrenia. Compr Psychiatry 2002;43(5):393–6.
7. Benson KL. Sleep in schizophrenia: pathology and treatment. Sleep Med Clin 2015;10(1):49–55.
8. Haffmans P, Hoencamp E, Knegtering HJ, et al. Sleep disturbance in schizophrenia. Br J Psychiatry 1994;165(5):697–8.
9. Hofstetter JR, Mayeda AR, Happel CR, et al. Sleep and daily activity preferences in schizophrenia: associations with neurocognition and symptoms. J Nerv Ment Dis 2003;191(6):408–10.
10. Ritsner M, Kurs R, Ponizovsky A, et al. Perceived quality of life in schizophrenia: relationships to sleep quality. Qual Life Res 2004;13(4):783–91.
11. Benca RM, Obermeyer WH, Thisted RA, et al. Sleep and psychiatric disorders: a meta-analysis. Arch Gen Psychiatry 1992;49:651–68.
12. Chouinard S, Poulin J, Stip E, et al. Sleep in untreated patients with schizophrenia: a meta-analysis. Schizophr Bull 2004;30(4):957–67.
13. Monti JM, Monti D. Sleep disturbance in schizophrenia. Int Rev Psychiatry 2005; 17(4):247–53.
14. Poulin J, Daoust AM, Forest G, et al. Sleep architecture and its clinical correlates in first episode and neuroleptic naive patients with schizophrenia. Schizophr Res 2003;62:147–53.
15. Keshavan MS, Reynolds CF, Kupfer DJ. Electroencephalographic sleep in schizophrenia: a critical review. Compr Psychiatry 1990;31:34–47.
16. Monti JM, BaHammam AS, Pandi-Perumal SR, et al. Sleep and circadian rhythm dysregulation in schizophrenia. Prog Neuropsychopharmacol Biol Psychiatry 2013;43(2):209–16.
17. Zarcone VP, Benson KL. BPRS symptom factors and sleep variables in schizophrenia. Psychiatry Res 1997;66(2–3):111–20.
18. Tekell JL, Hoffmann R, Hendrickse W, et al. High frequency EEG activity during sleep: characteristics in schizophrenia and depression. Clin EEG Neurosci 2005;36(1):25–35.
19. Taylor SF, Goldman RS, Tandon R, et al. Neuropsychological function and REM sleep in schizophrenic patients. Biol Psychiatry 1992;32(6):529–38.
20. Yang C, Winkelman JW. Clinical significance of sleep EEG abnormalities in chronic schizophrenia. Schizophr Res 2006;82:251–60.

21. Tandon R, Shipley JE, Taylor S, et al. Electroencephalographic sleep abnormalities in schizophrenia. Relationship to positive/negative symptoms and prior neuroleptic treatment. Arch Gen Psychiatry 1992;49:185–94.
22. Lauer CJ, Schreiber W, Pollmächer T, et al. Sleep in schizophrenia: a polysomnographic study of drug-naive patients. Neuropsychopharmacology 1997;16:51–60.
23. van Kammen DP, van Kammen WB, Peters J, et al. Decreased slow-wave sleep and enlarged lateral ventricles in schizophrenia. Neuropsychopharmacology 1988;1(4):265–71.
24. Tandon R, DeQuardo JR, Taylor SF, et al. Phasic and enduring negative symptoms in schizophrenia: biological markers and relationship to outcome. Schizophr Res 2000;45(3):191–201.
25. Keshavan MS, Pettegrew JW, Reynolds CF 3rd, et al. Biological correlates of slow wave sleep deficits in functional psychoses: 31P-magnetic resonance spectroscopy. Psychiatry Res 1995;57(2):91–100.
26. Riemann D, Hohagen F, Krieger S, et al. Cholinergic REM induction test: muscarinic supersensitivity underlies polysomnographic findings in both depression and schizophrenia. J Psychiatr Res 1994;28(3):195–210.
27. Malik S, Kanwar A, Sim LA, et al. The association between sleep disturbances and suicidal behaviors in patients with psychiatric diagnoses: a systematic review and meta-analysis. Syst Rev 2014;3:18.
28. Keshavan MS, Reynolds CF, Montrose D, et al. Sleep and suicidality in psychotic patients. Acta Psychiatr Scand 1994;89(2):122–5.
29. Wilson S, Argyropoulos S. Sleep in schizophrenia: time for closer attention. Br J Psychiatry 2012;200(4):273–4.
30. Manoach DS, Cain MS, Vangel MG, et al. A failure of sleep-dependent procedural learning in chronic, medicated schizophrenia. Biol Psychiatry 2004;56:951–6.
31. Goder R, Boigs M, Braun S, et al. Impairment of visuospatial memory is associated with decreased slow wave sleep in schizophrenia. J Psychiatr Res 2004;38:591–9.
32. Bódizs R, Lázár AS. Schizophrenia, slow wave sleep and visuospatial memory: sleep-dependent consolidation or trait-like correlation? J Psychiatr Res 2006; 40(1):89–90.
33. Forest GV, Poulin J, Daoust AM, et al. Attention and non-REM sleep in neuroleptic-naive persons with schizophrenia and control participants. Psychiatry Res 2007;149:33–40.
34. Taylor SF, Tandon R, Shipley JE, et al. Effect of neuroleptic treatment on polysomnographic measures in schizophrenia. Biol Psychiatry 1991;30(9):904–12.
35. Goldman M, Tandon R, DeQuardo JR, et al. Biological predictors of 1-year outcome in schizophrenia in males and females. Schizophr Res 1996;21(2):65–73.
36. Abi-Dargham A. Do we still believe in the dopamine hypothesis? New data bring new evidence. Int J Neuropsychopharmacol 2004;7(Suppl 1):S1–5.
37. Carlsson A, Waters N, Holm-Waters S, et al. Interactions between monoamines, glutamate, and GABA in schizophrenia: new evidence. Annu Rev Pharmacol Toxicol 2001;41:237–60.
38. Javitt DC. Glutamate as a therapeutic target in psychiatric disorders. Mol Psychiatry 2004;9(11):984–97.
39. Vacher CM, Gassmann M, Desrayaud S, et al. Hyperdopaminergia and altered locomotor activity in GABAB1-deficient mice. J Neurochem 2006; 97(4):979–91.
40. Monti JM, Hawkins M, Jantos H, et al. Biphasic effects of dopamine D-2 receptor agonists on sleep and wakefulness in the rat. Psychopharmacology (Berl) 1988; 95:395–400.

41. Monti JM, Jantos H, Fernandez M. Effects of the dopamine D-2 receptor agonist, quinpirole on sleep and wakefulness in the rat. Eur J Pharmacol 1989;169:61–6.
42. Wassef A, Baker J, Kochan LD. GABA and schizophrenia: a review of basic science and clinical studies. J Clin Psychopharmacol 2003;23:601–40.
43. Javitt DC. Intracortical mechanisms of mismatch negativity dysfunction in schizophrenia. Audiol Neurootol 2000;5(3–4):207–15.
44. Benson KL, Faull KF, Zarcone VP. Evidence for the role of serotonin in the regulation of slow wave sleep in schizophrenia. Sleep 1991;14(2):133–9.
45. van Kammen DP, Peters J, van Kammen WB, et al. CSF norepinephrine in schizophrenia is elevated prior to relapse after haloperidol withdrawal. Biol Psychiatry 1989;26(2):176–88.
46. Taheri S, Zeitzer JM, Mignot E. The role of hypocretins (orexins) in sleep regulation and narcolepsy. Annu Rev Neurosci 2002;25:283–313.
47. Nishino S, Ripley B, Mignot E, et al. CSF hypocretin-1 levels in schizophrenics and controls: relationship to sleep architecture. Psychiatry Res 2002;110(1):1–7.
48. Hobson JA, Stickgold R, Pace-Schott EF. The neuropsychology of REM sleep dreaming. Neuroreport 1998;9:R1–14.
49. Janowsky DS, Davis JM, El-Yousef MK, et al. A cholinergic–adrenergic hypothesis of mania and depression. Lancet 1972;2:632–5.
50. Benson KL, Sullivan EV, Lim KO, et al. Slow wave sleep and computed tomographic measures of brain morphology in schizophrenia. Psychiatry Res 1996;60(2–3):125–34.
51. Keshavan MS, Reynolds CF 3rd, Ganguli R, et al. Eletroencephalographic sleep and cerebral morphology in functional psychoses: a preliminary study with computed tomography. Psychiatry Res 1991;39(3):293–301.
52. Mazzoccoli G, Pazienza V, Vinciguerra M. Clock genes and clock-controlled genes in the regulation of metabolic rhythms. Chronobiol Int 2012;29:227–51.
53. Sollars PJ, Pickard GE. The Neurobiology of Circadian Rhythms. Psychiatr Clin N Am 2015. press.
54. Dibner C, Schibler U, Albrecht U. The mammalian circadian timing system: organization and coordination of central and peripheral clocks. Annu Rev Physiol 2010;72:517–49.
55. Takao T, Tachikawa H, Kawanishi Y, et al. CLOCK gene T3111C polymorphism is associated with Japanese schizophrenics: a preliminary study. Eur Neuropsychopharmacol 2007;17:273–6.
56. Mansour HA, Wood J, Logue T, et al. Association study of eight circadian genes with bipolar I disorder, schizoaffective disorder and schizophrenia. Genes Brain Behav 2006;5:150–7.
57. Yujnovsky I, Hirayama J, Doi M, et al. Signaling mediated by the dopamine D2 receptor potentiates circadian regulation by CLOCK: BMAL1. Proc Natl Acad Sci U S A 2006;103:6386–9.
58. DeMartinis NA, Winokur A. Effects of psychiatric medications on sleep and sleep disorders. CNS Neurol Disord Drug Targets 2006;6(1):17–29.
59. Winokur A, Kamath J. The effect of typical and atypical antipsychotic drugs on sleep of schizophrenic patients. In: Monti JM, Pandi-Perumal BL, Nutt JM, editors. Serotonin: molecular, functional and clinical aspects. Basel (Switzerland): Birkhauser, Verlag AG; 2008. p. 587–610.
60. Richelson E. Preclinical pharmacology of neuroleptics: focus on new generation compounds. J Clin Psychiatry 1996;57(1):4–11.

61. Richelson E, Souder T. Binding of antipsychotic drugs to human brain receptors: focus on newer generation compounds. Life Sci 2000;68(1):29–39.
62. Meltzer HY, Li Z, Kaneda Y, et al. Serotonin receptors: their key role in drugs to treat schizophrenia. Prog Neuropsychopharmacol Biol Psychiatry 2003;27(7):1159–72.
63. Dugovic C, Wauquier A. 5–HT2 receptors could be primarily involved in the regulation of slow-wave sleep in the rat. Eur J Pharmacol 1987;137(1):145–6.
64. Idzikowski C, Mills FJ, Glennard R. 5-hydroxytryptamine-2 antagonist increases human slow wave sleep. Brain Res 1986;378(1):164–8.
65. Declerck AL, Wauquier A, Van der Ham-Veltman PHM, et al. Increase in slow-wave sleep in humans with the serotonin-S2 antagonist ritanserin: the first exploratory polysomnographic study. Curr Ther Res Clin Exp 1987;41(6):427–32.
66. Katsuda Y, Walsh AE, Ware CJ, et al. meta-Chlorophenylpiperazine decreases slow-wave sleep in humans. Biol Psychiatry 1993;33(1):49–51.
67. Sharpley AL, Solomon RA, Fernando AL, et al. Dose-related effects of selective 5-HT2 receptor antagonists on slow-wave sleep in humans. Psychopharmacology (Berl) 1990;101(7):568–9.
68. Luthringer R, Staner L, Noel N, et al. A double-blind, placebo-controlled randomized study evaluating the effect of paliperidone extended release tablets on sleep architecture in patients with schizophrenia. Int Clin Psychopharmacol 2007;22(5): 299–308.
69. Cohrs S, Pohlmann K, Guan Z, et al. Sleep-promoting properties of quetiapine in healthy subjects. Psychopharmacology (Berl) 2004;174(3):421–9.
70. Cohrs S, Meier A, Neumann AC, et al. Improved sleep continuity and increased slow wave sleep and REM latency during ziprasidone treatment: a randomized, controlled crossover trial of 12 health male subjects. J Clin Psychiatry 2005; 66(8):989–96.
71. Miller DD. Atypical antipsychotics: sleep, sedation and efficacy. Prim Care Companion J Clin Psychiatry 2004;6(Suppl 2):3–7.
72. Winkelman JW. Schizophrenia, obesity, and obstructive sleep apnea. J Clin Psychiatry 2001;62:8–11.
73. Sharafkhaneh A, Giray N, Richardson P, et al. Association of psychiatric disorders and sleep apnea in a large cohort. Sleep 2005;28(11):1405–11.
74. Takahashi KI, Shimizu T, Sugita T, et al. Prevalence of sleep-related respiratory disorders in 101 schizophrenic inpatients. Psychiatry Clin Neurosci 1998;52(2): 229–31.
75. Surani SR. Diabetes, sleep apnea, obesity and cardiovascular disease: why not address them together? World J Diabetes 2014;5(3):381–4.
76. Stahl SM, Mignon L, Meyer JM. Which comes first: atypical antipsychotic treatment or cardiometabolic risk? Acta Psychiatr Scand 2009;119(3):171–9.
77. Allen RP, Earley CJ. Restless legs syndrome: a review of clinical and pathophysiologic features. J Clin Neurophysiol 2001;18:128–47.
78. Ancoli-Israel S, Martin J, Jones DW, et al. Sleep-disordered breathing and periodic limb movements in sleep in older patients with schizophrenia. Biol Psychiatry 1999;45(11):1426–32.
79. Waters F, Manoach DS. Sleep dysfunction in schizophrenia: a practical review. Open J Psychiatr 2012;2(4):384–92.
80. Shamir E, Laudon M, Barak Y, et al. Melatonin improves sleep quality of patients with chronic schizophrenia. J Clin Psychiatry 2000;61(5):373–7.
81. Shamir E, Rotenberg VS, Laudon M, et al. First-night effect of melatonin treatment in patients with chronic schizophrenia. J Clin Psychopharmacol 2000;20(6): 691–4.

82. Suresh Kumar PN, Andrade C, Bhakta SG, et al. Melatonin in schizophrenic outpatients: a double-blind, placebo-controlled study. J Clin Psychiatry 2007;68(2):237–41.

83. Andrade C, Suresh Kumar PN. Treating residual insomnia in schizophrenia: examining the options. Acta Psychiatr Scand 2013;127(1):11.

Sleep Disturbance in Substance Use Disorders

Timothy A. Roehrs, PhD*, Thomas Roth, PhD

KEYWORDS

- Insomnia • Daytime sleepiness • Alcoholism • Substance abuse
- Alertness disturbance

KEY POINTS

- All drugs of abuse and alcohol have disruptive effects on sleep, sleep stages, and consequent next-day alertness.
- These sleep and alertness disturbances may have a contributory role in the initiation, maintenance, and relapse in substance use disorders.
- Whether treatment of the sleep and alertness disturbances alters the risks is unclear.

INTRODUCTION

Drugs of abuse and alcohol have disruptive effects on sleep, in particular, interfering with the ease of falling asleep, increasing the difficulty in maintaining sleep, and altering the cycling of sleep stages from non–rapid eye movement (NREM) sleep to rapid eye movement (REM) sleep. These sleep effects then have a consequent impact on next-day function, including increasing daytime sleepiness and impairing alertness. The sleep and daytime sleepiness/alertness disturbances can be seen both during active substance use and during discontinuation of use. The specific characteristics of the sleep/alertness disturbances for various substances of abuse have been reviewed elsewhere and the reader is directed to these reviews for substance-specific information.[1,2] The purpose of this article is to discuss the modulatory role these sleep disturbances may play in substance use disorders (SUD).

It has been suggested that these sleep and alertness alterations, although not the primary reinforcing mechanism, function as contributing/modulatory factors in initiating and maintaining drug and alcohol abuse and as factors that increase the

Disclosures: T.A. Roehrs: speaker – Elsevier; grantee – Lundbeck; Grants: NIDA grants ROI DA038177, ROI DA017355, ROI DA011448 and NIAAA grants ROI AA013253, ROI AA011264. T. Roth: speaker – Merck; grantee – PG, Sunvion; consultant – AstraZeneca, Aventis, Bayer, BMS, Flamel, Intec, Jazz, Merck, Novartis, Pernix, Pfizer, Shire.
Department of Psychiatry and Behavioral Neuroscience, Sleep Disorders & Research Center, Henry Ford Health System, School of Medicine, Wayne State University, 2799 West Grand Boulevard, Detroit, MI 48202, USA
* Corresponding author.
E-mail address: troehrs1@hfhs.org

Psychiatr Clin N Am 38 (2015) 793–803
http://dx.doi.org/10.1016/j.psc.2015.07.008
0193-953X/15/$

Abbreviations

CBT-I	Cognitive–behavioral treatment for insomnia
DSM-5	*Diagnostic and Statistical Manual of Mental Disorders, fifth edition*
ICSD3	*International Classification of Sleep Disorders, third edition*
MSLT	Multiple Sleep Latency Test
NREM	Non–rapid eye movement
OSA	Obstructive sleep apnea
PLMD	Periodic Limb Movements Disorder
PSG	Polysomnography
REM	Rapid eye movement
RLS	Restless legs syndrome
SUD	Substance use disorders

---

risk for relapse. After briefly discussing diagnostic and measurement issues, this article discusses the role these sleep and alertness alterations play in initiating and maintaining alcohol and substance abuse and in relapse. We also discuss the extent to which treatment of sleep/alertness disturbances impact the risk of relapse. Finally, we briefly make note of the common hypothesized neurobiological pathophysiology underlying insomnia and SUD.

DIAGNOSTIC ISSUES
Sleep Disturbances

The 2 diagnostic systems for sleep disturbances are the *International Classification of Sleep Disorders, third edition* (ICSD3) of the American Academy of Sleep Medicine and the *Diagnostic and Statistical Manual of Mental Disorders, fifth edition* (DSM-5) of the American Psychiatric Association.[3,4] The most common sleep diagnosis associated with SUD is insomnia. Both the ICSD3 and DSM-5 define insomnia as difficulty initiating and maintaining sleep, and/or awakening early in the morning that occurs on 3 or more nights per week, endures for 3 months or more, and causes significant impairment in daytime functioning. Importantly, the sleep disturbance is present despite an adequate opportunity and circumstance to sleep. The diagnostic systems diverge slightly in classifying sleep disturbance in SUD. In DSM-5, insomnia is classified as comorbid with the specific SUD if it occurs beyond the immediate substance use (ie, before and after the discontinuation of substance use), whereas in ICSD3 one of the listed subtypes of insomnia is "insomnia due to drugs or substances." Note that the ICSD3 makes a somewhat stronger causal inference regarding the relation of sleep/alertness disturbance to substance use.

Substance Use Disorders

The generally accepted diagnostic classification system for substance-related disorders is the DSM-5. The DSM-5 reflects a major departure from the DSM-IV and DSM-IVR with regard to the diagnosis of SUD.[5] Substance-related disorders are divided into 2 major classes: (1) Substance Use Disorders and (2) Substance-Induced Disorders. SUD, formerly termed substance abuse and substance dependence (DSM-IVR), are characterized by behaviors and consequences (a total of 11 criteria are listed) in groupings that show impaired control, social impairment, risky use, and pharmacologic consequences (ie, tolerance, withdrawal) associated with the use of 10 classes of substances. Rather than distinguishing abuse and dependence as in DSM-IVR, in DSM-5 the severity of the disorder is rated by the number of symptoms present: mild 2 to 3, moderate 4 to 5, and severe 6 or more.

Substance-induced disorders are characterized by symptoms reflecting the presence of intoxication, withdrawal, or a mental disorder. As this category name implies, the disorder has to be associated with current or very recent use of the substance.

Although most drugs of abuse are disruptive of sleep and/or daytime alertness, such disturbances are not major criteria for SUD in DSM-5. They are mentioned as possible symptoms in a withdrawal syndrome, which is 1 of the 11 criteria for a SUD. DSM-5 emphasizes that symptoms of tolerance development and withdrawal, occurring only in the context of medical treatment (ie, prescribed medications), should not be diagnosed as SUD (distinguishing drug seeking from therapy seeking in clinical practice is discussed elsewhere in this article). Also as discussed elsewhere in this article, the role of disruptions of sleep and daytime alertness in SUD is not elaborated in DSM-5. One of the 11 major diagnostic criteria is "repeated attempts to quit/control use" (ie, relapse). Some of the strongest evidence regarding the role of sleep disturbance in substance abuse relates to the associated increased risk of relapse.[6]

ASSESSING SLEEP AND DAYTIME ALERTNESS DISTURBANCES

It should be noted that in both diagnostic systems, insomnia is a symptom based diagnosis. Objective markers such as polysomnographic (PSG) measures of sleep and sleep stages are not part of the diagnostic criteria. PSG refers to the continuous recording of multiple physiologic parameters during sleep that differentiate sleep and wake and the 2 distinct sleep states, NREM and REM sleep. Among insomnia patients, PSG-defined sleep often does not reflect insomnia symptoms.[7] On the other hand, as noted, in insomnia comorbid with SUD, PSG-defined disturbances of sleep, or more specifically alteration of sleep stages, have been shown for most all of the substances with abuse liability and have been shown to predict relapse (ie, slow wave sleep or REM sleep disturbance).[6]

An important diagnostic criterion for insomnia is that the sleep disturbance "causes significant impairment in daytime functioning." One of the most consistent findings of daytime impairment associated with insomnia is the presence of elevated latencies on the Multiple Sleep Latency Test (MSLT).[7] The MSLT uses standard PSG technology and scoring to assess the level of daytime sleepiness/alertness, calculated as the average time to fall asleep on 4 to 5 sleep opportunities conducted at 2-hour intervals across the day. People with insomnia have unusually high MSLT latencies compared with healthy volunteers, particularly given their disrupted and reduced nocturnal sleep times.[7] In healthy volunteers, decreasing sleep time and disrupting sleep continuity reduces MSLT latencies.[7] MSLT elevation (ie, hypervigilance) is consistent with neuroimaging, sympathetic nervous system, and hypothalamic–pituitary–adrenocortical axis monitoring findings that all show the presence of a state of "hyperarousal" associated with insomnia that is, present across the night and day.[7] We discuss the role "hyperarousal" may play in initiating and maintaining SUD elsewhere in this article.

An important qualification in diagnosing insomnia is that there be adequate opportunity and circumstances for sleep. That implies that there be adequate bedtime to express the full duration and compliment of sleep stages. NREM and REM sleep cycle across the night in 90- to 120-minute cycles. However, the relative presence of NREM and REM are not proportionally distributed over those cycles. The majority of slow wave sleep occurs during the first 2 cycles and the majority of REM sleep occurs during the last 2 cycles. Reducing sleep opportunity experimentally or by allowing patient/subject determination of the end of the sleep period may reduce artificially the amount of REM sleep. This distinction is particularly important given that 1 prominent sleep disturbance in SUD is early awakening with difficulty returning to sleep. Notably, a prominent effect of alcohol and many abused substances involves the suppression of REM sleep followed by a rebound and fragmentation of REM sleep during discontinuation.[6]

DISTINGUISHING THERAPY SEEKING AND DRUG SEEKING

The DSM-5 criteria for SUD involve an important caution that tolerance development and withdrawal symptoms occurring only in the context of medically indicated use of a prescribed drug should not lead to a SUD diagnosis. The sleep-specific signs during discontinuation may include REM sleep rebound or rebound insomnia, because many of the substances of abuse and alcohol alter these sleep parameters.[6] This rebound may lead to therapy seeking, making it difficult to differentiate drug-seeking from therapy-seeking behaviors.

In drug seeking, the drug and its effects, typically its "euphorogenic" effects, are the focus of the drug use, whereas in therapy seeking, the alleviation of the disease-related symptoms is the focus of the drug use. However, in the clinic, drug seeking and therapy seeking can become closely intertwined and what was once therapy seeking can shift to drug seeking. The challenge is to differentiate the 2 behaviors in making diagnoses and appropriately treating patients. The defining characteristic of drug seeking is evidence that the drug is taken in excessive amounts, in nontherapeutic contexts, and is preferred over other commodities (eg, money) and various social and occupational activities. The degree to which that the drug is chosen over other commodities or social activities provides evidence supporting its risk for abuse. The scientific literature for most drugs of abuse indicates that the drug is readily discriminated from placebo by behavioral and subjective assessments, which include ratings of the drug for it "euphorogenic" and drug-liking effects.[8] That is, the mood effects of the drug are the focus of its use.

In contrast, therapy seeking is evident if the drug has demonstrated efficacy for the disorder or condition being treated. Therapy seeking is also supported if the patient has the signs and symptoms of the appropriate diagnosis for the indicated use of the drug. The pattern of drug taking, including its dose, timing, and duration of use, should be consistent with its therapeutic effects. If the drug is no longer effective, its use is discontinued. Evidence supporting therapy-seeking behavior also includes that the patient believes that the drug is effective and readily experiences its therapeutic benefits.

The drug-seeking versus therapy-seeking distinction becomes difficult in situations where therapy seeking shifts to drug-seeking behavior. As noted, although presleep alcohol use may initially be effective in improving sleep onset for someone with insomnia, rapid tolerance development is likely, which may lead to dose escalation. Further, other of alcohol's reinforcing effects (ie, its "euphorogenic" effects) may be discovered by the person, especially as dose is escalated. At that point, its use may extend beyond the therapeutic context (ie, solely before sleep as a sleep inducer). A similar shifting pattern can be described for stimulant or opiate use. On the other hand, drug seeking may be maintained because the drug, in addition to its mood altering and "euphorogenic" effects, also has therapeutic effects (ie, the stimulant effects of cocaine or amphetamine do in fact reverse the excessive sleepiness that is experienced during drug discontinuation). Thus, the dependence is maintained by a combination of its mood-altering effects and its therapeutic effects, a circumstance that has been referred to as "self-medication."

ALERTNESS/SLEEP DISTURBANCE AND INITIATION OF SUBSTANCE ABUSE

Tetrahydrocannabinol, sedative-hypnotics, and alcohol may become reinforcers and lead to substance abuse through their capacity to induce sleep in persons with insomnia or to reverse a waking "hyperaroused" state. Volunteers with DSM-IVR–diagnosed insomnia and PSG-determined sleep disturbance, but no history of alcoholism or drug abuse, when given an opportunity to choose between previously experienced color-coded alcohol and placebo beverages at night before sleep, chose alcohol, whereas healthy volunteers with a similar level of self-reported social drinking chose placebo.[9] At baseline, the insomniacs had less slow wave sleep than the age-matched volunteers and the alcohol normalized their slow wave sleep. After 6 consecutive nights of the same alcohol dose, tolerance developed to the sleep effects. When given an opportunity to self-administer multiple doses before sleep after 6 nights of prior alcohol exposure, the insomniacs increased the dose compared with insomniacs randomized to take placebo for 6 nights.[10] A number of questions arise from these studies, including:

1. Would the insomniacs continue dose escalation in the face of the loss of hypnotic efficacy?
2. Would the hypnotic use lead to increased social drinking?
3. Would other of alcohol's effects such as its "euphorogenic" effects be discovered with increased dose or daytime use?

Studies have also assessed characteristics of sleep and responses to sleep challenges that reflect sleep regulatory processes in people with alcoholism or at risk for alcoholism. In children with a positive parental history of alcoholism compared with those that are family history negative, spectral analyses of the sleep electroencephalogram revealed less power in the slow wave sleep frequency bands and lower spindle frequency ranges.[11] In light of the fact that sleep is regulated by homeostatic processes, 1 approach to assessing the sleep homeostat is to assess slow wave activity in response to sleep challenges such as sleep restriction or sleep deprivation.[12] A study compared slow wave activity in alcohol-dependent adults with age-matched healthy volunteers at baseline and after sleep restriction. The alcohol-dependent group showed a blunted slow wave activity response (ie, decreased homeostatic sleep drive) to the sleep restriction.[12] These studies suggest that a slow wave sleep deficiency may be associated with the development of alcoholism. One of the known effects of alcohol on sleep is an enhancement of slow wave sleep with acute use.

Benzodiazepine receptor agonists are known to have a moderate abuse liability. In a series of studies of the abuse liability of benzodiazepine receptor agonists, subjects with DSM-IVR insomnia and PSG-determined sleep disturbance were randomized to 12 months of nightly zolpidem (10 mg) or placebo.[13] During 1-week probes in months 1, 4, and 12, they were given an opportunity to self-administer up to 15 mg of zolpidem (three 5-mg capsules) before sleep. In the subjects randomized to zolpidem, the dose was not escalated over the 12 months of nightly use. However, case reports of hypnotic abuse continue to appear in the literature and an analysis of the reports has identified 2 characteristic patterns in the cases: (1) the dose is escalated within 2 weeks of initiating use and (2) the nighttime hypnotic use extends to daytime use.[14] But 1 caution is to be made, stable daytime use does not always imply abuse. An earlier study not only showed nighttime self-administration of triazolam versus placebo by people with insomnia, but during separate daytime self-administration assessments in the same individuals, triazolam was also self-administered relative to placebo during the daytime. However, only those who showed evidence of daytime physiologic "hyperarousal" (ie, elevated latencies on the MSLT) self-administered during the day and triazolam normalized their MSLTs.[15] Whether these drug self-administration patterns reflect drug seeking or therapy seeking needs to be considered in the context of issues discussed herein.

ALERTNESS/SLEEP DISTURBANCE AND MAINTENANCE OF SUBSTANCE ABUSE

The alerting effects of stimulants are reinforcing for individuals who experience sleepiness, fatigue, or have difficulty functioning to a "normal" level. Healthy volunteers will self-administer a stimulant when they are sleepy, but not when alert.[16] Thus, self-administration of stimulants does not necessarily imply abuse. However, in substance abuse, sleepiness may be present as part of a withdrawal syndrome (ie, abstinence) after chronic nonmedical use of a stimulant. An early laboratory study assessed the disruptive effects of cocaine administration and discontinuation on sleep and daytime alertness.[17] Cocaine (600 mg/d) insufflated between 6 and 9 pm on 5 consecutive nights delayed sleep onset by 3 to 4 hours. During the first 2 discontinuation days, average daily sleep latency on the MSLT was less than 5 minutes (ie, a pathologic level of sleepiness), at least in part owing to the severely shortened sleep over the prior 5 days of cocaine use. The MSLT also showed multiple sleep onset REM periods, probably owing to a REM rebound secondary to the prior REM sleep suppression during the cocaine administration nights. After 14 days of abstinence, a nocturnal sleep disturbance and REM sleep rebound remained, although the MSLTs were free of sleep onset REM periods and the latencies returned to essentially normal levels.

It has been hypothesized that continued substance use, difficulty reducing use, and relapse may reflect "self-medication" to reverse the excessive sleepiness of the abstinence. In chronic caffeine or nicotine dependence, the 7- to 8-hour sleep period is functionally an enforced abstinence and given the pharmacokinetics of these drugs, the 8-hour abstinence during the sleep period is followed by enhanced sleepiness in the morning, and in extreme cases, smoking during the night. Caffeine or nicotine taken immediately when arising reverses the sleepy state. In amphetamine or cocaine abuse, excessive sleepiness during the initial drug abstinence has been consistently reported. Again, use of these stimulants will reverse the sleepiness.

During a period of chronic drug use, daytime sleepiness may also result from a drug-induced disturbance of nocturnal sleep, as illustrated. All the stimulants disrupt nocturnal sleep, with severity depending on dose and proximity of use to the sleep period. Disrupted and fragmented sleep produces daytime sleepiness. One could hypothesize that a drug-induced sleep disturbance at night leads to daytime sleepiness, which then enhances the likelihood of the self-administration of a stimulant during the day. This is a complex balance that always has to be dealt with in patients with excessive daytime sleepiness being prescribed stimulants. Also, this is the common vicious circle seen in heavy coffee drinkers. The vicious cycle raises questions as to how much dose escalation of stimulants, including coffee, is owing to tolerance versus an exacerbation of the daytime sleepiness associated with accumulated sleep loss.

The state of sleepiness may not necessarily be drug induced. It may also occur owing to chronic insufficient sleep in healthy people or owing to disturbed sleep efficiency and circadian dysrhythmia seen in persons with altered work and sleep–wake schedules, such as seen among shift workers or with "jet-lag". As noted, healthy volunteers will self-administer a stimulant when experiencing sleepiness[16]. Night workers and rotating shift workers have shortened and disturbed sleep when sleeping during the day, as well as increased sleepiness when awake at night. Rotating shift workers and night workers report a disproportionate use of sedating drugs, especially alcohol, to improve sleep and stimulants, especially caffeine, to improve alertness.[18,19] This substance use may increase risks of substance abuse.

Studies have shown that acute REM deprivation by awakening enhances pain sensitivity.[20] Thus, whether the known REM suppression of opiates is reducing their analgesic effect is a critical question. Additionally, whether the hypothesized reduced analgesic effect then leads to the need for higher opiate doses and to the development of physical dependence is also a critical issue.

ALERTNESS/SLEEP DISTURBANCE AND RELAPSE OF SUBSTANCE ABUSE

The majority of research on sleep disturbance as predictive of relapse in the substance abuse literature is reported for alcoholism.[6] Abnormal sleep patterns can persist for up to 3 years in alcoholism. Sleep remains shortened and REM sleep pressure elevated as reflected in increased REM percentages, shortened latencies to REM sleep and higher REM densities.[21] Although it is tempting to attribute these sleep abnormalities to the excessive alcohol drinking of the patients, the sleep problems could have preceded the development of the alcoholism (see Alertness/sleep disturbance and initiation of substance abuse) or they could be secondary to the development of other medical and psychiatric disorders that have developed during the excessive alcohol drinking.

Both objective and subjective measures of sleep after acute abstinence predict the likelihood of relapse during long-term abstinence. Early laboratory studies suggested that low levels of slow wave sleep are predictive of alcohol drinking relapse.[22] Other more recent studies have identified REM sleep disturbances, either increased REM sleep percent or shortened REM sleep latency as predictive of relapse.[23] Sleep-related relapse risk was greater than that associated with other variables such as age, marital status, employment, duration and severity of alcoholism, hepatic enzymes, and depression ratings.

A first of its kind study in cocaine-dependent individuals undergoing 12 days of inpatient abuse treatment and 6 weeks of outpatient behavioral treatment collected PSGs on weeks 1, 3, and 6 after discontinuation of cocaine.[24] Total sleep time was positively related to days of abstinence over the 6-week study. Other than alcohol, this is among the first studies in substance abusers that we are aware of relating PSG-defined sleep measures to relapse. These data raise the question whether insomnia-focused treatment would have a beneficial effect on substance use treatment.

TREATMENT OF SLEEP/ALERTNESS IN SUBSTANCE USE DISORDERS

The drug class of choice for insomnia treatment in patients without comorbid alcoholism is the benzodiazepine receptor agonists. However, although these drugs have a relatively moderate abuse liability in those without alcoholism or a history of sedative abuse, their risk in outpatients with alcoholism after acute inpatient withdrawal is unknown.[25] These drugs are effective for the immediate inpatient withdrawal syndrome, because they share the same mechanism of action as alcohol itself, promotion of gamma-aminobutyric acid inhibition.[26] A further caution to their outpatient use is that they have a high potential for toxicity and overdose when combined with alcohol,[26] thereby being dangerous for the people with the potential for alcoholism relapse.

Sedating antidepressant medications such as trazodone or doxepin are often used in the United States to treat insomnia and insomnia comorbid with depression. Trazodone (50–300 mg) has been used to treat sleep disturbance in patients with alcoholism in open-label, noncontrolled studies and has shown improved self-report measures of insomnia.[26] Drinking outcomes in trials with sleep promoting agents are mixed. A recently completed large placebo-controlled trial of the anticonvulsant, gabapentin (900 or 1800 mg), showed improvement in both sleep and drinking outcomes for both doses of gabapentin.[27] Currently, the 3 alcoholism treatments approved by the US Food and Drug Administration are disulfiram, naltrexone, and acamprostate. A placebo-controlled trial of acamprostate 666 mg for 15 days improved wake after sleep onset and stage 3 sleep on the 2 PSG nights, night 2 and night 15.[26] Unfortunately, drinking outcomes and their relation to sleep were not reported in this study.

Cognitive–behavioral treatment for insomnia (CBT-I) is an alternative to medications and several trials of CBT-I in patients with alcoholism associated with sleep disturbance have been conducted. A randomized, controlled trial of a brief CBT-I associated with alcoholism was conducted in 60 insomnia patients without comorbid depression.[28] The CBT-I treatment compared with wait-list controls improved sleep diary measures of sleep quality, sleep efficiency, awakenings, and time to fall asleep. However, CBT-I had no impact on drinking relapse rates over the 6-month follow-up period. An open trial of CBT-I in patients with alcoholism similarly found improved sleep, but not improved drinking outcomes.[29]

The literature on treating sleep disturbance in drug abuse is even more limited than that for alcoholism, but results reported for the few studies that have been carried out to date are provocative. A trial of CBT-I for insomnia and daytime sleepiness in adolescents reported improved sleep for those completing more than 4 sessions.[30] The improved sleep showed a trend toward reducing substance abuse problems at the 1-year follow-up. A treatment trial involving nicotine-dependent adults compared a 16- versus 24-hour nicotine patch during smoking abstinence.[31] The nicotine patch reduced smoking urges, with the 24-hour patch having a greater effect than the 16-hour patch. Interestingly, the 24-hour patch improved sleep, specifically the amount of slow wave sleep. This result in nicotine-dependent adults is in contrast with the sleep-disruptive effects of a nicotine patch on the sleep of nonsmokers. In the drug abuse treatment literature, sleep is rarely included as an outcome measure or considered a mediator of other outcome measures. A placebo-controlled trial of modafinil 400 mg/d in cocaine-dependent individuals improved the latency and sleep staging of sleep and reduced daytime sleepiness, but relapse outcomes were not measured.[32] The need for clinical trials that focus on treatment of sleep complaints in substance abuse is clearly evident. An inherent assumption in this discussion is that sleep disturbance is causally related to alcoholism or drug abuse, either as the precipitant or consequence. It should be noted that the sleep disturbance may be comorbid and independent or related to a third common factor. A recent review of the treatment literature concluded that the disorders are comorbid and treatment must be directed at both disorders.[33]

COMMON NEUROBIOLOGICAL DISTURBANCES

Insomnia and SUD may share a common neurobiological disturbance. A convergence of data from nighttime and daytime electrophysiology, event-related brain potential recordings, neuroimaging studies, sympathetic nervous system, and hypothalamic–pituitary–adrenal axis monitoring all suggest that insomnia is a disorder of "hyperarousal."[6] The pathology underlying this hyperarousal is in part an hypothalamic–pituitary–adrenocortical axis dysfunction involving corticotropin-releasing hormone and norepinephrine.[7] Many theories of addiction hypothesize that stress increases vulnerability to drug abuse.[34] Animal literature and human neuroimaging studies have identified brain circuits involved in stress that include release of corticotropin-releasing hormone from the paraventicular nucleus and norepinephrine activation initiated in locus coeruleus.[34] This corticotropin-releasing hormone/norepinephrine activation also activates dopaminergic brain motivational pathways known to be engaged by drugs of abuse including the ventral tegmental area and nucleus accumbens[34] (see Chapter 2). Thus, stress coactivates brain stress and reward circuits simultaneously. Therefore, at a behavioral level, stress enhances the positive, rewarding properties of drugs with abuse liability.

SUMMARY

The role of sleep/alertness disturbance in SUD is not understood fully. As this discussion indicates, sleep disturbances are at least contributory to SUD. From the epidemiologic literature it is known that insomnia is a risk factor for substance abuse.[17,18] However, the extent to which insomnia or daytime sleepiness leads to new cases of alcoholism or drug abuse is not known. Furthermore, the degree to which treatment of insomnia or daytime sleepiness in abstinent alcoholics and drug abusers reduces risk of relapse has yet to be determined. To date, the few alcoholism treatment trials have failed to demonstrate clearly that improved sleep reduces relapse, and the only available drug abuse treatment trial, although encouraging, is not conclusive.

Another important remaining question relates to the role of specific sleep stages on SUD and their treatment. In reviews of the sleep effects of alcohol and drugs of abuse, it is noted that most of the drugs of abuse suppress REM sleep, with tolerance to the REM-suppression developing rapidly.[1,2] The significance of these effects is not clear. Most antidepressants (tricyclics, monoamine oxidase inhibitors, and selective serotonin reuptake inhibitors) are highly potent REM suppressants, typically driving REM sleep to below 10% of the night and tolerance does not develop to the REM suppression produced by these antidepressant drugs, even with chronic use.[35] The degree of REM suppression in depressed patients is associated with improvement in mood.[35] Further, total sleep deprivation and REM sleep deprivation by awakening depressed patients on entry to REM sleep has antidepressant effects in patients with depression.[35]

At the very least, the REM effects may reflect the development of physical dependence and an altered central nervous system neurobiology. Chronic alcohol and drug use likely alters the neurobiology of sleep and the control of REM sleep, a predominately pontine cholinergeric phenomenon. As noted, in abstinent alcoholics, REM sleep disturbance remaining after acute discontinuation is predictive of relapse. We are unaware of studies regarding the presence of a REM disturbance after abstinence for other drugs of abuse and the predictive value of such a disturbance, if present, to relapse.

REFERENCES

1. Roehrs T, Roth T. Medication and substance abuse. In: Kryger M, Roth T, Dement WC, editors. Principles and practice of sleep medicine 5th edition. Part II, section 16. St Louis (MO): Elsevier Saunders; 2010. p. 1512–23.

2. Roehrs T, Roth T. Sleep and sleep disorders. In: Verster JC, Brady K, Galanter M, et al, editors. Drug abuse and addiction in medical illness. New York: Springer; 2012. p. 375–85.
3. American Academy of Sleep Medicine. International classification of sleep disorders. 3rd edition. Darian (IL): American Academy of Sleep Medicine; 2014.
4. American Psychiatric Association. Diagnostic and statistical manual of mental disorders. Washington, DC: American Psychiatric Association; 2013.
5. Hasin DS, O'Brien CP, Auriacombe M, et al. DSM-5 criteria for substance use disorders: recommendations and rationale. Am J Psychiatry 2013;170:834–51.
6. Brower KJ, Perron BE. Sleep disturbance as a universal risk factor for relapse in addictions to psychoactive substances. Med Hypotheses 2010;74:928–33.
7. Roehrs T, Gumenyuk V, Drake C, et al. Physiological correlates of insomnia. Curr Top Behav Neurosci 2014;21:277–90.
8. Rush CR, Madakasira S, Goldman NH, et al. Discriminative stimulus effects of xolpidem in pentobarbital-trained subjects: II. Comparison with triazolam and caffeine in humans. J Pharm Ex Ther 1997;280:174–280.
9. Roehrs T, Papineau K, Rosenthal L, et al. Ethanol as a hypnotic in insomniacs: self administration and effects on sleep and mood. Neuropsychopharmacololgy 1999;20:279–86.
10. Roehrs T, Blaisdell B, Cruz N, et al. Tolerance to hypnotic effects of ethanol in insomniacs. Sleep 2004;27:116ab.
11. Tarokh L, Carskadon MA. Sleep electroencephalogram in children with a parental history of alcohol abuse/dependence. J Sleep Res 2010;19:165–74.
12. Armitage R, Hoffman R, Conroy DA, et al. Effects of a 3-hour sleep delay on sleep homeostasis in alcohol dependent adults. Sleep 2012;35:273–8.
13. Roehrs TA, Randall S, Harris E, et al. Twelve months of nightly zolpidem does not lead to dose escalation: a prospective placebo-controlled study. Sleep 2011;34:1–6.
14. Vigneau-Victorri C, Dailly E, Veyrac G, et al. Evidence of zolpidem abuse and dependence: results of the French Centre for Evaluation and Information on Pharmacodependence (CEIP) network survey. Br J Clin Pharm 2007;64: 198–209.
15. Roehrs T, Bonahoom A, Pedrosi B, et al. Nighttime versus daytime hypnotic self-administration. Psychopharmacology 2002;2161:137–42.
16. Roehrs T, Papineau K, Rosenthal L, et al. Sleepiness and the reinforcing and subjective effects of methylphenidate. Exp Clin Psychopharm 1999;7:145–50.
17. Johanson CE, Roehrs T, Schuh K, et al. The effects of cocaine on mood and sleep in cocaine-dependent males. Exp Clin Psychopharm 1999;4:338–46.
18. Johnson EO, Roehrs T, Roth T, et al. Epidemiology of alcohol and medication as aids to sleep in early adulthood. Sleep 1998;21:178–86.
19. Johnson E, Roehrs T, Roth T, et al. Epidemiology of medication as aids to alertness in early adulthood. Sleep 1999;22:485–8.
20. Roehrs TA, Hyde M, Blaisdell B, et al. Sleep loss and REM sleep loss are hyperalgesic. Sleep 2006;29:145–51.
21. Drummond SPA, Gillin JC, Smith TL, et al. The sleep of abstinent pure primary alcoholic patients: natural course and relation to relapse. Alcohol Clin Exp Res 1998;22:1796–802.
22. Allen RP, Wagman AM, Funderburk FR, et al. Slow wave sleep: a predictor of individuals differences in response to drinking? Biol Psychiatry 1980;15:345–8.
23. Gillin JC, Smith TL, Irwin M, et al. Increased pressure for rapid eye movement sleep at time of hospital admission predicts relapse in nondepressed patients

with primary alcoholism at 3-month follow-up. Arch Gen Psychiatry 1994;51: 189–97.

24. Angarita GA, Canavan SV, Forselius E, et al. Abstinence-related changes in sleep during treatment for cocaine dependence. Drug Alcohol Dep 2014;134:343–7.

25. Brower KJ. Insomnia, alcoholism and relapse. Sleep Med Rev 2003;7:523–39.

26. Kolla BP, Mansukhani MP, Schneek T. Pharmacological treatment of insomnia in alcohol recovery: a systematic review. Alcohol Alcohol 2011;46:578–85.

27. Mason BJ, Quello S, Goodell V, et al. Gabapentin treatment for alcohol dependence. A randomized clinical trial. JAMA Intern Med 2014;174:70–7.

28. Currie SR, Clark S, Hodgins DC, et al. Randomized controlled trial of brief cognitive-behavioural interventions for insomnia in recovering alcoholics. Addiction 2004;99:1121–32.

29. Arnedt JT, Conroy D, Rutt J, et al. An open trial of cognitive-behavioral treatment for insomnia comorbid with alcohol dependence. Sleep Med 2007;8:176–80.

30. Bootzin RR, Stevens SJ. Adolescents, substance abuse, and the treatment of insomnia and daytime sleepiness. Clin Psychol Rev 2005;25:629–44.

31. Aubin HJ, Luthringer R, Demazieres A. Comparison of the effects of a 24-hour nicotine patch and a 16-hour nicotine patch on smoking urges and sleep. Nic Tobac Res 2006;8:193–201.

32. Morgan PT, Pace-Shott E, Pittman B, et al. Normalizing effects of modafinil on sleep in chronic cocaine users. Am J Psychiatry 2010;167:333–40.

33. Brower KJ. Assessment and treatment of insomnia in adult patients with alcohol use disorders. Alcohol 2015;49:417–27.

34. Sinha R. Chronic stress, drug use, and vulnerability to addiction. Ann NY Acad Sci 2008;1141:105–30.

35. Benca RM. Mood disorders. In: Kryger MH, Roth T, Dement WC, editors. Principles and practice of sleep medicine. 4th edition. Philadelphia: Elsevier Saunders; 2005. p. 1311–26.

Circadian Rhythm Sleep-Wake Disorders

Sabra M. Abbott, MD, PhD, Kathryn J. Reid, PhD, Phyllis C. Zee, MD, PhD*

KEYWORDS

- Circadian rhythm sleep-wake disorders • Delayed sleep phase type
- Advanced sleep phase type • Irregular sleep-wake type
- Non-24-hour sleep-wake type • Shift work type

KEY POINTS

- Circadian disruption is associated with adverse effects on physical and mental health.
- Circadian rhythm sleep-wake disorders (CRSWDs) frequently result in circadian misalignment and are often associated with an increased incidence of psychiatric disorders.
- There is a particularly high comorbidity between delayed sleep phase type and psychiatric disorders.
- Treatment of the CRSWDs focuses on a combination of appropriately timed light and melatonin, as well as on overall sleep hygiene.

INTRODUCTION

Disturbances in circadian timing can have profound effects on the quality and quantity of sleep as well as the expression and severity of neuropsychiatric and other medical disorders. It is now recognized that the high prevalence of circadian abnormalities in psychiatric disorders is not only a consequence of psychiatric symptoms but also due to alterations in the circadian regulatory system.[1] Circadian disruption, whether due to changes in the endogenous circadian system or through environmental and behavioral manipulations, can significantly impair sleep and wakefulness as well as mental and physical health.

Circadian (approximately 24-hour) rhythms are genetically regulated and are expressed in all tissues of the human body.[2] Thus, in addition to the sleep-wake cycle, nearly all physiologic and behavioral processes exhibit circadian rhythms, which are regulated by a central pacemaker located in the suprachiasmatic nucleus (SCN) of the anterior hypothalamus. Because the endogenous frequency of the circadian

Disclosure Statement: Drs S.M. Abbott and K.J. Reid have nothing to disclose. Dr P.C. Zee has served as a consultant for Vanda, Philips, and Merck and owns stock in Teva.
Department of Neurology, Northwestern University Feinberg School of Medicine, 710 North Lake Shore Drive, Suite 500, Chicago, IL 60611, USA
* Corresponding author.
E-mail address: p-zee@northwestern.edu

Psychiatr Clin N Am 38 (2015) 805–823
http://dx.doi.org/10.1016/j.psc.2015.07.012
0193-953X/15/$ – see front matter © 2015 Elsevier Inc. All rights reserved.

Abbreviations

AASM	American Academy of Sleep Medicine
CK1ε	Casein kinase 1ε
CRSWD	Circadian rhythm sleep-wake disorder
DLMO	Dim light melatonin onset
DSM-5	Diagnostic and Statistical Manual, Fifth Edition
FDA	US Food and Drug Administration
ICSD-3	International Classification of Sleep Disorders, Third Edition
SCN	Suprachiasmatic nucleus

oscillation in humans is slightly longer than 24 hours,[3] proper alignment with the external 24-hour physical environment and social and work-related activities requires daily adjustments to the internal clock. The light-dark cycle is the strongest synchronizing agent for the circadian system. In humans, light exposure before the core body temperature minimum (evening) produces delays, whereas light pulses after the core body temperature minimum (early morning) produces advances.[4] The SCN receives, in addition to light, internal signals from the pineal gland, via the nocturnal release of melatonin. Endogenous melatonin release begins to increase 2 to 3 hours before sleep onset and peaks in the middle of the night. Melatonin during the early morning delays the timing of circadian rhythms, whereas melatonin during the early evening induces advances in this timing, which is in contrast to the effects of light.[5] Secretion of melatonin from the pineal gland is regulated by the SCN through a projection from the hypothalamus to the superior cervical ganglion of the spinal cord.[6] Through timed exposure of these synchronizing agents (zeitgebers), the SCN makes daily adjustments to maintain synchronization (entrainment) with the external light-dark cycle and social and work schedules. Rhythmic information from the SCN is transmitted to other clocks in the brain and peripheral tissues to coordinate the function of the various organ systems.[7]

This article focuses on approaches to the diagnosis and management of CRSWDs. CRSWDs are characterized by a pattern of sleep disruption that is primarily due to an alteration of the endogenous circadian system or to a misalignment between the endogenous circadian rhythm and the sleep-wake schedule required by an individual's physical environment or social or professional schedule. In addition, the sleep disturbance is associated with symptoms of excessive sleepiness and/or insomnia and causes clinically significant distress or impairment of functioning.[8] The Diagnostic and Statistical Manual, Fifth Edition (DSM-5),[9] and International Classification of Sleep Disorders (ICSD-3)[8] are commonly used in clinical practice. Although the criteria for CRSWDs are similar between ICSD-3 and DSM-5, they do differ in 2 important ways. First, the DSM-5 includes 5 subtypes, delayed sleep phase, advanced sleep phase, non-24-hour sleep-wake, irregular sleep-wake, and shift work types, whereas the ICSD-3 describes 6 CRSWDs (including jet lag disorder). Second, the DSM-5 requires the presence of symptoms for at least 1 month and not for 3 months as in the ICSD-3. This article uses DSM-5 criteria and terminology. Although each of the disorders has its own specific treatments, cognitive and behavioral interventions aimed at maintaining a regular sleep-wake schedule, regular physical and social activities, and appropriate exposure to light are necessary for all patients.

DELAYED SLEEP PHASE TYPE

Delayed sleep phase type is a CRSWD in which an individual's required or preferred sleep and wake times are significantly delayed with respect to conventional times, with habitual bedtimes of typically of 2 to 6 AM or even later. These individuals often present with symptoms of insomnia related to difficulty initiating sleep and excessive daytime sleepiness, due to difficulty falling asleep and waking up earlier than the desired time. However, if patients are allowed to sleep during their preferred times, they exhibit normal sleep quality and duration for age. The DSM-5 also includes 2 sub-types, familial and overlapping with non-24-hour sleep-wake type.[9] Current diagnostic guidelines from the American Academy of Sleep Medicine (AASM) recommend obtaining sleep logs for at least 7 preferably 14 days, with actigraphy monitoring if possible (**Fig. 1**). Standardized chronotype questionnaires indicating the patient is an evening type and measurement of other circadian biomarkers such as the salivary dim light melatonin onset (DLMO) demonstrating a delayed circadian phase can be useful for confirming the diagnosis and for determining the optimal timing of treatment with light and or melatonin.[8]

The overall prevalence of delayed sleep phase type varies depending on the population being evaluated. It seems to be the highest among young adults, ranging from 7% to 16%, whereas it is estimated that approximately 10% of patients presenting to the sleep clinic with complaints of insomnia actually have delayed sleep phase type.[8] In a more recent population-based study of New Zealand adults, the prevalence of delayed sleep phase type ranged from 1.5% to 8.9%, depending on the definition used, and decreased with age.[10]

There are likely many factors contributing to the development of delayed sleep phase type, including genetic, environmental, and behavioral elements. Analysis of polymorphisms of core clock genes in relation to delayed sleep phase type has demonstrated an association between polymorphisms in the gene hPer3 and delayed sleep phase type.[11] These polymorphisms are located near the phosphorylation site for casein kinase Iε (CKIε) and likely play a role in the degradation rate of hPER3, which can affect the overall circadian period length in the individual.

Environmental factors proposed to contribute to the development of delayed sleep phase type include either increased exposure or sensitivity to the delaying effects of evening light or decreased exposure or sensitivity to the advancing effects of morning light. There is evidence in a small sample of patients with delayed sleep phase type demonstrating a greater degree of melatonin suppression in response to evening light, suggesting greater sensitivity to light at this time.[12] Although 2 adolescent studies have shown greater exposure to evening light and less exposure to morning light in evening-type individuals, when corrected for circadian time, there were no differences seen in the pattern of light exposure, suggesting it is not simply a matter of the timing of light exposure causing delayed sleep phase type.[13] Behavioral factors may also contribute to the development of delayed sleep phase type, with individuals choosing to stay up later, resulting in increased exposure to delaying light and decreased exposure to advancing light. Finally there is some evidence of individuals developing delayed sleep phase type after traumatic brain injury, possibly due to disruption of circadian regulatory systems, such as the normal melatonin secretion pathways.[14]

There is high comorbidity with psychiatric disease in individuals with delayed sleep phase type. In a population of 48 individuals with delayed sleep phase type, 75% had at least 1 past psychiatric diagnosis and 50% had a current psychiatric diagnosis, with the most common being substance abuse, mood disorders, or anxiety, alone or in combination.[15] In another study evaluating 90 patients with delayed sleep phase type, 64% had either moderate or severe depression.[16] Patients with delayed sleep phase type are also 3.3 times more likely to report symptoms of seasonal affective disorder.[17] It has also been demonstrated that there is a higher prevalence of delayed sleep phase type in individuals with obsessive-compulsive disorder than in controls.[18]

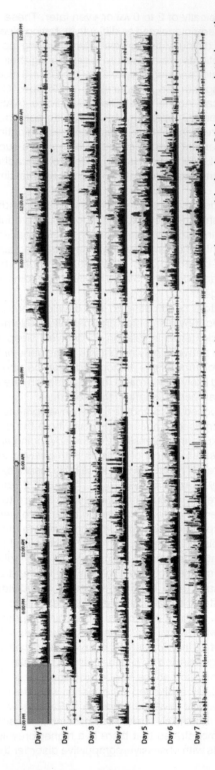

Fig. 1. Actigraphy data from an individual with delayed sleep phase type. Each line represents 48 hours, with the last 24 hours replotted on the following line. This patient went to bed on most days at approximately 6 AM, but on some days as late as 12 PM. Black bars indicate activity, yellow lines indicate light exposure, gray bars indicate the time before recording started, and blue triangles indicate when the patient pushed an event marker to indicate bed or wake time.

The treatment of delayed sleep phase type depends primarily on the timed administration of 2 key entraining signals, light and melatonin, along with maintaining regular sleep-wake times[19] (**Table 1**). Melatonin in the subjective evening and light during the subjective morning both advance the circadian clock; however, the key to treatment of delayed sleep phase type is to appropriately time the interventions with respect to an individual's biological clock rather than the environmental clock; this can be done by first assessing circadian phase markers, such as the timing of the salivary DLMO, or empirical treatment can be attempted based on the patient's current habitual sleep-wake timing.

Varying doses of melatonin have been tested. An early placebo-controlled crossover study demonstrated that 5 mg of melatonin administered 5 hours before DLMO

Table 1
Summary of the recommended diagnostic testing and treatments for the circadian rhythm sleep-wake disorders

Circadian Rhythm Sleep-Wake Disorder	Diagnosis	Treatment
Delayed sleep phase type	Recommended: Sleep logs and/or actigraphy for at least 7 d Optional: Biomarkers such as salivary DLMO. Morningness/eveningness questionnaires	Advance circadian phase: Low dose (0.5–3 mg) of melatonin, 5 h before habitual bedtime; bright light (at least 5000 lux) for 30 min to 2 h on awakening
Advanced sleep phase type	Recommended: Sleep logs and/or actigraphy for at least 7 d Optional: Biomarkers such as salivary DLMO. Morningness/eveningness questionnaires	Delay circadian phase: Bright light (at least 5000 lux) for 2 h in the evening (eg, 7–9 PM)
Irregular sleep-wake type	History and sleep diary (can be completed by caregiver) and/or actigraphy	Consolidate nocturnal sleep: Mixed modality therapy: daytime bright light, melatonin at bedtime (in children); structured activities
Non-24-h sleep-wake type	Recommended: Sleep logs and/or actigraphy for at least 14 d Optional: Sequential measurement of phase markers (eg, salivary DLMO or urine melatonin)	Entrainment: Blind: Melatonin (0.5 mg) or tasimelteon 1 h before habitual bedtime Sighted: Bright light on awakening, regular sleep wake schedule. ± melatonin
Shift work type (night)	Clinical history: Sleep logs and/or actigraphy may also be helpful	Align circadian rhythm to work schedule: Sleep hygiene; bright light intermittent exposure at work; avoid bright light in the early morning; low-dose melatonin sleep time. Excessive sleepiness: Modafinil/armodafinil, scheduled naps, caffeine, bright light Insomnia symptoms: Melatonin, hypnotics

resulted in a 1.5-hour phase advance, on average.[20] More recent studies have used lower doses of melatonin, in part given the concern that higher doses may result in high levels of melatonin persisting into the phase delay portion of the phase response curve. Comparing the effect of 0.5 mg with that of 3 mg of melatonin, the largest phase advances occurred after administration of 0.5 mg of melatonin, 2 to 4 hours before DLMO.[5] As DLMO usually occurs 2 to 3 hours before sleep onset, often treatment is empirically with 0.5 mg of melatonin, given 5 hours before habitual sleep onset. As an added benefit, melatonin has been demonstrated to improve overall depressive scores in patients with delayed sleep phase type.[21]

The treatment response to light has been primarily assessed in normal controls. Several smaller studies have demonstrated that a combination of evening light restriction and 2 hours of morning bright light therapy can successfully advance sleep and core body temperature rhythms.[22,23] However, to avoid inadvertently delaying the clock further, it is important to align the morning bright light therapy with the patient's biological morning, which may be several hours later than the environmental morning.

Several studies have evaluated the combined effects of light and melatonin. In one placebo-controlled trial, subjects were exposed to either bright or dim light and took either a placebo or a melatonin pill, in conjunction with a daily behavioral advance in schedule. All subjects advanced following treatment and showed improvements in daytime sleepiness and cognitive function, suggesting the behavioral change is an important component of treatment; however, only those receiving bright light and melatonin were able to maintain this advance in sleep pattern and the positive effects on sleepiness and cognitive function.[24,25] In another study, subjects were all given 0.5 mg of melatonin, 5 hours before habitual bedtime, along with 2 hours, 1 hour, or 30 minutes of bright (5000 lux) light. Subjects exposed to 2 hours of bright light showed the largest advances (2.4 hours), whereas those exposed to 30 minutes or 1 hour showed smaller but similar advances of 1.7 and 1.8 hours, respectively.[26]

ADVANCED SLEEP PHASE TYPE

Advanced sleep phase type is a CRSWD in which an individual's preferred sleep and wake times are significantly advanced with respect to conventional times. These individuals report an average sleep onset from 6 to 9 PM and wake time of 2 to 5 AM. However, if allowed to sleep during their preferred times, the sleep quality and duration are normal for age.[8] The DSM-5 also includes a subtype for familial cases.[9] Current guidelines from the AASM recommend obtaining sleep logs for at least 7 and preferably 14 days to confirm the diagnosis, with the addition of actigraphy monitoring if possible. Additional optional testing can include chronotype questionnaires, which should demonstrate a morningness preference and analysis of other circadian phase markers such as the salivary DLMO, which should show a significant advance in overall phase.[27] The differential diagnoses for advanced sleep phase type include chronic insomnia and major depressive disorder with early morning awakenings.

Overall, the prevalence of advanced sleep phase type is thought to be much lower than that of delayed sleep phase type, which may in part be because individuals generally experience fewer negative consequences from following an advanced schedule, as compared with the consequences of a delayed schedule. Prevalence estimates range from 1% to as high as 7% depending on the population sampled, with an overall higher prevalence observed in men and in older individuals.[10]

There is a strong hereditary component to advanced sleep phase type,[28] with several familial cohorts identified. Several different mutations have been identified, with the common factor being a mutation in either CKIε or the phosphorylation site for this kinase on the circadian clock protein hPER2.[29–31] Phosphorylation normally serves to stabilize this protein, and without it, the speed of the transcription-translation feedback loop increases, resulting in an overall shortened period.[32]

In individuals lacking a known genetic cause for the disorder, other alternative theories for potential causes include either increased sensitivity or exposure to the advancing effects of morning light or decreased sensitivity or exposure to the delayed effects of evening. In addition, the known familial cases have been reported to demonstrate a shorter overall circadian period,[29] resulting in entrainment at an earlier circadian phase.

There are fewer psychiatric comorbidities reported with advanced sleep phase type, when compared with delayed sleep phase type. However, it is important to distinguish the early morning awakening characteristic of advanced sleep phase type from the early morning awakenings associated with major depression.

Successful treatment of advanced sleep phase type depends primarily on the use of evening bright light, which delays the circadian clock (see **Table 1**). A pilot study using evening bright light in 9 individuals demonstrated a 1- to 2-hour delay in the onset of melatonin, a 2- to 4-hour delay in the core body temperature minimum, and an increase in total sleep time of greater than 1 hour.[33] Treating a larger cohort of 24 individuals with bright light from 7 to 9 PM resulted in a 2-hour phase delay in both temperature and melatonin.[34] Administration of melatonin early in the morning could theoretically also result in delays of the circadian clock. However, there are no large-scale trials demonstrating the safety and efficacy of early morning melatonin administration for the treatment of advanced sleep phase type, and there are some concerns that the sedating effects of melatonin may make its administration during the day undesirable.[35]

IRREGULAR SLEEP-WAKE TYPE

Irregular sleep-wake type is characterized by the absence of a clear single sleep and wake period, with an individual instead having at least 3 separate sleep bouts during a 24-hour period. Within this time frame, the total amount of sleep is normal for age, but it is spread throughout the day rather than occurring all at once.[8] The diagnosis is confirmed with sleep logs, ideally combined with actigraphy monitoring for at least 7 and preferably 14 days (**Fig. 2**). Data obtained by this approach demonstrate an absence of a clear major sleep period and the presence of at least 3 irregular sleep bouts within a 24-hour period, with the longest sleep bout usually occurring at night.[8]

Irregular sleep-wake type is thought to be due to either dysfunction of the central circadian pacemaker or an environmental disruption, resulting in decreased exposure to strong zeitgebers. As a result, the 2 populations in which irregular sleep-wake type is most frequently observed are children with developmental disabilities and adults with neurodegenerative disorders. These individuals often have degeneration of the SCN and are also often institutionalized, resulting in a loss of normal circadian zeitgebers, due to decreased activity and light exposure during the day and disrupted sleep at night.

There are several groups of children in whom irregular sleep phase type has been demonstrated. Children with Angelman syndrome, a disorder characterized by intellectual disability, gait and speech impairments, seizures, and craniofacial abnormalities, have been demonstrated by sleep logs to have an irregular sleep pattern, which correlates with a decreased amplitude of the melatonin rhythm.[36] Smith-Magenis syndrome is a genetic disorder characterized by craniofacial abnormalities, sleep disturbances, and behavioral problems. Although the most common circadian rhythm abnormality observed is an inversion of the sleep-wake cycle, irregular sleep

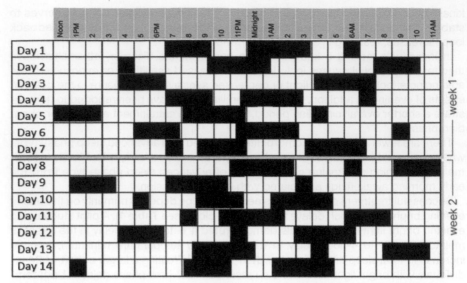

Fig. 2. Example sleep log data from an individual with irregular sleep-wake type. Each line represents 24 hours, with block boxes indicating the sleep period. Note that the individual has multiple sleep bouts throughout the 24-hour period, but total sleep time is within normal limits.

phase type can also be observed, along with a decreased amplitude of melatonin secretion.[37] Finally, autism is frequently associated with abnormalities in the sleep-wake pattern, including irregular sleep phase type.[38]

In the elderly, circadian and sleep-wake disturbances are common.[39] In a population of elderly patients with dementia, sleep diaries demonstrated either irregular or inverted sleep-wake schedules in most patients, with a corresponding alteration in the pattern of core body temperature.[40] There is growing evidence that circadian disruption is an early symptom in many neurodegenerative disorders.[41] A loss of SCN neurons has been demonstrated in individuals with Alzheimer disease with circadian rhythm abnormalities.[42]

External factors can also contribute to the development of irregular sleep phase type. Traumatic brain injury is frequently associated with sleep and circadian disorders. Although the most frequently reported is either insomnia or delayed sleep phase type, irregular sleep phase type has also been reported.[43] The underlying mechanism is presumably related to disruption of the normal melatonin signaling pathways or to damage to the SCN as was seen in a case report of an individual with SCN damage following a gunshot wound to the head, who then developed irregular sleep phase type.[44] Irregular sleep phase type has also been reported in individuals with cranial tumors, such as pituitary adenomas that impinge on the SCN.[45]

Although there has been limited success in some populations with the use of timed light or melatonin alone, the primary treatment of irregular sleep phase type focuses on mixed modality therapy. Daytime bright light exposure in the elderly[46] and in children[47] has been demonstrated to increase nighttime sleep. Melatonin given at bedtime has been demonstrated to improve sleep efficiency in developmentally impaired children[48] but not in elderly patients with dementia.[49] In the elderly with irregular sleep phase type, mixed modality therapy, consisting of a combination of daily light exposure and behavioral strategies to reduce time in bed and increase activity during the day, has been most effective[50] (see **Table 1**).

NON-24-HOUR SLEEP-WAKE TYPE

Non-24-hour sleep-wake type is a CRSWD in which individuals are unable to entrain to the 24-hour day and instead follow their endogenous circadian period, which is usually slightly longer than 24 hours. Their sleep-wake pattern moves progressively later each day, eventually alternating between sleeping during the night and sleeping during the day. Because of this pattern, sleep complaints may consist of insomnia, excessive daytime sleepiness, or both.[8] Diagnostic recommendations from the AASM include obtaining sleep logs and actigraphy for at least 14 days to confirm the presence of a non-24-hour pattern (**Fig. 3**).[27] However, in some cases, monitoring for even longer than 14 days may be necessary. Other markers of circadian phase may be obtained, such as salivary melatonin or urinary 6-sulfatoxy melatonin levels. However, these need to be obtained at 2 time points, at least 2 to 4 weeks apart, to confirm a nonentrained rhythm.[8]

There are 2 primary populations in which non-24-hour sleep-wake type can be observed. This disorder was first described in individuals lacking all light perception. More recently, it has been increasingly recognized in individuals with normal vision. Although not all blind individuals are affected, those lacking light input to the SCN, either through loss of the melanopsin containing retinal ganglion cells or through loss of the retinohypothalamic projections from the eye to the SCN, are more likely to not be entrained.[51] In a recent study of 127 blind individuals, 63% of those with no light perception were not entrained, whereas only 21% of those with light perception were not entrained.[52] In sighted individuals the underlying cause is still unclear. However, possibilities include a decreased sensitivity to the circadian effects of light, despite normal visual perception, or a longer circadian period, making it more difficult to entrain to a 24-hour cycle. There is some support for the latter hypothesis, with a recent study demonstrating that, under forced desynchrony conditions, individuals with sighted non-24-hour sleep-wake type have a significantly longer free-running period than controls (24.3–24.6 hours vs 23.95–24.3 hours).[53]

Individuals with non-24-hour sleep-wake type often have comorbid depression or bipolar disorder, similar to those with delayed sleep phase type. In one large case series, psychiatric disease preceded the sleep-wake disorder in 28% of patients, whereas an additional 34% developed major depression following the onset of the sleep disorder.[54] Social isolation seems to contribute to the development of, and result from, this disorder.

Successful treatment of non-24-hour sleep-wake type depends on the underlying cause of the disorder (see **Table 1**). For blind individuals, several studies have demonstrated that taking a low dose of melatonin at a fixed time, approximately 1 hour before the desired bedtime, can result in effective entrainment and improved sleep. Doses have ranged from 10 mg[55] to 0.5 mg,[56] with lower doses generally preferred. A melatonin agonist, tasimelteon, has been developed as the first US Food and Drug Administration (FDA)-approved medication for non-24-hour sleep-wake type.[57] In sighted individuals, there is less data available on treatment options, but current recommendations include enforcing strong social cues through fixed sleep-wake schedules and timed light exposure. Although there are case reports of melatonin being effective in this population, it has not been as well studied as in blind individuals.[19]

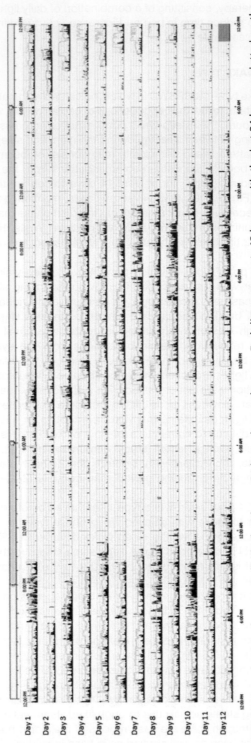

Fig. 3. Actigraphy data from an individual with non-24-hour sleep-wake type. Each line represents 48 hours, with the last 24 hours replotted on the following line. Black bars indicate activity, yellow lines indicate light exposure and grey bar indicates time when recording stopped. Each day the sleep-wake pattern moves about 1 hour later.

SHIFT WORK TYPE

Shift work type is characterized by symptoms of insomnia and/or excessive sleepiness when required to work during usual sleep times.[9] Shift work can be considered as any work schedule that is outside of conventional 8 AM to 6 PM work hours. Most of the data on shift work type come from studies of night shift workers. It is estimated that at least 20% of the workforce in the United States is employed in shift work.[58] Although sleep-wake disruption is common in shift workers,[59] it is estimated that only 5% to 10% of shift workers have a shift work type sleep disorder.[60]

Diagnosis of shift work type is based primarily on history. The use of actigraphy (**Fig. 4**) and/or a sleep diary may be helpful for diagnosis, particularly if the person has an irregular work schedule. Other primary sleep disorders, such as narcolepsy, obstructive sleep apnea, and restless legs, should be considered in the differential diagnosis of excessive sleepiness and sleep disturbance in shift workers.

The pathogenesis of shift work type and the reason only some individuals are affected are not entirely clear. It is thought that individual differences in susceptibility to circadian disruption, including age, sex, and circadian chronotype, contribute to the expression of the disorder.[61–63] Several studies suggest that there are differences in sleep-wake physiology in those who develop shift work type compared with shift workers without the disorder.[62,64–66] Compared with shift workers without the disorder, those with shift work type have shorter sleep duration, shorter sleep latency on the multiple sleep latency test, hyperreactivity to novel stimuli, and reduced brain response to auditory stimuli as measured by brain event-related potentials. Within shift work type, there seem to be 2 phenotypes, those with insomnia and sleepiness and those with insomnia but no sleepiness. A recent study reported data supporting a genetic basis for these different phenotypes. Those with insomnia and sleepiness were found to be more likely to have a long tandem repeat on PER3 than those with insomnia but no sleepiness.[62]

Shift workers are also more likely to have dysfunction in other areas of daily functioning, such as alcohol use disorder, substance abuse disorders, and depression, although it is not necessarily specific to those with shift work type.[9,60,67–70] Drake and colleagues[60] have shown that shift workers with shift work type are more likely to have depression than shift workers without the sleep disorder. For example, in a patient with bipolar disorder, night work was reported to trigger depression and labile mood that improved within a few days of returning to the day shift.[70]

Shift work can also place a burden on relationships with family and friends. For example, the schedule may cause conflict related to responsibilities with family life and child rearing, reduced marital happiness, greater sexual problems, and divorce.[69,71] Shift workers are also at higher risk for other health-related conditions, including obesity, cardiometabolic disorders, gastrointestinal disorders, altered reproductive health, and cancer.[60,72,73] These comorbidities are thought to result from one or perhaps a combination of the consequences of shift work schedules, including short sleep duration, circadian misalignment, and increased light exposure at night.

Treatment of shift work type aims to improve alertness at work, sleep quality during the required sleep time, and overall quality of life (see **Table 1**). Realignment of the timing of endogenous circadian rhythms with the required sleep-wake and work schedules is ideal but is often challenging because of social factors that can interfere with stable circadian adjustment. This realignment is typically achieved with timed light-dark exposure and/or melatonin administration. Bright light exposure can be used in the short term to improve alertness and/or to phase shift the circadian clock. Several studies have shown that bright light (3000–5000 lux), even intermittently

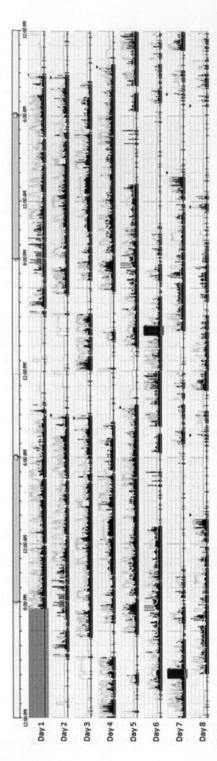

Fig. 4. Actigraphy data from an individual with shift work type. Each line represents 48 hours, with the last 24 hours replotted on the following line. This patient worked 5 consecutive night shifts and was in bed between 7:30 to 8:00 AM following the shifts, whereas the patient went to bed between 10 PM and midnight on the days off. Black bars indicate activity, yellow lines indicate light exposure, blue bars indicate off-wrist, gray bars indicate the time before recording started, and blue triangles indicate when the patient pushed an event marker to indicate bed or wake time.

applied during the first half of the night shift, improves alertness immediately and over time speeds up the alignment of the sleep-wake and circadian systems.[74-81] Avoidance of bright light in the morning after the night shift is also recommended and has been shown to aid in phase delaying the circadian clock.[77,81] However, there has been some criticism of this approach given that morning is a time of increased sleepiness and light is alerting. If workers avoid light at this time when driving home, they may be at an increased risk for a drowsy driving incident. Finally, melatonin given before sleep after the night shift may help phase delay the circadian clock and improve sleep quality. However, melatonin has not been shown to improve alertness during the night shift.[77,82-84]

If the person reverts to sleeping at night and being awake during the day on nonwork days, circadian adjustment to the shift work schedule can be adversely affected. Because of this, a compromised phase position approach in which the worker remains partially aligned to the night shift on the nonwork days is recommended. For night shift workers, they would schedule their sleep and wake time so that it falls in between their work day sleep schedule and a more traditional sleep schedule. For example, they would sleep from 3 AM to 11 AM. Although this approach has only been reported in a simulated night shift schedule in nonshift workers,[85-87] it has potential for clinical application.

Some patients may also require treatments that address insomnia symptoms during scheduled sleep times and residual sleepiness while at work. Short-acting hypnotic medications or melatonin have been used to treat insomnia,[88-90] whereas modafinil, armodafinil, caffeine, acute bright light exposure, or prophylactic napping can improve alertness.[91-93] Although caffeine is effective in reducing sleepiness and improving performance,[27,94-96] tolerance can develop. Modafinil and armodafinil are both FDA approved for the treatment of hypersomnia associated with shift work type. Modafinil, 200 mg, or armodafinil, 150 mg, is typically administered at the beginning of the shift, and the dose can be titrated as required to optimize alertness. However, improvements in sleepiness are generally modest.[97-99] All patients should be counseled on being aware of the signs of excessive sleepiness and fatigue and the potential of increased risk of sleepiness-related accidents.

A multimodal approach is recommended in the treatment of the symptoms of shift work type. For example, sleep hygiene should be a key component of any treatment approach, including maintaining a regular sleep time (when feasible based on work times) that allows for an adequate amount of time in bed each day; keeping the sleeping environment cool, dark, and quiet; and having a routine that allows the patient to wind down before going to bed.[27] This routine is of particular importance because shift workers are often instructed to attempt to sleep as soon as possible after completing their shift, which, unlike day workers, leaves little time for relaxation before bedtime. Obtaining adequate sleep before the work shift improves alertness, but if this is not possible, then a combination of the therapies discussed earlier can be used to improve alertness (phase shifting the circadian clock, bright light during work, napping, caffeine, modafinil/armodafinil). However, phase shifting the circadian clock is not always feasible or even recommended if the patient only works the night shift sporadically or on an irregular schedule. In this case, strategies to improve alertness while at work would be most beneficial.

Given the variety of shift work schedules that are used at present, it is useful to tailor treatment approaches based on the individual and their work schedule. There is a lack of well-designed and controlled experiments testing treatment approaches in those with shift work type. The majority of studies to date have been in nonshift workers or in shift workers regardless of whether they meet criteria for shift work type or not.

Although there is some evidence, it is yet to be determined whether, among shift workers, those with shift work type are more prone to the poor health outcomes associated with long-term shift work exposure, such as obesity, gastrointestinal disorders, cancer, and cardiometabolic disorders.[72,73,100]

SUMMARY

The CRSWDs encompass a wide spectrum of disorders, all of which are associated with dysregulation of the internal circadian system with respect to the external environment. This dysregulation can have a significant impact on physical and mental health, and there is a high comorbidity of psychiatric disease with many of these disorders. CRSWDs should be considered in the differential diagnosis of sleep-wake disturbances. Thus, questions regarding the timing of sleep-wake pattern and work schedules should be part of the routine history of all patients with symptoms of insomnia and excessive sleepiness, particularly in the practice of psychiatry.

REFERENCES

1. Landgraf D, McCarthy MJ, Welsh DK. Circadian clock and stress interactions in the molecular biology of psychiatric disorders. Curr Psychiatry Rep 2014; 16(10):483.
2. Yamazaki S, Numano R, Abe M, et al. Resetting central and peripheral circadian oscillators in transgenic rats. Science 2000;288(5466):682–5.
3. Duffy JF, Cain SW, Chang AM, et al. Sex difference in the near-24-hour intrinsic period of the human circadian timing system. Proc Natl Acad Sci U S A 2011; 108(Suppl 3):15602–8.
4. St Hilaire MA, Gooley JJ, Khalsa SB, et al. Human phase response curve to a 1 h pulse of bright white light. J Physiol 2012;590(Pt 13):3035–45.
5. Burgess HJ, Revell VL, Molina TA, et al. Human phase response curves to three days of daily melatonin: 0.5 mg versus 3.0 mg. J Clin Endocrinol Metab 2010; 95(7):3325–31.
6. Teclemariam-Mesbah R, Kalsbeek A, Pevet P, et al. Direct vasoactive intestinal polypeptide-containing projection from the suprachiasmatic nucleus to spinal projecting hypothalamic paraventricular neurons. Brain Res 1997;748(1–2): 71–6.
7. Buijs RM, Scheer FA, Kreier F, et al. Organization of circadian functions: interaction with the body. Prog Brain Res 2006;153:341–60.
8. ICSD-3. The international classification of sleep disorders: diagnostic and coding manual. 2nd edition. Darien (IL): American Academy of Sleep Medicine; 2014.
9. American Psychiatric Association. DSM-5 Task Force. Diagnostic and statistical manual of mental disorders: DSM-5. 5th edition. Washington, DC: American Psychiatric Association; 2013.
10. Paine SJ, Fink J, Gander PH, et al. Identifying advanced and delayed sleep phase disorders in the general population: a national survey of New Zealand adults. Chronobiol Int 2014;31(5):627–36.
11. Ebisawa T, Uchiyama M, Kajimura N, et al. Association of structural polymorphisms in the human period3 gene with delayed sleep phase syndrome. EMBO Rep 2001;2(4):342–6.
12. Aoki H, Ozeki Y, Yamada N. Hypersensitivity of melatonin suppression in response to light in patients with delayed sleep phase syndrome. Chronobiol Int 2001;18(2):263–71.

13. Auger RR, Burgess HJ, Dierkhising RA, et al. Light exposure among adolescents with delayed sleep phase disorder: a prospective cohort study. Chronobiol Int 2011;28(10):911–20.
14. Ayalon L, Borodkin K, Dishon L, et al. Circadian rhythm sleep disorders following mild traumatic brain injury. Neurology 2007;68(14):1136–40.
15. Reid KJ, Jaksa AA, Eisengart JB, et al. Systematic evaluation of axis-I DSM diagnoses in delayed sleep phase disorder and evening-type circadian preference. Sleep Med 2012;13(9):1171–7.
16. Abe T, Inoue Y, Komada Y, et al. Relation between morningness-eveningness score and depressive symptoms among patients with delayed sleep phase syndrome. Sleep Med 2011;12(7):680–4.
17. Lee HJ, Rex KM, Nievergelt CM, et al. Delayed sleep phase syndrome is related to seasonal affective disorder. J Affect Disord 2011;133(3):573–9.
18. Nota JA, Sharkey KM, Coles ME. Sleep, arousal, and circadian rhythms in adults with obsessive-compulsive disorder: a meta-analysis. Neurosci Biobehav Rev 2015;51:100–7.
19. Sack RL, Auckley D, Auger RR, et al. Circadian rhythm sleep disorders: part II, advanced sleep phase disorder, delayed sleep phase disorder, free-running disorder, and irregular sleep-wake rhythm. An American Academy of Sleep Medicine review. Sleep 2007;30(11):1484–501.
20. Nagtegaal JE, Kerkhof GA, Smits MG, et al. Delayed sleep phase syndrome: a placebo-controlled cross-over study on the effects of melatonin administered five hours before the individual dim light melatonin onset. J Sleep Res 1998; 7(2):135–43.
21. Rahman SA, Kayumov L, Shapiro CM. Antidepressant action of melatonin in the treatment of delayed sleep phase syndrome. Sleep Med 2010;11(2): 131–6.
22. Rosenthal NE, Joseph-Vanderpool JR, Levendosky AA, et al. Phase-shifting effects of bright morning light as treatment for delayed sleep phase syndrome. Sleep 1990;13(4):354–61.
23. Gradisar M, Dohnt H, Gardner G, et al. A randomized controlled trial of cognitive-behavior therapy plus bright light therapy for adolescent delayed sleep phase disorder. Sleep 2011;34(12):1671–80.
24. Saxvig IW, Wilhelmsen-Langeland A, Pallesen S, et al. A randomized controlled trial with bright light and melatonin for delayed sleep phase disorder: effects on subjective and objective sleep. Chronobiol Int 2014;31(1):72–86.
25. Wilhelmsen-Langeland A, Saxvig IW, Pallesen S, et al. A randomized controlled trial with bright light and melatonin for the treatment of delayed sleep phase disorder: effects on subjective and objective sleepiness and cognitive function. J Biol Rhythms 2013;28(5):306–21.
26. Crowley SJ, Eastman CI. Phase advancing human circadian rhythms with morning bright light, afternoon melatonin, and gradually shifted sleep: can we reduce morning bright-light duration? Sleep Med 2015;16(2):288–97.
27. Morgenthaler TI, Lee-Chiong T, Alessi C, et al. Practice parameters for the clinical evaluation and treatment of circadian rhythm sleep disorders. An American Academy of Sleep Medicine report. Sleep 2007;30(11):1445–59.
28. Reid KJ, Chang AM, Dubocovich ML, et al. Familial advanced sleep phase syndrome. Arch Neurol 2001;58(7):1089–94.
29. Jones CR, Campbell SS, Zone SE, et al. Familial advanced sleep-phase syndrome: a short-period circadian rhythm variant in humans. Nat Med 1999; 5(9):1062–5.

30. Toh KL, Jones CR, He Y, et al. An hPer2 phosphorylation site mutation in familial advanced sleep phase syndrome. Science 2001;291(5506):1040–3.
31. Xu Y, Padiath QS, Shapiro RE, et al. Functional consequences of a CKIdelta mutation causing familial advanced sleep phase syndrome. Nature 2005; 434(7033):640–4.
32. Shanware NP, Hutchinson JA, Kim SH, et al. Casein kinase 1-dependent phosphorylation of familial advanced sleep phase syndrome-associated residues controls PERIOD 2 stability. J Biol Chem 2011;286(14):12766–74.
33. Lack L, Wright H. The effect of evening bright light in delaying the circadian rhythms and lengthening the sleep of early morning awakening insomniacs. Sleep 1993;16(5):436–43.
34. Lack L, Wright H, Kemp K, et al. The treatment of early-morning awakening insomnia with 2 evenings of bright light. Sleep 2005;28(5):616–23.
35. Zee PC. Melatonin for the treatment of advanced sleep phase disorder. Sleep 2008;31(7):923 [author reply: 5].
36. Takaesu Y, Komada Y, Inoue Y. Melatonin profile and its relation to circadian rhythm sleep disorders in Angelman syndrome patients. Sleep Med 2012; 13(9):1164–70.
37. Potocki L, Glaze D, Tan DX, et al. Circadian rhythm abnormalities of melatonin in Smith-Magenis syndrome. J Med Genet 2000;37(6):428–33.
38. Cortesi F, Giannotti F, Ivanenko A, et al. Sleep in children with autistic spectrum disorder. Sleep Med 2010;11(7):659–64.
39. Kristina F, Zdanys KF, Steffens DC. Sleep Disturbances in the Elderly. Psychiatr Clin N Am 2015, in press.
40. Okawa M, Mishima K, Hishikawa Y, et al. Circadian rhythm disorders in sleep-waking and body temperature in elderly patients with dementia and their treatment. Sleep 1991;14(6):478–85.
41. Lim AS, Yu L, Costa MD, et al. Increased fragmentation of rest-activity patterns is associated with a characteristic pattern of cognitive impairment in older individuals. Sleep 2012;35(5):633–640B.
42. Wang JL, Lim AS, Chiang WY, et al. Suprachiasmatic neuron numbers and rest-activity circadian rhythms in older humans. Ann Neurol 2015;78(2): 317–22.
43. Gardani M, Morfiri E, Thomson A, et al. Evaluation of sleep disorders in patients with severe traumatic brain injury during rehabilitation. Arch Phys Med Rehabil 2015. [Epub ahead of print].
44. DelRosso LM, Hoque R, James S, et al. Sleep-wake pattern following gunshot suprachiasmatic damage. J Clin Sleep Med 2014;10(4):443–5.
45. Borodkin K, Ayalon L, Kanety H, et al. Dysregulation of circadian rhythms following prolactin-secreting pituitary microadenoma. Chronobiol Int 2005; 22(1):145–56.
46. Mishima K, Okawa M, Hishikawa Y, et al. Morning bright light therapy for sleep and behavior disorders in elderly patients with dementia. Acta Psychiatr Scand 1994;89(1):1–7.
47. Guilleminault C, McCann CC, Quera-Salva M, et al. Light therapy as treatment of dyschronosis in brain impaired children. Eur J Pediatr 1993; 152(9):754–9.
48. Wasdell MB, Jan JE, Bomben MM, et al. A randomized, placebo-controlled trial of controlled release melatonin treatment of delayed sleep phase syndrome and impaired sleep maintenance in children with neurodevelopmental disabilities. J Pineal Res 2008;44(1):57–64.

49. Serfaty M, Kennell-Webb S, Warner J, et al. Double blind randomised placebo controlled trial of low dose melatonin for sleep disorders in dementia. Int J Geriatr Psychiatry 2002;17(12):1120–7.

50. Alessi CA, Martin JL, Webber AP, et al. Randomized, controlled trial of a non-pharmacological intervention to improve abnormal sleep/wake patterns in nursing home residents. J Am Geriatr Soc 2005;53(5):803–10.

51. Sollars PJ, Pickard GE. The Neurobiology of Circadian Rhythms. Psychiatr Clin N Am 2015, in press.

52. Flynn-Evans EE, Tabandeh H, Skene DJ, et al. Circadian rhythm disorders and melatonin production in 127 blind women with and without light perception. J Biol rhythms 2014;29(3):215–24.

53. Kitamura S, Hida A, Enomoto M, et al. Intrinsic circadian period of sighted patients with circadian rhythm sleep disorder, free-running type. Biol Psychiatry 2013;73(1):63–9.

54. Hayakawa T, Uchiyama M, Kamei Y, et al. Clinical analyses of sighted patients with non-24-hour sleep-wake syndrome: a study of 57 consecutively diagnosed cases. Sleep 2005;28(8):945–52.

55. Sack RL, Brandes RW, Kendall AR, et al. Entrainment of free-running circadian rhythms by melatonin in blind people. N Engl J Med 2000;343(15):1070–7.

56. Lewy AJ, Bauer VK, Hasler BP, et al. Capturing the circadian rhythms of free-running blind people with 0.5 mg melatonin. Brain Res 2001;918(1–2):96–100.

57. Tasimelteon (Hetlioz) for non-24-hour sleep-wake disorder. Med Lett Drugs Ther 2014;56(1441):34–5.

58. Workers on flexible and shift schedules in 2004 summary. 2004. Available at: http://www.bls.gov/news.release/flex.nr0.htm. Accessed July 10, 2015.

59. Akerstedt T. Work hours, sleepiness and the underlying mechanisms. J Sleep Res 1995;4(S2):15–22.

60. Drake CL, Roehrs T, Richardson G, et al. Shift work sleep disorder: prevalence and consequences beyond that of symptomatic day workers. Sleep 2004;27(8): 1453–62.

61. Folkard S, Monk TH, Lobban MC. Short and long-term adjustment of circadian rhythms in 'permanent' night nurses. Ergonomics 1978;21(10):785–99.

62. Gumenyuk V, Belcher R, Drake CL, et al. Differential sleep, sleepiness, and neurophysiology in the insomnia phenotypes of shift work disorder. Sleep 2015;38(1):119–26.

63. Harma MI, Hakola T, Akerstedt T, et al. Age and adjustment to night work. Occup Environ Med 1994;51(8):568–73.

64. Gumenyuk V, Howard R, Roth T, et al. Sleep loss, circadian mismatch, and abnormalities in reorienting of attention in night workers with shift work disorder. Sleep 2014;37(3):545–56.

65. Gumenyuk V, Roth T, Drake CL. Circadian phase, sleepiness, and light exposure assessment in night workers with and without shift work disorder. Chronobiol Int 2012;29(7):928–36.

66. Gumenyuk V, Roth T, Korzyukov O, et al. Shift work sleep disorder is associated with an attenuated brain response of sensory memory and an increased brain response to novelty: an ERP study. Sleep 2010;33(5):703–13.

67. Perry-Jenkins M, Goldberg AE, Pierce CP, et al. Shift work, role overload, and the transition to parenthood. J Marriage Fam 2007;69(1):123–38.

68. Lee HY, Kim MS, Kim O, et al. Association between shift work and severity of depressive symptoms among female nurses: the Korea Nurses' Health Study. J Nurs Manag 2015. [Epub ahead of print].

69. White L, Keith B. The effect of shift work on the quality and stability of marital relations. J Marriage Fam 1990;52(2):453–62.
70. Meyrer R, Demling J, Kornhuber J, et al. Effects of night shifts in bipolar disorders and extreme morningness. Bipolar Disord 2009;11(8):897–9.
71. Presser H. Working in a 24/7 economy: challenges for American families. New York: Russell Sage Foundation; 2003.
72. Brum MC, Filho FF, Schnorr CC, et al. Shift work and its association with metabolic disorders. Diabetol Metab Syndr 2015;7:45.
73. He C, Anand ST, Ebell MH, et al. Circadian disrupting exposures and breast cancer risk: a meta-analysis. Int Arch Occup Environ Health 2015;88(5):533–47.
74. Boivin DB, James FO. Circadian adaptation to night-shift work by judicious light and darkness exposure. J Biol rhythms 2002;17(6):556–67.
75. Burgess HJ, Sharkey KM, Eastman CI. Bright light, dark and melatonin can promote circadian adaptation in night shift workers. Sleep Med Rev 2002;6(5):407–20.
76. Campbell SS, Dijk DJ, Boulos Z, et al. Light treatment for sleep disorders: consensus report. III. Alerting and activating effects. J Biol rhythms 1995;10(2):129–32.
77. Crowley SJ, Lee C, Tseng CY, et al. Combinations of bright light, scheduled dark, sunglasses, and melatonin to facilitate circadian entrainment to night shift work. J Biol Rhythms 2003;18(6):513–23.
78. Dawson D, Campbell SS. Timed exposure to bright light improves sleep and alertness during simulated night shifts. Sleep 1991;14(6):511–6.
79. Dawson D, Encel N, Lushington K. Improving adaptation to simulated night shift: timed exposure to bright light versus daytime melatonin administration. Sleep 1995;18(1):11–21.
80. Eastman CI, Liu L, Fogg LF. Circadian rhythm adaptation to simulated night shift work: effect of nocturnal bright-light duration. Sleep 1995;18(6):399–407.
81. Eastman CI, Stewart KT, Mahoney MP, et al. Dark goggles and bright light improve circadian rhythm adaptation to night-shift work. Sleep 1994;17(6):535–43.
82. Sharkey KM, Eastman CI. Melatonin phase shifts human circadian rhythms in a placebo-controlled simulated night-work study. Am J Physiol Regul Integr Comp Physiol 2002;282(2):R454–63.
83. Sharkey KM, Fogg LF, Eastman CI. Effects of melatonin administration on daytime sleep after simulated night shift work. J Sleep Res 2001;10(3):181–92.
84. Smith MR, Lee C, Crowley SJ, et al. Morning melatonin has limited benefit as a soporific for daytime sleep after night work. Chronobiol Int 2005;22(5):873–88.
85. Smith MR, Fogg LF, Eastman CI. A compromise circadian phase position for permanent night work improves mood, fatigue, and performance. Sleep 2009;32(11):1481–9.
86. Smith MR, Fogg LF, Eastman CI. Practical interventions to promote circadian adaptation to permanent night shift work: study 4. J Biol rhythms 2009;24(2):161–72.
87. Smith MR, Cullnan EE, Eastman CI. Shaping the light/dark pattern for circadian adaptation to night shift work. Physiol Behav 2008;95(3):449–56.
88. Walsh JK, Schweitzer PK, Anch AM, et al. Sleepiness/alertness on a simulated night shift following sleep at home with triazolam. Sleep 1991;14(2):140–6.
89. Hart CL, Haney M, Nasser J, et al. Combined effects of methamphetamine and zolpidem on performance and mood during simulated night shift work. Pharmacol Biochem Behav 2005;81(3):559–68.

90. Hart CL, Ward AS, Haney M, et al. Zolpidem-related effects on performance and mood during simulated night-shift work. Exp Clin Psychopharmacol 2003;11(4): 259–68.
91. Garbarino S, Mascialino B, Penco MA, et al. Professional shift-work drivers who adopt prophylactic naps can reduce the risk of car accidents during night work. Sleep 2004;27(7):1295–302.
92. Purnell MT, Feyer AM, Herbison GP. The impact of a nap opportunity during the night shift on the performance and alertness of 12-h shift workers. J Sleep Res 2002;11(3):219–27.
93. Sallinen M, Harma M, Akerstedt T, et al. Promoting alertness with a short nap during a night shift. J Sleep Res 1998;7(4):240–7.
94. Akerstedt T, Ficca G. Alertness-enhancing drugs as a countermeasure to fatigue in irregular work hours. Chronobiol Int 1997;14(2):145–58.
95. Babkoff H, French J, Whitmore J, et al. Single-dose bright light and/or caffeine effect on nocturnal performance. Aviat Space Environ Med 2002;73(4):341–50.
96. Muehlbach MJ, Walsh JK. The effects of caffeine on simulated night-shift work and subsequent daytime sleep. Sleep 1995;18(1):22–9.
97. Czeisler CA, Walsh JK, Roth T, et al. Modafinil for excessive sleepiness associated with shift-work sleep disorder. N Engl J Med 2005;353(5):476–86.
98. Czeisler CA, Walsh JK, Wesnes KA, et al. Armodafinil for treatment of excessive sleepiness associated with shift work disorder: a randomized controlled study. Mayo Clin Proc 2009;84(11):958–72.
99. Erman MK, Rosenberg R, Modafinil Shift Work Sleep Disorder Study Group. Modafinil for excessive sleepiness associated with chronic shift work sleep disorder: effects on patient functioning and health-related quality of life. Prim Care Companion J Clin Psychiatry 2007;9(3):188–94.
100. Ramin C, Devore EE, Wang W, et al. Night shift work at specific age ranges and chronic disease risk factors. Occup Environ Med 2015;72(2):100–7.

Sleep Disturbances in Patients with Medical Conditions

Jayesh Kamath, MD, PhD*, Galina Prpich, MS, Sarah Jillani, MBBS

KEYWORDS

- Sleep disturbances • Insomnia • Medical conditions • Comorbidities
- Symptom cluster • Cancer • Inflammation • Cognitive behavioral therapy

KEY POINTS

- Sleep disorders occur at higher rates in patients with medical conditions than in the general population.
- Sleep disturbances frequently present as part of a symptom cluster with medical and psychiatric comorbidities in these patients.
- Immune and neuroendocrine alterations play a role in the pathophysiology of sleep disorders in these patients and may share a common pathway with other comorbidities.
- Assessment and treatment of medical and psychiatric comorbidities is a crucial first step in the management of sleep disturbances in patients with medical conditions.
- Treatment includes cognitive–behavioral therapy and pharmacologic treatments directed toward the sleep disturbances as well as comorbidities.

OVERVIEW

Patients with medical conditions commonly experience sleep disturbances, at much higher rates than in the general population.[1,2] Sleep disruptions are often overlooked in these patients owing to other, more urgent concerns, such as the diagnosis and treatment of primary medical conditions.[3] Additionally, sleep–wake disturbances are often part of symptom clusters complicating diagnoses and management of patients with medical conditions.[4] Both experimental evidence and clinical experience demonstrate that sleep–wake cycle disturbances in patient with medical conditions include insomnia, hypersomnia, sleep-disordered breathing, restless legs syndrome, periodic

Disclosure: The authors have nothing to disclose.
Department of Psychiatry, University of Connecticut School of Medicine, 263 Farmington Avenue, Farmington, CT 06030-6415, USA
* Corresponding author.
E-mail address: jkamath@uchc.edu

Psychiatr Clin N Am 38 (2015) 825–841
http://dx.doi.org/10.1016/j.psc.2015.07.011
0193-953X/15/$ – see front matter © 2015 Elsevier Inc. All rights reserved.

Abbreviations	
CBT	Cognitive–behavioral therapy
CBT-I	Cognitive–behavioral therapy for insomnia
DSM	Diagnostic and Statistical Manual of Mental Disorders
MS	Multiple sclerosis
OSA	Obstructive sleep apnea
PLMD	Periodic limb movements disorder
REM	Rapid eye movement
RLS	Restless legs syndrome

limb movements disorder (PLMD), rapid eye movement (REM) behavior disorders, and narcolepsy.[5] A large body of literature has documented sleep disturbances in patients with cancer.[6] Studies evaluating sleep problems have also been conducted in patients with other medical conditions, for example, in patients with cardiovascular events,[7] neurologic disorders,[5,8] respiratory disorders,[9] gastrointestinal disorders,[10] pain disorders,[11] and in many other medical conditions. However, a limited number of studies have been conducted in patients with medical conditions other than cancer. The present article reviews evidence on sleep–wake disturbances in patients with diverse medical conditions, with a primary focus on the existing extensive literature in cancer. Evidence and conclusions drawn from the cancer and noncancer literature is applied to discuss pathophysiology, assessment, and management of sleep disruptions in patients with medical conditions in general.

The fourth edition of the Diagnostic and Statistical Manual of Mental Disorders (DSM IV) included sleep disorders owing to medical conditions as a subcategory under the umbrella of secondary sleep disorders.[12] The DSM V workgroup added major changes to the nosology of sleep–wake disorders in DSM V to simplify the classification of sleep disorders and to enhance its clinical utility, reliability, and validity.[13] The subcategories of sleep disorders owing to medical and mental conditions are eliminated in the DSM V.[12,14] Instead the diagnoses of primary insomnia and hypersomnia are changed to the insomnia and hypersomnia disorder and their relationship to medical or mental conditions (when present) are now indicated, with specification of the comorbid clinical conditions. These changes capture the dynamic relationship between sleep–wake disorders and medical/mental conditions, with greater emphasis on how they interact and impact each other. Furthermore, these changes underscore that the patient has a sleep disorder that warrants independent clinical attention and that the treatment of medical/psychiatric disorders may not improve the comorbid sleep disorder.[12] The DSM V continues to emphasize that, to diagnose any sleep–wake disorder, it has to meet the threshold of impairment in functioning as well as causing psychological distress to the individual.[14]

SLEEP–WAKE CYCLE DISTURBANCES IN PATIENTS WITH MAJOR MEDICAL CONDITIONS
Sleep–Wake Cycle Disturbances in Patients with Cancer

Several studies have investigated sleep–wake cycle disturbances along the continuum of cancer care.[2] These studies have documented the epidemiology, pathophysiology, assessment, and management of sleep disruptions in patients with cancer.[6] Evidence has also accumulated supporting the significant negative impact of sleep disturbances on quality of life, functioning, and morbidity in these patients.[15] Rates of sleep disturbances in patients with cancer range between 25% and 60% depending on the cancer type, stage, cancer treatments, treatment-related side effects, and medical/psychiatric comorbidities.[2] Evidence suggests that the most frequent sleep–wake disorder in this patient population is insomnia.[16] Insomnia can present as a transient inability to initiate or maintain sleep or as an insomnia syndrome, with repeated experiences of insomnia occurring more than 3 nights per week, including difficulty falling asleep or night time awakenings (>30 minutes), a reduced ratio of sleep time to time spent in bed (<85% sleep efficiency), associated with impaired daytime functioning and marked distress.[17] Insomnia in cancer patients is most often secondary to physical and/or psychological factors associated with cancer and cancer treatments.[6]

Sleep–Wake Cycle Disturbances in Medical Conditions Other than Cancer

The following is a summary of the sleep–wake cycle disturbances in other major medical conditions.

Sleep–wake cycle disturbances in patients with neurologic disorders

In patients with multiple sclerosis (MS), sleep disorders are more common than in the general population, ranging from 25% to 62%.[18–21] Sleep disorders are among the most critical factors in the development of fatigue, the most common debilitating symptom of MS.[19,22] Decreased sleep efficiency on polysomnography has been correlated with fatigue in patient with MS compared with controls.[22] Sleep disturbances in these patients have also been associated with depression, anxiety, and disability, associated with a negative impact on quality of life.[18] The sleep disorders that are highly prevalent in patients with MS include insomnia, restless legs syndrome, and sleep-disordered breathing.[5] Preliminary evidence suggests that inflammation and disruption of melatonin pathways may play a role in the pathophysiology of sleep disorders in patients with MS.[5]

Another major neurologic disorder with high prevalence of sleep disorders is epilepsy. Evidence suggests that sleep disorders in patients with epilepsy are partially owing to the occurrence of seizures, which are known to disrupt sleep architecture beyond the periictal period. An additional complicating factor related to sleep disturbances in patients with epilepsy involves effects of antiepileptic drugs on sleep.[8,23] In a recent study, patients with seizures had significant decreases in REM sleep and increases in stage I sleep during overnight polysomnography, as compared with sleep findings during seizure-free nights.[8] Evidence suggests that sleep disturbances in certain subtypes of epilepsy (partial seizures) may be inherent to the disorder, independent of all other factors.[8] Sleep disturbances in these patients have been associated with impaired quality of life and impaired seizure control.[8] The most common sleep disorders seen in patients with epilepsy include insomnia, sleep-disordered breathing, and periodic limb movement disorder.[24]

Sleep-related breathing disorders are common in neuromuscular diseases such as amyotrophic lateral sclerosis and myasthenia gravis, in inherited myopathies such as myotonic dystrophy, and in neurodegenerative diseases such as multiple systemic atrophy and Alzheimer's dementia.[25]

Sleep–wake cycle disturbances in patients with disorders associated with pain syndromes

Multiple rheumatic disorders with pain syndromes have been associated with sleep disturbances.[26] These include rheumatoid arthritis, ankylosing spondylitis, osteoarthritis, scleroderma, systemic lupus erythematosus, and Sjögren syndrome.[11] Pain and sleep disorders in these patients have been associated with depression, anxiety, and fatigue.[11] Neurons located in the nucleus raphe magnus facilitate and inhibit nociceptive impulses to thalamocortical pathways. These neurons are influenced by the sleep–wake cycle, with inhibitory pain-off neurons activated during deep sleep and excitatory pain-on neurons activated during wakefulness.[27] Sleep deprivation, especially REM sleep deprivation, has been associated with a reduced pain threshold.[28]

Sleep–Wake Cycle Disturbances in Patients with Other Medical Conditions

In patients recovering from cardiac events, such as acute myocardial infarction, coronary artery bypass graft surgery, or percutaneous intervention, the prevalence of sleep disorders is higher than in the general population.[7,29] Sleep disorders in these patients are associated with depression and anxiety, and have been reported to interfere with treatment adherence, recovery, and cardiac rehabilitation.[7,29]

Sleep disorders are common in patients with several gastrointestinal disorders including gastroesophageal reflux disease, peptic ulcer disease, inflammatory bowel disease, irritable bowel syndrome, and liver disorders.[10] Evidence suggests that sleep disturbances in these patients may share a common inflammatory pathophysiologic pathway with the primary medical condition.[10]

RISK FACTORS FOR SLEEP DISTURBANCES IN PATIENTS WITH MEDICAL CONDITIONS

Risk factors for sleep disturbances in patients with medical conditions are frequently multifactorial (**Fig. 1**). These can include predisposing, precipitating, and perpetuating factors.[30–32] Certain biological factors such as personal and family history of mood or anxiety disorders as well as a history of headaches can increase vulnerability to sleep disruptions in the context of medical conditions.[33] Personal or family history of substance use disorders with legal or illegal substances (eg, alcohol, nicotine, amphetamines) can play a major role in increasing vulnerability to sleep disturbances.[33] Psychological and social factors such as heightened stress response, hyperarousability, increased sleep reactivity, and relationship conflicts can also predispose patients to sleep–wake cycle disruptions when struggling with stress related to active medical issues.[30]

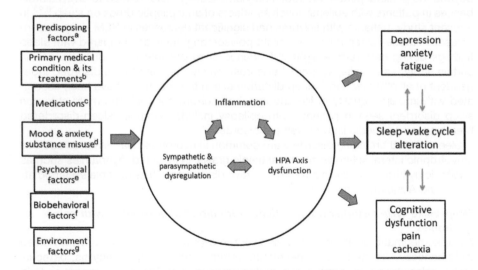

Fig. 1. Underlying mechanisms and comorbidities of sleep disturbance in patients with medical conditions. [a] Example: increased sleep reactivity. [b] Example: cancer and cancer treatments. [c] Example: corticosteroids. [d] Example: alcohol. [e] Example: job loss, relationship conflicts. [f] Example: maladaptive sleep behaviors. [g] Example: hospital setting. HPA, hypothalamic–pituitary–adrenal.

Precipitating factors can include disruption of the sleep–wake cycle owing to the primary medical condition, which can happen via multiple pathways. Examples of precipitating influences include increased levels of proinflammatory cytokines or cooccurring symptoms and comorbidities related to the primary medical condition.[10,31] In the context of primary medical conditions or comorbidities such as cardiopulmonary disorders as a result of cancer/cancer treatments, symptoms such as pain, fatigue, and gastrointestinal disturbances can frequently cause or exacerbate sleep disturbances.[34,35] Certain medications used to treat the primary medical conditions can also cause disruption of the sleep–wake cycle, either directly or indirectly owing to their side effects, for example, corticosteroids for autoimmune disorders, and chemotherapeutic or biological agents for treatment of cancer.[16] Psychosocial factors such as frequent hospitalizations, distress owing to unstable/active medical issues, uncertainty about treatment and prognosis, and resulting social issues (eg, job loss) can exacerbate sleep disturbances.[16]

Persistent difficulties with sleep and comorbid symptoms can lead to maladaptive sleep behaviors, all of which may further perpetuate sleep disturbances such as cognitive distortions, as well as long-term and/or inappropriate use of medications.[35] Abrupt withdrawal from certain medications can also exacerbate sleep disturbances, including both benzodiazepines and nonbenzodiazepine hypnotic drugs, as well as other central nervous system depressants such as opioids, tricyclic antidepressants, and antihistamine sedatives.[32] Patients often attempt to discontinue the use of legal or illegal substances, such as alcohol, nicotine, and opioids when diagnosed with medical conditions such as cancer, diabetes, or cardiopulmonary illnesses. Withdrawal associated with the discontinued use of such substances can also contribute to sleep disruptions.[35] Additionally, environmental factors can contribute to sleep disturbances in patients with medical conditions. For example, the sleep of hospitalized patients is frequently interrupted by hospital routines, treatment schedules, roommates, and other factors such as noise and room temperature in the hospital setting.[36]

Sleep–wake cycle disturbances can have a significant negative impact on the overall well-being of patients with medical conditions.[18,29] These factors include heightened distress, impairment in social/occupational functioning, negative impact on relationships, and decreased quality of life.[37,38] Furthermore, sleep disturbances and their consequences such as daytime fatigue, dysphoric states with anger and irritability, and cognitive impairment can have a negative impact on patients' decision making and on their ability to engage in treatments for their primary medical condition.[38] This, in turn, can increase morbidity and mortality, and can lead to worse health outcomes owing to noncompliance with treatment recommendations.[38,39]

UNDERLYING MECHANISMS AND THE PATHOPHYSIOLOGY OF SLEEP DISTURBANCES IN PATIENTS WITH MEDICAL CONDITIONS

Increasing evidence suggests that chronic inflammation with unregulated activation of the innate immune system contributes to the development of dysfunctional behavioral alternations resembling alterations seen in patients with medical conditions.[40] Evidence from both animal and human studies shows that administration of selected proinflammatory cytokines induces a "sickness syndrome" that has many overlapping features with behavioral comorbidities commonly seen in patients with medical conditions, including depression, fatigue, cognitive dysfunction, and impaired sleep.[40] These cytokine-induced behavioral changes have also been associated with dysregulation of the hypothalamic–pituitary–adrenal axis as well as alterations in neurotransmitters such as serotonin, norepinephrine, and dopamine, all of which play a critical role in the regulation of a number of behaviors including regulation of sleep.[41] Evidence also indicates that psychological stress can activate proinflammatory cytokines and their signaling pathways.[42] Activation of proinflammatory pathways may be mediated by the activation of the sympathetic nervous system[43] and enhanced owing to disruption of hypothalamic–pituitary–adrenal axis functioning.[44]

In patients with medical conditions, especially in patients with cancer or cardiovascular illness, several behavioral comorbidities have been associated with increased inflammation and alterations in neuroendocrine functioning and regulation.[45] Behavioral comorbidities in these patients, such as fatigue, depression, cognitive dysfunction, and sleep impairment have been associated with increased levels proinflammatory cytokines and signaling, flattening of circadian cortisol rhythms, activation of the sympathetic nervous system, and alterations in neurotransmitter systems (see **Fig. 1**).[45] These behavioral comorbidities, which frequently coexist as symptom clusters in patients with medical conditions, seem to share common pathophysiologic pathways.[45] These pathways contributing to the behavioral alterations (including sleep impairment) may be activated by the medical conditions, by their treatments, by psychological stress associated with the medical illness, and by other psychosocial factors, and they are exacerbated by the negative impact of these comorbidities on each other, for example, worsening of fatigue or depression associated with sleep disturbances.[45,46]

SCREENING AND ASSESSMENT OF SLEEP DISTURBANCES IN PATIENTS WITH MEDICAL CONDITIONS

As noted, sleep–wake disturbances in patients with medical conditions occur in the context of multiple factors. In patients with medical conditions, sleep disturbances are frequently part of a symptom cluster associated with the primary and secondary medical conditions, as well as with the consequences of their medical treatments. Investigation of these symptom clusters and their interrelationship with sleep disturbances is critical when assessing sleep disruptions in patients with medical conditions.[33] Sleep disturbances may not always resolve with the resolution or treatment of the cooccurring symptoms or disorders, such as pain, depression, or fatigue. Furthermore, it is well-established that persistent sleep disturbances can increase the vulnerability to both medical (eg, cardiometabolic) and psychiatric (eg, depression/anxiety) disorders, emphasizing the importance of treatment of sleep disturbances in association with other medical/psychiatric symptoms in these patients.[47]

Screening

Given the negative impact that sleep disruption can have on patients' medical and/or psychiatric conditions and their quality of life, all patients with medical conditions should be screened for sleep disturbances by their health care providers at every visit. Identification of sleep disturbances can be accomplished in a 2-step process—an initial screening evaluation followed by a comprehensive assessment (**Fig. 2**).[48] The initial screen includes 2 questions: (1) is the sleep disturbance present on average 3 or more nights per week? and (2) does the sleep problem negatively affect the daytime functioning and quality of life of the patient?[48] Some guidelines recommend the use of scales or questionnaires such as the Epworth Sleepiness Scale,[49] PROMIS sleep thermometer tool,[48] and the Insomnia Severity Index.[33]

Assessment

A positive screen should be followed by a comprehensive assessment (see **Fig. 2**). The comprehensive assessment should include careful review of sleep patterns,

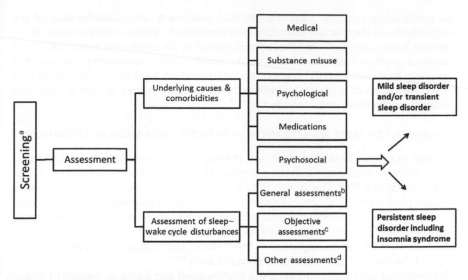

Fig. 2. Screening and assessment of sleep disturbance in patients with medical conditions. [a] Consists of the following questions: (1) "Are sleep disturbances present 3+ nights/week on average?" (2) "Do sleep problems negatively affect daytime functioning and quality of life?" [b] Includes nature and extent of sleep problem, impact on functioning, and quality of life. [c] Includes sleep diary and validated questionnaires. [d] Includes polysomnography and actigraphy. Sleep parameters: total sleep time, sleep latency, sleep efficiency, wake time after sleep onset, napping during the day, circadian rhythm, excessive daytime sleepiness, and quality of perceived sleep.

medical conditions, and medications, psychological evaluation, substance use status, diet, exercise and activity levels, and caregiver routines, if applicable.[33] A detailed assessment of predisposing risk factors, including a review of medical, psychiatric, and substance use history, other psychosocial and relevant environmental factors, and a physical examination is critical both from a diagnostic and management perspective. Assessment can be divided into 2 key aspects as follows:

1. Focused assessment of symptoms of sleep disturbances using validated questionnaires such as the Insomnia Severity Index and sleep logs or a sleep diary maintained over at least a 2-week period.[33] Assessment of the following parameters should be included in sleep logs or a sleep diary: total sleep time, sleep latency, sleep efficiency, wake time after sleep onset, napping during the day, circadian rhythm, excessive daytime sleepiness, and perceived quality of sleep.[50] This assessment should also include an evaluation of the impact of the sleep disturbance on daytime functioning, quality of life, relationships, and employment.[50] Beliefs and perceptions about sleep and sleep disturbances should be included in the assessments.[33] Such assessment should also include a review of risk factors including assessment of preexisting sleep disturbances (before medical conditions), sleep issues owing to psychiatric/substance use issues, and environmental and psychosocial risk factors contributing to sleep disruptions.[50] Polysomnography, an objective tool, is considered when sleep-related breathing disorders and periodic limb movement disorder are suspected.[33]

2. Unique aspects of the assessment of sleep disturbances in patients with medical conditions include assessment of medical conditions and their treatments, review

of medications used to treat the medical conditions, and consideration of the contribution of the medical condition and associated treatment on the sleep problems in these patients.[33] Another unique aspect of the assessment involves evaluation of medical and psychiatric comorbidities (pain, depression, fatigue, etc) resulting from the primary medical condition and its treatments. Assessment of the contribution of such comorbidities to sleep disturbances is critical both with respect to diagnosis and management.[33]

MANAGEMENT OF SLEEP DISTURBANCES IN PATIENTS WITH MEDICAL CONDITIONS

In general, principles of the management of sleep disturbances in patients with medical condition are similar to the management of sleep disturbances in patients without medical conditions.[33,50] The major difference in the management of sleep disturbances in patients with medical conditions involves the assessment and management of the primary medical condition, related comorbidities, and medications used to treat these conditions in terms of their contribution to sleep–wake disturbances.[33,50] This includes evaluation and management of the medical, psychological, and psychosocial impact of the medical conditions and comorbidities.[33,50]

The treatment plan should address the multifactorial and treatable causes of sleep–wake disturbances (**Fig. 3**). Identification and treatment of comorbidities such as pain, fatigue, depression/anxiety, nausea, and shortness of breath that directly or indirectly contribute to sleep problems is a critical first step in the management of sleep disturbances in these patients.[33,50] Addressing certain behavioral issues and environmental/psychosocial factors that contribute to sleep disruptions such as alcohol use, life stressors, worries, and negative thoughts about prognosis is another important aspect of the treatment plan.[33,50] Identification of medications (eg, antiepileptic medications, corticosteroids) that can disrupt sleep architecture and exacerbate sleep issues and seeking alternatives or alternate dosing (eg, nighttime dosing) represents another critical step in management.[33,50] However, sleep disturbances frequently persist despite addressing comorbidities, behavioral/psychosocial factors, medications, and other

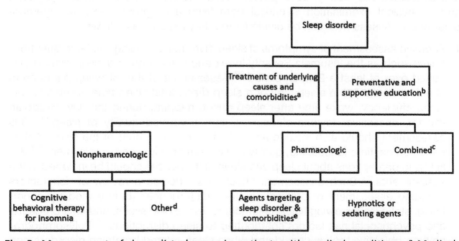

Fig. 3. Management of sleep disturbances in patients with medical conditions. [a] Medical, psychological, psychosocial, substance use, medications. [b] Sleep hygiene. [c] Nonpharmacologic and pharmacologic simultaneously. [d] Exercise and complimentary therapies such as yoga. [e] For example, mirtazapine for treating insomnia, depression, and loss of appetite.

factors that can exacerbate sleep disturbances. It is recommended that a combined approach be used to target the triggering/contributing factors (eg, pain, nocturia) as well as factors that maintain and reinforce sleep disruptions over time, such as dysfunctional beliefs about sleep and maladaptive sleep behaviors.[33,50]

When sleep disturbances persist despite addressing the contributing factors mentioned, other treatment options should be explored. These include both nonpharmacologic and pharmacologic treatment options.

Nonpharmacologic Management

Established guidelines recommend that sleep hygiene education should be included as a standard part of best practices in the management of sleep disturbances in patients with or without medical conditions.[51] Sleep hygiene education/intervention includes consistent bedtime and wake time; regular exercise, but not within 2 to 4 hours of bedtime, avoiding caffeine, alcohol, or stimulating activities for at least 6 hours before bedtime; a quiet bedroom with regulated temperature; and avoiding naps during the day.[51] It should be noted that evidence supporting the efficacy of sleep hygiene education as a single intervention for sleep disturbance remains limited. Furthermore, sleep hygiene as a single intervention is usually inadequate in patients with medical conditions owing to the multifactorial nature of sleep disturbances in these patients.[33]

A prominent role for cognitive–behavioral therapy (CBT) in the management of sleep-disturbances has been supported by evidence reported in several recent studies.[52] Studies establishing the effectiveness of CBT for insomnia (CBT-I), a specialized CBT targeting insomnia, have been conducted in patients with cancer.[30,53] The CBT-I uses a multimodal approach including sleep hygiene education, cognitive restructuring, behavioral strategies, and relaxation therapy.[54] Cognitive restructuring includes restructuring negative thoughts, dysfunctional beliefs and attitudes about sleep, addressing excessive worrying, and monitoring the adequacy of sleep.[54] Behavioral strategies include sleep restriction, stimulus control, and addressing maladaptive behaviors related to sleep.[54] Relaxation therapy, especially when combined with imagery, can be helpful to achieve cognitive and behavioral objectives.[30] In cancer survivors, randomized controlled studies using CBT-I have shown positive results with improvement in several sleep parameters and continued benefit over a 6- to 12-month period.[30,53,55] CBT principles and strategies can also be helpful to manage other factors contributing to and exacerbating sleep disturbances, such as distress associated with primary medical conditions, comorbidities (eg, pain, fatigue, depression), and medication side effects. Other nonpharmacologic treatments that have shown some preliminary efficacy in the management of sleep disturbances in patients with cancer include exercise intervention[56,57] and complementary therapies such as Mindfulness-Based Stress Reduction and yoga-based intervention.[58,59]

Pharmacologic Management

Pharmacologic treatments are commonly used to treat sleep–wake cycle disturbances in patients with medical conditions. However, evidence for their efficacy and safety remains limited in this patient population.[16] Beneficial and harmful effects of medications should be weighed carefully in terms of primary medical conditions, comorbidities, concomitant medications, and other patient factors.[33] When pharmacotherapy is used, selection of agents is guided by medical/psychiatric comorbidities, symptom patterns, drug–drug interactions, and treatment goals. One of the distinguishing features of pharmacotherapeutic management of sleep disturbances in patients with medical conditions involves selection of agents targeting both sleep problems and comorbid medical conditions as a first step. For example, mirtazapine can be considered when patients with cancer report insomnia, depression, and loss of appetite, and gabapentin can be considered for insomnia with hot flashes. Other medication classes, such as benzodiazepines or nonbenzodiazepine hypnotic agents, antihistamines, and other sedating antidepressants can also be used when necessary. However, pharmacologic treatments should be used with extreme caution owing to the higher risk of adverse effects in this patient population owing to the comorbidities and potential for interactions with other medications.[33]

Combined Treatment

Studies combining CBT-I with pharmacologic treatments report greater benefit with the combined approach than with either CBT-I or pharmacotherapy alone.[60,61] The combined approach may be even more beneficial in patients with medical conditions, because it may help to limit the dose and duration of pharmacotherapy, decreasing the risk of potential adverse effects.[33]

SPECIAL ISSUES
Multidirectional Interactions Between Sleep Disturbances, Obstructive Sleep Apnea, and Cardiometabolic and Respiratory Disorders

Several common sleep problems that cause sleep deprivation, such as poor sleep schedules, shift work, obstructive sleep apnea (OSA), narcolepsy, and other insomnias, are likely to contribute to the burden of metabolic and cardiovascular disease.[62] Sleep influences several physiologic functions, including hypothalamic–pituitary–adrenal axis activity, glucose metabolism, modulation of the autonomic nervous system, ventilation, and nocturnal oxygen saturation.[63–65] Sleep also influences diet and physical activity.[66] Sleep deprivation causes release of hormones such as ghrelin and leptin,[63] which are known to increase hunger and caloric intake, increasing the risk of obesity, impaired glucose regulation, and cardiometabolic disorders.[63] Sleep disturbances may also contribute to cardiovascular disorders via effects on periodic alterations in blood pressure and heart rate, autonomic system activity, and insulin sensitivity.[64,67]

OSA, a highly prevalent condition,[68] has been associated with insulin resistance and changes in respiration, leading to hypoxemia and hypercapnia.[47,64,65,69] OSA is characterized by periodic upper airway collapse and decrease in airflow during sleep.[70] Etiologic factors associated with OSA are divided into structural and nonstructural abnormalities. Structural abnormalities related to craniofacial bony anatomy include tonsillar hypertrophy,[71] inferior displacement of the hyoid bone, and jaw deformities such as retrognathia and micrognathia.[72] Structural abnormalities related to nasal obstruction include deviated nasal septum and nasal obstruction.[73] The most common nonstructural risk factors that predispose individuals to OSA are obesity, central fat distribution, smoking, and alcohol and sedative use before bed.[47,74] According to the Wisconsin Sleep Cohort study, the prevalence of OSA in adult women is 9% and almost 3 times higher in adult men at 24%.[75] Patients with overlapping chronic obstructive pulmonary disease and OSA experience heightened oxygen desaturation, which can cause cardiac arrhythmias, pulmonary hypertension, and nocturnal death.[65] OSA also leads to disturbances in the normal sleep cycle, including restless sleep, frequent middle of the night awakenings, snoring, and sensations of choking, which cause arousal and insomnia.[74] Subsequently patients may experience nonrestorative sleep and excessive daytime sleepiness, which can lead to changes in mood and personality, including depression, fatigue, and anxiety.[68]

Sleep disturbances and OSA have been linked with cardiovascular disorders,[69,76] respiratory disorders,[9,77] metabolic disorders such as diabetes mellitus,[64] and depression.[78] Evidence suggests multidirectional interactions and a shared patho-physiology between OSA, sleep disturbances, and these disorders (**Fig. 4**). Treatment of OSA and other sleep disturbances may help to prevent or manage these disorders.[47]

The treatment of OSA includes measures to treat the underlying cause, such as obesity with diet and exercise, and treatment of cardiovascular illness, for example, heart failure therapy such as β-blockers and diuretics.[70] Other treatment modalities include continuous positive airway pressure, and nocturnal oxygen supplementation.[70] Symptomatic treatment for excessive daytime sleepiness involves the use of modafinil or armodafinil.[79] Pharmacologic agents used to treat insomnia (eg, benzodiazepines and nonbenzodiazepine hypnotics) should generally be avoided in patients with OSA, because they can exacerbate respiratory problems. The role of treatment of OSA in remitting insomnia symptoms independent of CBT remains to be established.[80]

Sleep-Related Movement Disorders

Restless legs syndrome (RLS), also known as Willis–Ekbom disease,[81] is a common sleep-related movement disorder that occurs in 15% of the population.[82] Studies have suggested that RLS may have a strong genetic component and be autosomal dominant.[83] Other studies have suggested a disturbance in dopaminergic[84] and iron function, such as in patients with iron-deficiency anemia[85] and low dopamine.[86]

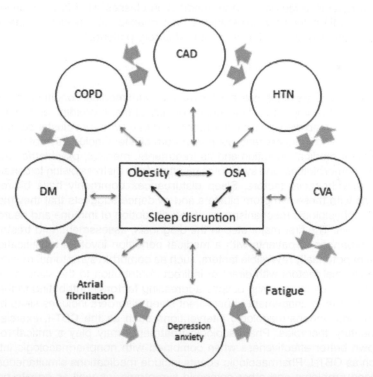

Fig. 4. Multidirectional interactions between OSA, sleep disturbances, and associated medical conditions. CAD, coronary artery disease; COPD, chronic obstructive pulmonary disease; CVA, cerebrovascular accident; DM, diabetes mellitus; HTN, hypertension; OSA, obstructive sleep apnea.

Secondary causes of RLS include acquired chronic renal diseases, peripheral neuropathy, and medications such as serotonergic antidepressants and dopamine antagonists.[81] RLS has been associated with several other medical conditions, including diabetes, Parkinson's disease, celiac disease, rheumatoid arthritis, and pregnancy.[87] The onset of RLS may range from childhood to adulthood.[88] RLS presents with symptoms such as an urge or need to constantly move one's legs.[81] Other symptoms of RLS include sensations such as aching, pulling, and creeping.[81] The symptoms are reported to worsen during periods of inactivity and rest, especially at night.[81]

PLMD is commonly seen in association with RLS.[81] It is thought to occur in 80% of patients with RLS and narcolepsy.[81] It is also associated with REM sleep behavior disorder.[89] Patients often present with symptoms of disturbed sleep, daytime fatigue, and reports of multiple middle of the night awakenings.[87] Often, a bed partner describes involuntary leg kicking by the patient with PLMD or the leg movements are captured on the sleep study.[87] Similar to RLS, PLMD is associated with diverse medical conditions including anemia, uremia, chronic lung disease, myelopathies, and peripheral neuropathy.[87]

A careful review of medical conditions, comorbidities, and medications is necessary when diagnosing RLS and PLMD. Polysomnography plays a critical role in the diagnostic assessment of PLMD.[87] The treatment of RLS and PLMD includes adjustment of aggravating medications, such as dopamine antagonists, iron supplementation in iron-deficient patients, and treatment with dopaminergic agonists such as pramipexole and ropinirol.[87] Dopamine agonists are considered first-line medications after addressing reversible factors.[87] Other medication classes used in the management of RLS and PLMD include benzodiazepines (eg, clonazepam), calcium channel ligands (eg, pregabalin), and opioids for treatment refractory patients.[81]

SUMMARY

Sleep disturbances are highly prevalent in patients with medical conditions and have a significant negative impact on functioning, quality of life, morbidity, and mortality in these patients. Sleep disorders are frequently part of a symptom cluster complicating their diagnosis and management. Such symptom clusters include symptoms related to the primary medical condition and its treatments, medical, psychiatric, and substance use comorbidities, and symptoms resulting from distress owing to certain environmental/psychosocial factors. Sleep disturbances commonly have bidirectional interactions with these symptom clusters and evidence suggests that they may also share pathophysiologic mechanisms involving disruption of immune and neuroendocrine pathways. The first major step in the diagnosis, assessment, and treatment of sleep disturbances in patients with a medical condition involves identification and treatment of potentially reversible factors, such as comorbid symptoms, medications, and psychosocial factors with direct or indirect contribution to the sleep disruption. Sleep disturbances may persist despite addressing factors contributing to the sleep problems. Further management of persistent sleep disorders includes sleep hygiene education, and nonpharmacologic interventions such as the CBT-I, exercise, and complementary therapies. Pharmacologic treatments may play a critical role and have shown better effectiveness when combined with nonpharmacologic interventions such as CBT-I. Pharmacologic agents include medications simultaneously targeting sleep problems and other comorbid symptoms, as well as agents primarily targeting sleep disruption.

Most of the studies investigating sleep–wake cycle disturbances associated with medical conditions have been conducted in patients with cancer. Studies in patients with other medical conditions are limited and are primarily epidemiologic in nature, despite the high prevalence of sleep problems in these patients. Therefore, studies investigating the diagnosis, assessment, and management of sleep disturbances are needed in patients with other major medical conditions. Such studies should also evaluate the contribution of sleep disturbances to morbidity and mortality, their relationship with medical and psychiatric comorbidities, and their impact on functioning, and the quality of life in patients with medical conditions.

REFERENCES

1. Sleep disorders problems. In: National Sleep Foundation Web site. Available at: http://sleepfoundation.org/sleep-disorders-problems. Accessed May 1, 2015.
2. Palesh OG, Roscoe JA, Mustian KM, et al. Prevalence, demographics, and psychological associations of sleep disruption in patients with cancer: University of Rochester Cancer Center-Community Clinical Oncology Program. J Clin Oncol 2010;28(2):292–8.
3. Dickerson SS, Sabbah EA, Ziegler P, et al. The experience of a diagnosis of advanced lung cancer: sleep is not a priority when living my life. Oncol Nurs Forum 2012;39(5):492–9.
4. Fiorentino L, Rissling M, Liu L, et al. The symptom cluster of sleep, fatigue and depressive symptoms in breast cancer patients: severity of the problem and treatment options. Drug Discov Today Dis Models 2011;8(4):167–73.
5. Barun B. Pathophysiological background and clinical characteristics of sleep disorders in multiple sclerosis. Clin Neurol Neurosurg 2013;115(Suppl 1): S82–5.
6. Fiorentino L, Ancoli-Israel S. Sleep dysfunction in patients with cancer. Curr Treat Options Neurol 2007;9(5):337–46.
7. Le Grande MR, Jackson AC, Murphy BM, et al. Relationship between sleep disturbance, depression and anxiety in the 12 months following a cardiac event. Psychol Health Med 2015;11:1–8.
8. Bazil CW. Epilepsy and sleep disturbance. Epilepsy Behav 2003;4(Suppl 2):S39–45.
9. Collop N. Sleep and sleep disorders in chronic obstructive pulmonary disease. Respiration 2010;80(1):78–86.
10. Ali T, Choe J, Awab A, et al. Sleep, immunity and inflammation in gastrointestinal disorders. World J Gastroenterol 2013;19(48):9231–9.
11. Roizenblatt M, Rosa Neto NS, Tufik S, et al. Pain-related diseases and sleep disorders. Braz J Med Biol Res 2012;45(9):792–8.
12. Reynolds CF 3rd, Redline S, DSM-V Sleep-Wake Disorders Workgroup and Advisors. The DSM-V sleep-wake disorders nosology: an update and an invitation to the sleep community. J Clin Sleep Med 2010;6(1):9–10.
13. Winokur A. The Relationship between sleep disturbances and psychiatric disorders: Introduction and Overview. Psychiatr Clin N Am 2015. in press.
14. Reynolds CF 3rd, O'Hara R. DSM-5 sleep-wake disorders classification: overview for use in clinical practice. Am J Psychiatry 2013;170(10):1099–101.
15. Guzman-Marin R, Avidan AY. Sleep disorders in patients with cancer. J Community Support Oncol 2015;13(4):148–55.
16. Howell D, Oliver TK, Keller-Olaman S, et al. Sleep disturbance in adults with cancer: a systematic review of evidence for best practices in assessment and management for clinical practice. Ann Oncol 2014;25(4):791–800.
17. Harsora P, Kessmann J. Nonpharmacologic management of chronic insomnia. Am Fam Physician 2009;79(2):125–30.

18. Lobentanz IS, Asenbaum S, Vass K, et al. Factors influencing quality of life in multiple sclerosis patients: disability, depressive mood, fatigue and sleep quality. Acta Neurol Scand 2004;110(1):6–13.

19. Attarian HP, Brown KM, Duntley SP, et al. The relationship of sleep disturbances and fatigue in multiple sclerosis. Arch Neurol 2004;61(4):525–8.

20. Merlino G, Fratticci L, Lenchig C, et al. Prevalence of 'poor sleep' among patients with multiple sclerosis: an independent predictor of mental and physical status. Sleep Med 2009;10(1):26–34.

21. Bamer AM, Johnson KL, Amtmann D, et al. Prevalence of sleep problems in individuals with multiple sclerosis. Mult Scler 2008;14(8):1127–30.

22. Braley TJ, Chervin RD, Segal BM. Fatigue, tiredness, lack of energy, and sleepiness in multiple sclerosis patients referred for clinical polysomnography. Mult Scler Int 2012;2012:673936.

23. Placidi F, Diomedi M, Scalise A, et al. Effect of anticonvulsants on nocturnal sleep in epilepsy. Neurology 2000;54(5 Suppl 1):S25–32.

24. Beran RG, Plunkett MJ, Holland GJ. Interface of epilepsy and sleep disorders. Seizure 1999;8(2):97–102.

25. Deak MC, Kirsch DB. Sleep-disordered breathing in neurologic conditions. Clin Chest Med 2014;35(3):547–56.

26. Moldofsky H. Rheumatic manifestations of sleep disorders. Curr Opin Rheumatol 2010;22(1):59–63.

27. Foo H, Mason P. Brainstem modulation of pain during sleep and waking. Sleep Med Rev 2003;7(2):145–54.

28. Roehrs T, Hyde M, Blaisdell B, et al. Sleep loss and REM sleep loss are hyperalgesic. Sleep 2006;29(2):145–51.

29. Banack HR, Holly CD, Lowensteyn I, et al. The association between sleep disturbance, depressive symptoms, and health-related quality of life among cardiac rehabilitation participants. J Cardiopulm Rehabil Prev 2014;34(3):188–94.

30. Berger AM. Update on the state of the science: sleep-wake disturbances in adult patients with cancer. Oncol Nurs Forum 2009;36(4):E165–77.

31. Savard J, Morin CM. Insomnia in the context of cancer: a review of a neglected problem. J Clin Oncol 2001;19(3):895–908.

32. Bastien CH, Vallières A, Morin CM. Precipitating factors of insomnia. Behav Sleep Med 2004;2(1):50–62.

33. Howell D, Oliver TK, Keller-Olaman S, et al. A Pan-Canadian practice guideline: prevention, screening, assessment, and treatment of sleep disturbances in adults with cancer. Support Care Cancer 2013;21(10):2695–706.

34. Bower JE, Ganz PA, Irwin MR, et al. Inflammation and behavioral symptoms after breast cancer treatment: do fatigue, depression, and sleep disturbance share a common underlying mechanism? J Clin Oncol 2011;29(26):3517–22.

35. Graci G. Pathogenesis and management of cancer-related insomnia. J Support Oncol 2005;3(5):349–59.

36. Boonstra L, Harden K, Jarvis S, et al. Sleep disturbance in hospitalized recipients of stem cell transplantation. Clin J Oncol Nurs 2011;15(3):271–6.

37. Dickerson SS, Connors LM, Fayad A, et al. Sleep-wake disturbances in cancer patients: narrative review of literature focusing on improving quality of life outcomes. Nat Sci Sleep 2014;6:85–100.

38. Fleming L, Gillespie S, Espie CA. The development and impact of insomnia on cancer survivors: a qualitative analysis. Psychooncology 2010;19(9):991–6.

39. Cappuccio FP, D'Elia L, Strazzullo P, et al. Sleep duration and all-cause mortality: a systematic review and meta-analysis of prospective studies. Sleep 2010;33(5):585–92.

40. Dantzer R, Kelley KW. Twenty years of research on cytokine-induced sickness behavior. Brain Behav Immun 2007;21(2):153–60.
41. Besedovsky HO, del Rey A. Immune-neuro-endocrine interactions: facts and hypotheses. Endocr Rev 1996;17(1):64–102.
42. Frank MG, Baratta MV, Sprunger DB, et al. Microglia serve as a neuroimmune substrate for stress-induced potentiation of CNS pro-inflammatory cytokine responses. Brain Behav Immun 2007;21(1):47–59.
43. Godbout JP, Chen J, Abraham J, et al. Exaggerated neuroinflammation and sickness behavior in aged mice following activation of the peripheral innate immune system. FASEB J 2005;19(10):1329–31.
44. Pace TW, Hu F, Miller AH. Cytokine-effects on glucocorticoid receptor function: relevance to glucocorticoid resistance and the pathophysiology and treatment of major depression. Brain Behav Immun 2007;21(1):9–19.
45. Miller AH, Ancoli-Israel S, Bower JE, et al. Neuroendocrine-immune mechanisms of behavioral comorbidities in patients with cancer. J Clin Oncol 2008;26(6): 971–82.
46. Irwin MR. Inflammation at the intersection of behavior and somatic symptoms. Psychiatr Clin North Am 2011;34(3):605–20.
47. Surani SR. Diabetes, sleep apnea, obesity and cardiovascular disease: why not address them together? World J Diabetes 2014;5(3):381–4.
48. Vernon MK, Dugar A, Revicki D, et al. Measurement of non-restorative sleep in insomnia: a review of the literature. Sleep Med Rev 2010;14(3):205–12.
49. Johns MW. A new method for measuring daytime sleepiness: the Epworth sleepiness scale. Sleep 1991;14(6):540–5.
50. Sleep disorders – for health professionals (PDQ). In: National Cancer Institute Website. 2014. Available at: www.cancer.gov/about-cancer/treatment/side-effects/sleep-disorders-hp-pdq. Accessed June 10, 2015.
51. Schutte-Rodin S, Broch L, Buysse D, et al. Clinical guideline for the evaluation and management of chronic insomnia in adults. J Clin Sleep Med 2008;4(5): 487–504.
52. Morin CM, Bootzin RR, Buysse DJ, et al. Psychological and behavioral treatment of insomnia: update of the recent evidence (1998-2004). Sleep 2006;29(11): 1398–414.
53. Epstein DR, Dirksen SR. Randomized trial of a cognitive-behavioral intervention for insomnia in breast cancer survivors. Oncol Nurs Forum 2007;34(5):E51–9.
54. Garland SN, Johnson JA, Savard J, et al. Sleeping well with cancer: a systematic review of cognitive behavioral therapy for insomnia in cancer patients. Neuropsychiatr Dis Treat 2014;10:1113–24.
55. Espie CA. "Stepped care": a health technology solution for delivering cognitive behavioral therapy as a first line insomnia treatment. Sleep 2009;32(12): 1549–58.
56. Mustian KM, Sprod LK, Janelsins M, et al. Exercise recommendations for cancer-related fatigue, cognitive impairment, sleep problems, depression, pain, anxiety, and physical dysfunction: a review. Oncol Hematol Rev 2012; 8(2):81–8.
57. Payne JK, Held J, Thorpe J, et al. Effect of exercise on biomarkers, fatigue, sleep disturbances, and depressive symptoms in older women with breast cancer receiving hormonal therapy. Oncol Nurs Forum 2008;35(4):635–42.
58. Carlson LE, Garland SN. Impact of mindfulness-based stress reduction (MBSR) on sleep, mood, stress and fatigue symptoms in cancer outpatients. Int J Behav Med 2005;12(4):278–85.

59. Mustian KM, Sprod LK, Janelsins M. Multicenter, randomized controlled trial of yoga for sleep quality among cancer survivors. J Clin Oncol 2013;31(26): 3233–41.

60. Jacobs GD, Pace-Schott EF, Stickgold R, et al. Cognitive behavior therapy and pharmacotherapy for insomnia: a randomized controlled trial and direct comparison. Arch Intern Med 2004;164(17):1888–96.

61. Morin CM, Colecchi C, Stone J, et al. Behavioral and pharmacological therapies for late-life insomnia: a randomized controlled trial. JAMA 1999;281(11):991–9.

62. Depner CM, Stothard ER, Wright KP Jr. Metabolic consequences of sleep and circadian disorders. Curr Diab Rep 2014;14(7):507.

63. Jackson CL, Redline S, Emmons KM. Sleep as a potential fundamental contributor to disparities in cardiovascular health. Annu Rev Public Health 2015;36:417–40.

64. Reutrakul S, Van Cauter E. Interactions between sleep, circadian function, and glucose metabolism: implications for risk and severity of diabetes. Ann N Y Acad Sci 2014;1311:151–73.

65. McNicholas WT, Verbraecken J, Marin JM. Sleep disorders in COPD: the forgotten dimension. Eur Respir Rev 2013;22(129):365–75.

66. Mozaffarian D, Hao T, Rimm EB, et al. Changes in diet and lifestyle and long-term weight gain in women and men. N Engl J Med 2011;364(25):2392–404.

67. Spiegelhalder K, Fuchs L, Ladwig J, et al. Heart rate and heart rate variability in subjectively reported insomnia. J Sleep Res 2011;20(1 Pt 2):137–45.

68. Macey PM, Woo MA, Kumar R, et al. Relationship between obstructive sleep apnea severity and sleep, depression and anxiety symptoms in newly-diagnosed patients. PLoS One 2010;5(4):e10211.

69. Genta-Pereira DC, Pedrosa RP, Lorenzi-Filho G, et al. Sleep disturbances and resistant hypertension: association or causality? Curr Hypertens Rep 2014; 16(8):459.

70. Costanzo MR, Khayat R, Ponikowski P, et al. Mechanisms and clinical consequences of untreated central sleep apnea in heart failure. J Am Coll Cardiol 2015;65(1):72–84.

71. Moser RJ 3rd, Rajagopal KR. Obstructive sleep apnea in adults with tonsillar hypertrophy. Arch Intern Med 1987;147(7):1265–7.

72. Watanabe T, Isono S, Tanaka A, et al. Contribution of body habitus and craniofacial characteristics to segmental closing pressures of the passive pharynx in patients with sleep-disordered breathing. Am J Respir Crit Care Med 2002; 165(2):260–5.

73. Young T, Skatrud J, Peppard PE. Risk factors for obstructive sleep apnea in adults. JAMA 2004;291(16):2013–6.

74. Patil SP, Schneider H, Schwartz AR, et al. Adult obstructive sleep apnea: pathophysiology and diagnosis. Chest 2007;132(1):325–37.

75. Dancey DR, Hanly PJ, Soong C, et al. Gender differences in sleep apnea: the role of neck circumference. Chest 2003;123(5):1544–50.

76. Grandner MA. Addressing sleep disturbances: an opportunity to prevent cardiometabolic disease? Int Rev Psychiatry 2014;26(2):155–76.

77. Böing S, Randerath WJ. Sleep disorders in asthma and chronic obstructive pulmonary disease (COPD). Ther Umsch 2014;71(5):301–8.

78. Gilat H, Vinker S, Buda I, et al. Obstructive sleep apnea and cardiovascular comorbidities: a large epidemiologic study. Medicine (Baltimore) 2014;93(9):e45.

79. Pack AI, Black JE, Schwartz JR, et al. Modafinil as adjunct therapy for daytime sleepiness in obstructive sleep apnea. Am J Respir Crit Care Med 2001; 164(9):1675–81.

80. Krakow B, Melendrez D, Lee SA, et al. Refractory insomnia and sleep-disordered breathing: a pilot study. Sleep Breath 2004;8(1):15–29.
81. Silber MH, Becker PM, Earley C, et al. Willis-Ekbom Disease Foundation revised consensus statement on the management of restless legs syndrome. Mayo Clin Proc 2013;88(9):977–86.
82. Malhotra A, Orr JE, Owens RL. On the cutting edge of obstructive sleep apnoea: where next? Lancet Respir Med 2015;3(5):397–403.
83. Trenkwalder C, Högl B, Winkelmann J. Recent advances in the diagnosis, genetics and treatment of restless legs syndrome. J Neurol 2009;256(4):539–53.
84. Connor JR, Wang XS, Allen RP, et al. Altered dopaminergic profile in the putamen and substantia nigra in restless leg syndrome. Brain 2009;132(Pt 9):2403–12.
85. Connor JR, Boyer PJ, Menzies SL, et al. Neuropathological examination suggests impaired brain iron acquisition in restless legs syndrome. Neurology 2003;61(3): 304–9.
86. Cervenka S, Pålhagen SE, Comley RA, et al. Support for dopaminergic hypoactivity in restless legs syndrome: a PET study on D2-receptor binding. Brain 2006; 129(Pt 8):2017–28.
87. Salas RE, Rasquinha R, Gamaldo CE. All the wrong moves: a clinical review of restless legs syndrome, periodic limb movements of sleep and wake, and periodic limb movement disorder. Clin Chest Med 2010;31(2):383–95.
88. Gamaldo CE, Benbrook AR, Allen RP, et al. Childhood and adult factors associated with restless legs syndrome (RLS) diagnosis. Sleep Med 2007;8(7–8): 716–22.
89. Mendelson WB. Are periodic leg movements associated with clinical sleep disturbance? Sleep 1996;19(3):219–23.

New Developments in Insomnia Medications of Relevance to Mental Health Disorders

Andrew D. Krystal, MD, MS*

KEYWORDS

- Personalization • Insomnia • Comorbid psychiatric disorders • Suvorexant
- Doxepin • Prazosin • Eszopiclone

KEY POINTS

- There are a number of insomnia medications with high specificity of effects, many of which have recently become available.
- Such agents pave the way for a new paradigm for insomnia therapy where specific interventions are selected to target a specific type of sleep.
- This approach promises an improved risk–benefit ratio over the traditional "one-size-fits-all" approach to insomnia therapy.
- This article reviews insomnia medications and discusses the implications for optimizing the treatment of insomnia occurring comorbid with psychiatric conditions.

INTRODUCTION

There are a number of different medications available for treating patients with insomnia. However, consistent with guidelines, these interventions are generally not administered with any degree of personalization.[1] The treatment of insomnia has long been carried out without subtyping insomnia patients and customizing the choice of treatment to match patient subtype.

The primary reason for this has been that, for many years, we have had only a limited set of interventions to administer and there has not been any evidence that these differ fundamentally in the nature of their therapeutic effects. Treatment was long dominated by a group of medications which bind to the benzodiazepine binding

Grants/Research Support: NIH (HHS-N271-2012-000006-I, R01 MH095780, R01 MH091053, R01HL096492, R01 MH078961, R01 MH076856), Teva, Sunovion, Neosynch, Brainsway, Janssen, Novartis, Eisai. Consultant: Attentiv, Teva, Eisai, Jazz, Janssen, Merck, Neurocrine, Novartis, Otsuka, Pfizer, Lundbeck, Roche, Sunovion, Paladin, Pernix, Transcept.
Duke Clinical Research Institute, Duke University School of Medicine, Durham, NC 27705, USA
* Box 3309 DUMC, Durham, NC 27710.
E-mail address: andrew.krystal@duke.edu

Psychiatr Clin N Am 38 (2015) 843–860
http://dx.doi.org/10.1016/j.psc.2015.08.001
0193-953X/15/$ – see front matter © 2015 Elsevier Inc. All rights reserved.

Abbreviations	
α_1	α_1 adrenergic receptor
5-HT	Serotonin
5-HT-2	Serotonin 5-HT-2 receptor
FDA	Food and drug administration
GABA	Gamma-aminobutyric acid
GABA-A	Gamma-aminobutyric acid type A receptor
H1	Histamine H1 receptors
MT1	Melatonin type 1 receptor
MT2	Melatonin type 2 receptor
NE	Norepinephrine
OX1	Orexin type 1 receptor
OX2	Orexin type 2 receptor

site of the gamma-aminobutyric acid (GABA) type A (GABA-A) receptor complex.[2] Examples include triazolam, temazepam, flurazepam, zolpidem, zaleplon, and eszopiclone. These medications have been believed to differ only in their pharmacokinetic profiles that, along with medication dosage, determine the timing and duration of clinical effects. As a result, the personalization of therapy that has been possible has been limited to matching the time of night of effect of medications to the time of night of a given patient's sleep difficulty as specified in the US Food and Drug Administration (FDA) indications for these medications.[1–3] For example, zolpidem and zaleplon are indicated only for the treatment of problems falling asleep, whereas eszopiclone and the extended release formulation of zolpidem are indicated for the treatment of patients with sleep onset problems, sleep maintenance problems, or both.[2,3]

A greater degree of personalization is increasingly becoming possible in the clinical management of insomnia based on new research on insomnia therapies and the existence of medications with high specificity, many of which have become available recently.[3] These agents include drugs that act with high specificity at particular receptors and have a relatively focused impact on particular brain circuits. Such agents pave the way for a new paradigm for insomnia therapy where specific medications are selected to target the specific type of sleep difficulty experienced by each patient. This paradigm includes specific agents for patients with insomnia cooccurring with particular psychiatric disorders.

For example, evidence indicates that some insomnia medications have greater therapeutic effects in patients with insomnia occurring with major depression and generalized anxiety disorder than others.[3–8] This approach promises an improved risk–benefit ratio over the traditional "one-size-fits-all" model of insomnia therapy based on drugs without pharmacologic specificity and on drugs that have relatively global effects impacting many areas of the brain other than those needed to improve a patient's particular sleep problem. There are times when high effect specificity is not desirable, including instances where a medication is being used to treat more than 1 condition, such as insomnia and depression. Another instance where high specificity may not be optimal is when there are several processes driving insomnia, such as stress, pain, and depression.

The critical point is that we now have tools available with varying specificity of effects and different types of specific effects that provide us with unprecedented ability to target therapy to the particular needs of each patient. Taking advantage of this opportunity so as to optimize care requires that we understand the particular characteristics of each of our treatment options and the relative merits of administering these options to the various types of patients encountered in clinical practice. To this end, this article reviews the insomnia medications in light of the new paradigm of personalization, with special emphasis on implications for optimizing the treatment of insomnia cooccurring with psychiatric conditions.

OVERVIEW OF INSOMNIA THERAPIES

The current primary treatment options for insomnia include nonmedication therapies, most notably cognitive–behavioral therapy for insomnia and a number of types of pharmacologic therapies. The scope of this article is limited to considering the medication therapies for insomnia. Pharmacologic therapies are composed of the benzodiazepines, the nonbenzodiazepines, the selective melatonin receptor agonists, the selective histamine H1 antagonists, the selective adrenergic α_1 antagonists, the selective hypocretin/orexin antagonists, antidepressants, antipsychotics, and over-the-counter nonselective H1 antagonists. These agents vary in the specificity of their effects (**Table 1**). Some agents have high pharmacologic specificity in terms of having effects at a single receptor. Of these agents, some have nonspecific clinical effects because the receptor that they affect has a broad impact on brain function. Others have very specific clinical effects because binding to their target receptor has a relatively limited effect on the brain, mainly impacting specific sleep–wake modulating circuitry.[9] Insomnia medications are reviewed in the following sections, focusing on the degree of specificity of their effects and the implications for optimizing insomnia therapy.

INSOMNIA MEDICATIONS WITH RELATIVELY LOW SPECIFICITY OF EFFECTS

Medications with low specificity of effects include the benzodiazepines, the nonbenzodiazepines, antidepressants, antipsychotics, and over-the-counter antihistamines. Their low specificity is owing to either having clinically significant effects on multiple receptors or because the receptor that they bind to has a broad impact on brain function. These agents have long dominated the clinical treatment of insomnia and are the foundation upon which our current one-size-fits-all model of insomnia pharmacotherapy was built.

Benzodiazepines

Distinguishing characteristics
The benzodiazepines are a group of medications that share a common chemical structure.[3]

Agents used to treat insomnia
Agents approved by the FDA for insomnia include triazolam, flurazepam, temazepam, estazolam, and quazepam.[2] Agents approved by the US FDA for an indication other than insomnia include clonazepam (approved for seizures, anxiety), alprazolam (approved for anxiety), and lorazepam (approved for anxiety).[2]

Mechanism of action
The benzodiazepines are positive allosteric modulators of the GABA-A receptor complex. They bind to a site on the receptor complex, referred to as the "benzodiazepine binding site" and create a conformational change that enhances the inhibition that occurs when GABA binding activates the receptor.[10] The effects on sleep derive from enhancing the GABA-A–mediated inhibition of wake promoting regions of the brain such as the lateral hypothalamus, the tuberomammillary nucleus, and the locus coeruleus.

Table 1
Specificity of insomnia therapies

Treatment	Pharmacologic Specificity	Specificity of Effect on Brain Function	Target
Suvorexant	Highly specific	Highly specific	Antagonism of orexin receptors
Doxepin 3–6 mg	Highly specific	Highly specific	Antagonism of H1 histamine receptors
Prazosin	Highly specific	Highly specific	Antagonism of α_1 adrenergic receptors
Ramelteon	Highly specific	Highly specific	Agonism of melatonin MT1/MT2 receptors
Benzodiazepines	Highly specific	Nonspecific	Binding to benzodiazepine binding site on GABA-A receptor complex leads to broad CNS inhibition
Nonbenzodiazepines	Highly specific	Nonspecific	Binding to benzodiazepine binding site on GABA-A receptor complex leads to broad CNS inhibition
Antidepressants	Nonspecific	Nonspecific	Antagonism of 5HT and NE transporters, 5HT2, α_1, adrenergic, H1 histaminergic, and muscarinic cholinergic antagonism
Antipsychotics	Nonspecific	Nonspecific	Dopamine type 2, dopamine type 1, 5HT2, α_1, adrenergic, H1 histaminergic, and muscarinic cholinergic antagonism
OTC "antihistamines"	Nonspecific	Nonspecific	Antagonism of H1 histamine receptors and cholinergic receptors

Abbreviations: 5HT2, 5-hydroxytryptamine 2; CNS, central nervous system; GABA, gamma-aminobutyric acid; MT1, melatonin type 1 receptor; MT2, melatonin type 2 receptor; NE, norepinephrine; OTC, over the counter.

Pharmacologic specificity

The benzodiazepines have high pharmacologic specificity in dosages used to treat insomnia. At these dosages, all of the clinical effects of these agents are believed to be owing to positive allosteric modulation of the GABA-A receptor complex at the benzodiazepine binding site. However, it should be noted that, among agents that bind to the benzodiazepine binding site of the GABA-A receptor complex, the benzodiazepines are relatively nonspecific. They cause clinically significant effects through binding to 4 different types of GABA-A receptors, each of which has a different distribution in the brain.[11,12]

Specificity of effects on brain functions (effects other than sleep–wake systems)
Benzodiazepines have broad inhibitory effects on brain function. This is because GABA is the predominant inhibitory neurotransmitter in the brain. As a result, enhancement of GABA-A–mediated inhibition has the potential to have extremely broad effects. By exerting effects at 4 major GABA-A receptor types, the benzodiazepines produce widespread inhibition of brain activity.[9,11–13] The result of this widespread inhibition is that these medications have a number of clinical effects other than sleep enhancement. Such effects include anxiolytic effects, cognitive impairment, motor impairment, myorelaxation, antiseizure effects, and rewarding effects associated with abuse potential.

Clinical implications for personalization of therapy
Based on the nonspecific clinical effects of the benzodiazepines, they are well-suited for use in patients who have insomnia occurring in the setting of 1 or more conditions that can be improved by the nonsleep effects of these medications. Examples include patients with insomnia occurring with significant anxiety or pain, for which the anxiolytic and myorelaxant effects of these medications are highly desirable. Patients without such cooccurring conditions are best treated with another type of medication because of the non–sleep-related effects of these agents, such as cognitive impairment, motor impairment, and abuse potential, which result in a risk–benefit ratio that is less favorable than that of other options for patients without cooccurring conditions, such as severe anxiety. The 1 exception to this is that, compared with other available options, the benzodiazepines and nonbenzodiazepines administered in the dosages routinely used to treat insomnia have the most robust effects on sleep onset.[2] As a result, there may be some patients with severe sleep onset difficulty for whom a benzodiazepine may constitute the agent with the best risk–benefit ratio of available medications, even where there is not an associated condition that is also being targeted for therapy.

Nonbenzodiazepines

Distinguishing characteristics
The nonbenzodiazepines are a heterogenous group of medications that do not have the chemical structure common to benzodiazepines but act via the same mechanism as the benzodiazepines.[3]

Agents used to treat insomnia
Agents approved nu the FDA for insomnia include zolpidem and zaleplon (approved for the treatment of sleep onset difficulties only) and zolpidem modified release and eszopiclone (approved for the treatment of sleep onset and maintenance difficulties).[2]

Mechanism of action
The nonbenzodiazepines, like the benzodiazepines, are positive allosteric modulators of the GABA-A receptor complex, promoting sleep by enhancing GABA-A–mediated inhibition of wake promoting regions of the brain, such as the lateral hypothalamus, the tuberomammillary nucleus, and the locus coeruleus.

Pharmacologic specificity
The nonbenzodiazepines have high pharmacologic specificity in dosages used to treat insomnia. At these dosages, all of the clinical effects of these agents are believed to be owing to positive allosteric modulation of the GABA-A receptor complex at the benzodiazepine binding site. However, they have greater pharmacologic specificity than the benzodiazepines. Although the benzodiazepines have clinically significant

effects at 4 major types of GABA-A receptors, the nonbenzodiazepines tend to bind preferentially to a subset of these GABA-A receptors.[11,12]

Specificity of effects on brain functions (effects on systems other than sleep–wake systems)

The nonbenzodiazepines, like the benzodiazepines, have relatively broad inhibitory effects on brain function owing to the wide distribution of GABA in the brain. However, the clinical effects of the nonbenzodiazepines are believed to be relatively more focused than the benzodiazepines.[11,12] Zolpidem and zaleplon have effects predominantly at GABA-A receptors, which enhance sleep but also lead to impairment of cognition and motor function.[11,12] Eszopiclone binding to GABA-A receptors has relatively greater anxiolytic, myorelxant, and perhaps antidepressant effects in addition to sleep enhancing effects. Indeed, when eszopiclone/fluoxetine cotherapy was compared with placebo/fluoxetine treatment of patients with depression and insomnia, eszopiclone was found not only to improve sleep but also to enhance the antidepressant response (eszopiclone led to improvement in nonsleep depression symptoms).[4,5] Eszopiclone similarly improved not only sleep, but also symptoms of generalized anxiety disorder compared with placebo when administered with escitalopram.[6] However, when equivalent studies were carried out with zolpidem modified release, improvement in sleep compared with placebo was noted but not improvement in depression or symptoms of generalized anxiety disorder.[7,8]

Clinical implications for personalization of therapy

The differences among the nonbenzodiazepines dictate different uses for these medications. Based on the available evidence, eszopiclone stands as the treatment of choice for combination with selective serotonin (5-HT) reuptake inhibitor therapy in the treatment of patients with insomnia cooccurring with major depression and generalized anxiety disorder.[4–6] Zolpidem and zaleplon have robust effects on sleep onset like the benzodiazepines. However, they are preferred over the benzodiazepines owing to their relatively limited duration of effects and less broad clinical impact, which together represent an improved risk–benefit profile for those with severe sleep onset difficulties.[2] In those with severe sleep onset problems who also have sleep maintenance difficulties, it is necessary to turn to eszopiclone and zolpidem modified release, which have both robust onset effects and therapeutic effects on sleep maintenance.[2] Note that these agents are preferred only where severe sleep onset problems occur along with maintenance difficulties. If it is not the case that onset problems are substantial, then there are other agents with more favorable risk–benefit ratios than the nonbenzodiazepines (see below).

Antidepressants

Distinguishing characteristics

The antidepressants are a heterogenous group of agents of a number of chemical classes which have been approved by the US FDA for the treatment of major depression. Despite their relatively widespread use for the treatment of insomnia, limited data exist regarding the treatment of insomnia with these agents.

Agents used to treat insomnia

There are no antidepressants approved by the US FDA for the treatment of insomnia in the dosage range used to treat depression.[2] The antidepressants most frequently used "off-label" to treat insomnia include trazodone, mirtazapine, amitriptyline, and doxepin.[2] These agents are generally used in dosages below their antidepressant dosages when used to treat insomnia. Doxepin, in dosages of 3 to 6 mg (antidepressant dosage range 75–150 mg), is approved by the US FDA for insomnia treatment.

Mechanism of action

The mechanism by which antidepressants are believed to have therapeutic effects on depression primarily involves inhibition of the 5-HT and norepinephrine (NE) reuptake transporters. The mechanisms underlying their effects on sleep differ but derive from antagonism of 1 or more wake promoting systems mediated by blockade of the serotonin 5-HT-2 receptor (5-HT-2), α_1 adrenergic, H1 histaminergic, and muscarinic cholinergic receptors.[2]

Pharmacologic specificity

The antidepressants are nonselective agents pharmacologically with varying degrees of antagonism of 5-HT and NE transporters, and 5-HT-2, α_1, adrenergic, H1 histaminergic, and muscarinic cholinergic antagonism.[2]

Specificity of effects on brain functions (effects on systems other than sleep–wake systems)

Because of the pharmacologic nonselectivity of these agents, they have relatively widespread effects on brain function, inhibiting a number of key neural systems. This results in effects other than sleep enhancement that vary among these agents and leads to a relatively unfavorable side effect profile in many cases. Given the lack of trials of insomnia treatment with these agents, the side effect profiles generally have to be inferred from trials of these patients carried out in patients with mood or anxiety disorders. Their side effects may include weight gain, orthostatic hypotension, dry mouth, constipation, blurred vision, urinary retention, cognitive impairment, cardiotoxicity, sexual dysfunction, and potentially delirium.[2]

Clinical implications for personalization of therapy

Given the lack of data from controlled trials, it is not possible to reliably determine the risk–benefit ratio of these agents when used to treat insomnia. However, in theory, these agents would be expected to be particularly useful in cases where nonspecific effects are advantageous. This would include patients with insomnia cooccurring with depression, anxiety, pain, stress. In this regard, there have been 3 small, double-blind, controlled studies of the treatment of insomnia cooccurring mood disorders with trazodone 50 to 100 mg.[14–16] These studies provided some evidence that trazodone improves sleep (primary benefit seen in sleep maintenance) when administered in this setting. However, benefit was offset by significant next-day morning impairment, which was detected with objective testing. It is reasonable to consider the use of these agents in treatment-resistant insomnia patients in whom it might be advantageous to block multiple wake-promoting systems.

Antipsychotics

Distinguishing characteristics

The antipsychotics, much like the antidepressants, are a heterogenous group of agents from a number of different chemical classes that have been approved by the US FDA for the treatment of psychotic disorders. Like the antidepressants, they have a relatively widespread use for the treatment of insomnia despite the fact that minimal data exist regarding the treatment of insomnia with these agents.[2]

Agents used to treat insomnia

No antipsychotics are approved by the US FDA for the treatment of insomnia.[2] The antipsychotics most frequently used off-label to treat insomnia include quetiapine, olanzapine, lurasidone, and risperidone.[2] These agents are generally used in dosages below their antipsychotic dosages when used to treat insomnia.

Mechanism of action

The mechanism by which antipsychotic drugs are believed to have therapeutic effects on psychosis involves primarily blockade of the dopamine type 2 receptor. The mechanisms underlying their effects on sleep differ, but derive from antagonism of 1 or more wake-promoting systems mediated by blockade of 5-HT-2, α_1 adrenergic, H1 histaminergic, dopaminergic, and muscarinic cholinergic receptors.[2]

Pharmacologic specificity

The antipsychotics are nonselective agents pharmacologically with varying degrees of antagonism of 5-HT-2, serotonin 5-HT-7 receptor, α_1, adrenergic, H1 histaminergic, dopaminergic (dopamine type 1 and dopamine type 2), and muscarinic cholinergic antagonism.[2]

Specificity of effects on brain functions (effects on systems other than sleep–wake systems)

Because of the pharmacologic nonselectivity of these agents, they have relatively widespread effects on brain function, inhibiting a number of key neural systems. This results in effects other than sleep enhancement that vary among these agents and leads to a relatively unfavorable side effect profile in many cases. Given the lack of trials of insomnia treatment with these agents, the side effect profiles generally have to be inferred from trials of these patients carried out in patients with schizophrenia and bipolar disorder. The side effects may include weight gain, insulin resistance, orthostatic hypotension, dry mouth, constipation, blurred vision, urinary retention, cognitive impairment, extrapyramidal side effects such as tardive dyskinesia and parkinsonism, and sexual dysfunction.[2]

Clinical implications for personalization of therapy

As with antidepressants, given the lack of data from controlled trials, it is not possible to reliably determine the risk–benefit ratio of antipsychotic drugs when used to treat insomnia. However, in theory, these agents would be expected to be particularly useful in cases where nonspecific effects are advantageous. This would include patients with insomnia cooccurring with mania, schizophrenia, depression, anxiety, pain, or stress. It is also reasonable to consider these agents in treatment-resistant insomnia patients where it might be advantageous to block multiple wake-promoting systems.

Nonselective Antihistamines

Distinguishing characteristics

Medications referred to as "antihistamines" are generally those that were developed for the treatment of allergies.[3] Among these agents are a group that are available over the counter and used to treat sleep problems. We refer to them as nonselective antihistamines in that they have clinically significant effects at receptors other than H1 receptors in doses used for insomnia treatment. Like the antidepressants and antipsychotics, these agents are used by many people suffering from disturbed sleep despite the fact that minimal data exist on their risk–benefit profile in the treatment of insomnia patients.[2,9]

Agents used to treat insomnia

The agents available over the counter with significant histamine H1 receptor antagonism that are most commonly used to treat insomnia are diphenhydramine, doxylamine, and chlorpheniramine.[2,3]

Mechanism of action

The mechanisms underlying the sleep enhancing effects of these agents is believed to be antagonism of H1 histamine receptors and muscarinic cholinergic receptors.[2,9] This antagonism blocks the wake-promoting effects of histamine neurons in the tuberomammillary nucleus and mitigates the wake promotion mediated by acetylcholine.[2,9]

Pharmacologic specificity

These agents, in the dosages used to treat sleep disturbance, are relatively nonselective among those that block H1 receptors because of their clinically significant effects at both H1 and muscarinic cholinergic receptors.[2,9]

Specificity of effects on brain functions (effects on systems other than sleep–wake systems)

The cholinergic antagonism of these agents results in effects other than sleep enhancement, which leads to a relatively unfavorable side effect profile compared with the selective H1 antagonists in many cases. The associated side effects may include dry mouth, blurred vision, constipation, urinary retention, cognitive impairment, and delirium.[2,3,9]

Clinical implications for personalization of therapy

The limited data on insomnia treatment with these agents limits estimating their risk–benefit profile. No data exist for chlorpheniramine. Doxylamine has only been studied in a double-blind, placebo-controlled trial in patients experiencing sleep disturbance after surgery and found some benefit in self-reported sleep with this agent.[17] A few trials have been carried out with diphenhydramine, which preliminarily indicate that this agent has more benefit for sleep maintenance than onset, although in 1 study, sleep enhancing effects were lost over several days of dosing.[18–23] Because more selective H1 antagonists have robust effects on sleep maintenance, a better side effect profile, and have been definitively found not to lose benefit in up to 3 months of nightly use, they should be preferred for use over these nonselective H1 antagonists. The only exception to this is the treatment of insomnia occurring in patients with rhinitis, where the anticholinergic effects of these agents would be of benefit.[9,24,25]

INSOMNIA MEDICATIONS WITH HIGHLY SPECIFIC EFFECTS

There are a number of medications available for treating patients with insomnia that have highly specific pharmacologic effects that lead to relatively focused effects on brain function. These agents provide us, for the first time, with a window into the varying clinical effects of modulating specific brain systems. They establish a new guiding principal for conceptualizing insomnia medications: "mechanism matters" and open the door to a new paradigm for insomnia therapy, where medications are chosen to address the specific type of problem experienced by subgroups of insomnia patients. In this section, these medications are discussed, reviewing the support for this new paradigm and outlining how each drug fits into this paradigm in terms of clinical indications for their optimal use.

Selective H1 Histamine Receptor Antagonists

Distinguishing characteristics

This group of agents is distinguished from the nonspecific histamine H1 antagonists by having greater pharmacologic specificity.[2,9] The nonspecific antihistamines reviewed have relatively greater effects at muscarinic cholinergic receptors than the agents considered to be highly selective.

Agents used to treat insomnia

Doxepin, in dosages of 3 to 6 mg, is the only highly selective H1 antagonist that is available for use in the treatment of insomnia patients.[2,9] Doxepin is referred to as a "tricyclic antidepressant" and in dosages from 75 to 300 mg this agent has broad pharmacologic effects and is FDA approved for the treatment of depression.[2,9] However, in dosages of 3 to 6 mg doxepin becomes a highly selective and potent H1 antagonist and is FDA approved for the treatment of insomnia.

Mechanism of action

Selective H1 antagonists enhance sleep by preventing the arousing effect of histamine mediated by binding to H1 receptors.[9]

Pharmacologic specificity

Although many agents are referred to as antihistamines, doxepin, in the 3 to 6 mg range, is actually a more potent and selective H1 antagonist than any agent available in the United States that is referred to as an antihistamine.[9] Doxepin's most potent effect is H1 antagonism and its affinity for this receptor is more than 7 times greater than its affinity for any other receptor.[9] The consequence of this relatively greater H1 affinity is that there should be a dosage where doxepin has clinically relevant effects at H1 and at no other receptors.[9] This seems to be the case for the 3- to 6-mg range, whereas in dosages from 75 to 300 mg, doxepin has clinically important effects at multiple receptors including the 5-HT and NE transporters, which are believed to represent the mechanisms responsible for its robust antidepressant effects.[9] Thus, doxepin, in the 3- to 6-mg range, is an intervention with high pharmacologic specificity for antagonism of histamine H1 receptors. The trials carried out with low-dose doxepin administration provide our first glimpse into the clinical effects associated with highly specific H1 antagonism.

Specificity of effects on brain functions (effects on systems other than sleep–wake systems)

As a consequence of the pharmacologic specificity of doxepin 3 to 6 mg for histamine H1 receptors and the relatively limited impact of the histamine system, this agent has relatively circumscribed effects on brain function.[9] Because histamine H1 receptor activation plays a limited role in functions other than enhancing arousal, the clinical effects of doxepin in the 3- to 6-mg range are also limited primarily to preventing arousal, as evidenced by the relative absence of side effects observed in clinical trials.[9,24–27] Further, given that histamine is only 1 of a set of wake-promoting systems that function in parallel and can maintain the arousal level even if histamine H1 receptors are blocked (NE, hypocretin/orexin, acetylcholine, 5-HT, etc), the clinical effects of doxepin 3 to 6 mg are limited to situations where histamine release is significant and activity in the other wake-promoting systems is relatively minimal.[9] This occurs primarily in the middle and end of the night. At other times, blocking histamine is of relatively minimal consequence; arousal is maintained by the other parallel wake promoting systems. As a result, doxepin 3 to 6 mg has a highly circumscribed effect that is limited to enhancing sleep during the middle and end of the night. The clinical manifestation of having such a focal impact is an improved risk–benefit ratio over other options for treating sleep maintenance problems.[9,24–27]

Clinical implications for personalization of therapy

Based on the relatively favorable risk–benefit ratio of doxepin 3 to 6 mg for treating patients with sleep maintenance insomnia, this agent should be considered for patients experiencing difficulty staying asleep in the relative absence of problems falling asleep. Of particular note, this agent, along with the hypocretin/orexin antagonists are the only drugs that can improve sleep in the last third of the night without substantially increasing the risk of morning impairment.[9] In fact, doxepin 3 to 6 mg is unique in having its greatest therapeutic effect size in the last hour of the night.[24,25] As such, it is the treatment of choice for those whose sleep difficulties are predominantly problems with early morning awakening, a group that includes many patients with psychiatric disorders (**Table 2**). The robust therapeutic effect such individuals have in response to treatment with such focused H1 antagonism suggests that they represent a subgroup of insomnia patients who have histamine overactivity underlying their insomnia. This is consistent with preclinical data on the physiology of the histamine system, which indicate that the primary effect of this system is to increase arousal at the end of the night.[9,28] This subgroup of patients who experiences sleep disturbance predominantly in the last third of the night, includes many older adults and defines the target phenotype for this medication. By identifying this subgroup and treating them with the specific intervention that best targets their type of sleep difficulty, that is, doxepin 3 to 6 mg, it is possible to improve the risk–benefit ratio as compared with providing insomnia therapy, which is not personalized in this way.

Selective Hypocretin/Orexin Antagonists

Distinguishing characteristics
This group of agents is distinguished by having as their predominant pharmacologic effect antagonism of receptors of the peptide hypocretin/orexin (hereafter referred to as orexin).

Agents used to treat insomnia
There is currently only 1 orexin antagonist available for the treatment of insomnia. This agent, suvorexant, blocks both types of orexin receptors (orexin type 1 receptor [OX1]

Table 2
Personalizing insomnia therapies for patients with psychiatric disorders

Condition Associated with Insomnia	Most Specific Agents Suited for Use	Nonspecific Agents Best-Suited for Use
Generalized anxiety disorder	Suvorexant (theoretic basis)	Eszopiclone
Posttraumatic stress disorder	Prazosin	—
Major depression	—	Eszopiclone
Substance dependence/ discontinuation	Suvorexant (theoretic basis)	—
Psychosis	—	Antipsychotic
Any condition associated only with early morning awakening or early morning awaking and sleep maintenance difficulty	Doxepin 3–6 mg	—
Any condition associated only with problems falling asleep	Ramelteon/melatonin	Zolpidem/zaleplon
Any condition associated with problems falling asleep and staying asleep	Suvorexant	Eszopiclone, zolpidem extended release
Delayed sleep phase syndrome	Melatonin	—
Autism and other neurodevelopmental disorders	Melatonin	—

and orexin type 2 receptor [OX2]) and is approved by the FDA for treatment of problems falling asleep and staying asleep in dosages of 10 to 20 mg.[29–31]

Mechanism of action

Orexins are peptides released by the lateral hypothalamus that play an important role in maintaining wakefulness. Support for this role derives in part from evidence that loss of orexin neurons is associated with narcolepsy in humans and a number of different animals.[32] Selective orexin antagonists enhance sleep by preventing the arousing effects of orexin peptides, which are mediated by their binding to OX1 and OX2 receptors.[32]

Pharmacologic specificity

There are a number of orexin antagonists with high pharmacologic specificity, including suvorexant, which is potent and selective in terms of having orexin receptor antagonism as its predominant effect.[31]

Specificity of effects on brain functions (effects on systems other than sleep–wake systems)

Orexin receptor antagonists have highly focused effects on the brain. Remarkably, there are only 10,000 to 20,000 neurons in the entire brain that release orexins.[32,33] The orexin antagonists block only the receptors targeted by these neurons. However, the orexin receptors modulate the activity of a number of key brain areas that are responsible for their arousing effects but also would be expected to affect motivation, reward function, feeding behavior, locomotion, and sympathetic nervous system tone.[34] This occurs because of the presence of orexin receptors on neurons in the cortex, basal forebrain, tuberomammillary nucleus, periaqueductal gray, dorsal raphe, locus coeruleus, nucleus accumbens, substantia nigra, nucleus of the solitary tract, and ventromedial medulla.[34] So, although the orexin receptors have highly limited effects on brain function, in addition to promoting arousal, these agents would be expected to modulate several other functions that may be of clinical relevance. However, these modulatory effects do not manifest in adverse effects clinically. The side effect profile observed in clinical trials with suvorexant suggests a quite favorable risk–benefit ratio, with limited adverse effects, consistent with a medication that is highly specific, having effects predominantly on arousal systems.[30,31] Of particular interest with respect to the adverse effects of these agents, there is no evidence that suvorexant causes narcolepsy-like symptoms, such as cataplexy, hallucinations, and paralysis, that might have been expected based on the fact that loss of orexin neurons is associated with narcolepsy.[30–32]

Clinical implications for personalization of therapy

The clinical effects of orexin receptor antagonists have been evaluated primarily in patients with primary insomnia.[30,31] Although 1 study included patients with medical and psychiatric conditions cooccurring with insomnia, the sizes of the groups of subjects with these conditions was insufficient to allow subgroup analyses.[31] As a result, relatively little is known about the effects of orexin antagonists on the various presentations of insomnia patients encountered in clinical practice. However, we can infer that insomnia subgroups likely to improve with treatment with orexin receptor antagonists on the basis of information regarding the anatomy and physiology of the orexin system. As discussed, consideration of the outputs of the orexin neurons indicates a primary effect of promoting arousal but also modulation of motivation, reward function, feeding behavior, locomotion, and sympathetic nervous system tone.[34] Consideration of the inputs to orexin neurons can provide insight about what triggers orexin neurons to increase the arousal level and modulate motivation, reward, and other functions. A key input to the orexin neurons comes from the circadian clock, the suprachiasmatic nucleus of the hypothalamus.[34] The input from the clock is responsible for what is believed to be among the most important functions of orexin neurons, which is to maintain arousal during the biological day so as to allow long, consolidated periods of wakefulness.[34] Orexin-mediated arousal increases over the course of the day to counteract the increasing homeostatic sleep drive, which would otherwise lead to periodic sleep episodes, as seen in patients with narcolepsy who lack orexin neurons.[32–34] On this basis, orexin antagonists would seem to be particularly well-suited for individuals attempting to sleep at an adverse circadian time (eg, shift workers, jet lag), where wakefulness is being maintained at least to a degree by clock-driven, orexin-mediated arousal.[33] Individuals who seem to get a "second wind" in the late evening and cannot shut down and sleep would also be prime candidates for a selective orexin receptor antagonist.[33] Other key inputs to orexin neurons include the lateral septum, amygdala, periaqueductal gray, and parabrachial nucleus.[34] These inputs to orexin neurons are believed to mediate stress/anxiety–associated increases in arousal.[34] On this basis, it would be reasonable to consider the use of orexin antagonists in those patients experiencing difficulty sleeping in the setting of stress and/or anxiety.[33] Inputs from the nucleus accumbens and the ventral tegmental area are believed to trigger arousal in the context of loss of rewarding stimuli via orexin neurons.[34] As such, it would be reasonable to consider using orexin receptor antagonists in individuals with disturbed sleep in the context of recently discontinuing substances of abuse or who are driven by low reward states to pursue goal-directed behavior and have difficulty sleeping in that context.[33] Given our limited experience with orexin receptor antagonists, future research studies are needed to test the proposed hypotheses that orexin receptor antagonists are particularly well-suited for use in these insomnia subgroups. However, this very specific intervention illustrates the potential for achieving an improved risk–benefit ratio by using a medication that targets insomnia occurring in specific contexts with a therapy that has specific effects on the key neural system underlying the symptoms.

Selective α_1 Adrenergic Antagonists

Distinguishing characteristics
This group of agents is distinguished by having as their predominant pharmacologic effect antagonism of α_1 adrenergic receptors.

Agents used to treat insomnia
The only selective α_1 adrenergic receptors that has been used to any significant degree in the treatment of insomnia is prazosin. This agent is approved by the FDA for treatment of hypertension but is used off-label for the treatment of insomnia in dosages from 1 to 12 mg.[29,35–39]

Mechanism of action
NE plays an important role in mediating arousal, particularly in the context of stress, anxiety, and novelty.[40,41] Selective α_1 adrenergic antagonists enhance sleep by preventing the arousal that occurs when NE binds to α_1 adrenergic receptors.

Pharmacologic specificity
Prazosin has high pharmacologic specificity for α_1 adrenergic receptors.[40]

Specificity of effects on brain functions (effects on systems other than sleep–wake systems)
Prazosin also has highly specific clinical effects. The effects are limited to modifying sleep and blood pressure. In terms of effects on sleep, there have been no trials evaluating the treatment of primary insomnia patients with prazosin. However, 4 placebo-controlled trials have provided data indicating that prazosin has significant effects on nightmares and sleep maintenance in patients with posttraumatic stress disorder.[35–39] The studies also suggest that the only nonsleep adverse effects of significance with prazosin administration are orthostatic hypotension and dizziness.[35–39]

Clinical implications for personalization of therapy
The available data on the risks and benefits of using prazosin as a treatment for patients with sleep disturbance suggest that prazosin should be the treatment of choice for treating nightmares and problems with sleep maintenance in patients with posttraumatic stress disorder.[35–39] Using this highly specific intervention in posttraumatic stress disorder patients promises an improved risk–benefit ratio over less selective options. Whether prazosin has therapeutic effects on insomnia occurring in other settings remains unknown, because no studies of its use for treating insomnia in other settings have been carried out. However, potentially relevant to the clinical use of prazosin is evidence that many patients with insomnia have elevated serum levels of NE.[42,43] Although peripheral elevation of NE may occur independent of elevation in central nervous system NE, it seems of interest to investigate whether individuals with increased serum NE might represent an increased NE insomnia subtype and might respond preferentially to treatment with a selective adrenergic antagonist like prazosin.

Selective Melatonin Receptor Agonists

Distinguishing characteristics
This group of medications is distinguished by having as their predominant pharmacologic effect agonism of melatonin receptors.

Agents used to treat insomnia
The hormone melatonin is available over the counter and ramelteon, a substantially more potent agonist at melatonin melatonin type 1 receptor (MT1) and melatonin type 2 receptor (MT2) receptors is approved by the US FDA for treatment of sleep onset difficulties.[2]

Mechanism of action
These agents promote sleep onset by binding to neuronal membrane-bound MT1-type melatonin receptors.

Pharmacologic specificity
Melatonin has effects at all 3 types of melatonin receptors.[44] Ramelteon has high specificity for MT1 and MT2 receptors.[44]

Specificity of effects on brain functions (effects on systems other than sleep–wake systems)
Both melatonin and ramelteon also have very specific effects on brain function that is primarily limited to modulation of sleep, as evidenced by the results of clinical trials with these agents. Both agents have been found to have therapeutic effects only on sleep onset difficulties.[2,45,46] Adverse effects have been relatively limited and both are without abuse potential. Studies of melatonin are somewhat difficult to interpret because they have involved a variety of dosages, preparations, and timing of

dosing.[45,46] These studies indicate that melatonin has a greater effect on patients with delayed sleep phase syndrome than on patients with insomnia, although meta-analyses suggest that melatonin has some therapeutic effect on sleep onset in insomnia patients.[45,46] Available evidence suggests that ramelteon is safe for use in patients with sleep apnea and chronic obstructive pulmonary disease.[47,48]

Clinical implications for personalization of therapy

Given the relatively favorable side effect profile of these agents and the fact that they have clinical effects only on sleep onset, they should be considered for treating individuals with sleep onset difficulty in the absence of sleep maintenance problems or when sleep onset problems are the predominant type of sleep difficulty. It should be noted that patients who have been treated previously with benzodiazepines and nonbenzodiazepines may be less satisfied with the effects of these agents. Melatonin is the treatment of choice for patients with sleep onset problems in the setting of delayed sleep phase syndrome.[45,46] Melatonin has also been found to have therapeutic effects on sleep difficulties in patients with autism and other neurodevelopmental disorders and should be considered for use in these populations.[49,50]

SUMMARY

Recent developments in research on insomnia treatments and the emergence of treatments with high pharmacologic specificity allow an unprecedented degree of personalization of insomnia therapy. By tailoring the mechanism and characteristics of the chosen insomnia therapy to the specific nature of each patient's insomnia, the clinician can achieve an improved risk–benefit ratio over providing treatment according to the traditional model of insomnia therapy, where little to no tailoring of therapy to the specifics of patients occurs. To facilitate having practitioners provide this type of improved care, this article has reviewed the available insomnia medications, pointing out where data support targeting treatment to particular subtypes of insomnia patients, with a focus on patients with psychiatric disorders. However, it must be understood that this is a work in progress. We have only limited evidence to guide how to best match specific treatment options to specific patient subgroups. Nevertheless, once considered "pie in the sky," this approach already allows improving the risk–benefit ratio for many patients with insomnia. The emergence of new data and new agents will bring an expanding capacity to personalize insomnia therapy and better allow us to improve the lives of the many patients suffering from insomnia.

REFERENCES

1. Schutte-Rodin S, Broch L, Buysse D, et al. Clinical guideline for the evaluation and management of chronic insomnia in adults. J Clin Sleep Med 2008;4(5): 487–504.
2. Krystal AD. A compendium of placebo-controlled trials of the risks/benefits of pharmacological treatments for insomnia: the empirical basis for U.S. clinical practice. Sleep Med Rev 2009;13(4):265–74.
3. Minkel J, Krystal AD. Optimizing the pharmacologic treatment of insomnia: current status and future horizons. Sleep Med Clin 2013;8(3):333–50.
4. Fava M, McCall WV, Krystal A, et al. Eszopiclone co-administered with fluoxetine in patients with insomnia coexisting with major depressive disorder. Biol Psychiatry 2006;59(11):1052–60.

5. Krystal A, Fava M, Rubens R, et al. Evaluation of eszopiclone discontinuation after cotherapy with fluoxetine for insomnia with coexisting depression. J Clin Sleep Med 2007;3(1):48–55.
6. Pollack M, Kinrys G, Krystal A, et al. Eszopiclone coadministered with escitalopram in patients with insomnia and comorbid generalized anxiety disorder. Arch Gen Psychiatry 2008;65(5):551–62.
7. Fava M, Asnis GM, Shrivastava RK, et al. Improved insomnia symptoms and sleep-related next-day functioning in patients with comorbid major depressive disorder and insomnia following concomitant zolpidem extended-release 12.5 mg and escitalopram treatment: a randomized controlled trial. J Clin Psychiatry 2011;72(7):914–28.
8. Fava M, Asnis GM, Shrivastava R, et al. Zolpidem extended-release improves sleep and next-day symptoms in comorbid insomnia and generalized anxiety disorder. J Clin Psychopharmacol 2009;29(3):222–30.
9. Krystal AD, Richelson E, Roth T. Review of the histamine system and the clinical effects of H1 antagonists: basis for a new model for understanding the effects of insomnia medications. Sleep Med Rev 2013;17(4):263–72.
10. Sieghart W, Sperk G. Subunit composition, distribution and function of GABA(A) receptor subtypes. Curr Top Med Chem 2002;2:795–816.
11. Sanna E, Busonero F, Talani G, et al. Comparison of the effects of zaleplon, zolpidem, and triazolam at various GABA(A) receptor subtypes. Eur J Pharmacol 2002;451(2):103–10.
12. Jia F, Goldstein PA, Harrison NL. The modulation of synaptic GABA(A) receptors in the thalamus by eszopiclone and zolpidem. J Pharmacol Exp Ther 2009; 328(3):1000–6.
13. Lancel M. Role of GABAA receptors in the regulation of sleep: initial sleep responses to peripherally administered modulators and agonists. Sleep 1999;22: 33e42.
14. Nierenberg AA, Adler LA, Peselow E, et al. Trazodone for antidepressant-associated insomnia. Am J Psychiatry 1994;151(7):1069–72.
15. Saletu-Zyhlarz GM, Abu-Bakr MH, Anderer P, et al. Insomnia related to dysthymia: polysomnographic and psychometric comparison with normal controls and acute therapeutic trials with trazodone. Neuropsychobiology 2001;44:139–49.
16. Saletu-Zyhlarz GM, Abu-Bakr MH, Anderer P, et al. Insomnia in depression: differences in objective and subjective sleep and awakening quality to normal controls and acute effects of trazodone. Prog Neuropsychopharmacol Biol Psychiatry 2002;26:249–60.
17. Smith G, Smith PH. Effects of doxylamine and acetaminophen on postoperative sleep. Clin Pharmacol Ther 1985;37(5):549–57.
18. Kudo Y, Kurihara M. Clinical evaluation of diphenhydramine hydrochloride for the treatment of insomnia in psychiatric patients: a double-blind study. J Clin Pharmacol 1990;30(11):1041–8.
19. Rickels K, Morris RJ, Newman H, et al. Diphenhydramine in insomniac family practice patients: a double- blind study. J Clin Pharmacol 1983;23(5–6): 234–42.
20. Morin C, Koetter U, Bastien C, et al. Valerian-hops combination and diphenhydramine for treating insomnia: a randomized placebo-controlled clinical trial. Sleep 2005;28(11):1465–71.
21. Meuleman J, Nelson RC, Clark RL. Evaluation of temazepam and diphenhydramine as hypnotics in a nursing-home population. Drug Intell Clin Pharm 1987; 21(9):716–20.

22. Glass JR, Herrmann N, Busto UE, et al. Effects of 2-week treatment with temaze-pam and diphenhydramine in elderly insomniacs: a randomized, placebo-controlled trial. J Clin Psychopharmacol 2008;28(2):182–8.
23. Richardson G, Roehrs TA, Rosenthal L, et al. Tolerance to daytime sedative effects of H1 antihistamines. J Clin Psychopharmacol 2002;22(5):511–5.
24. Krystal AD, Durrence HH, Scharf M, et al. Efficacy and safety of Doxepin 1 mg and 3 mg in a 12-week sleep laboratory and outpatient trial of elderly subjects with chronic primary insomnia. Sleep 2010;33:1553–61.
25. Krystal AD, Lankford A, Durrence HH, et al. Efficacy and safety of doxepin 3 and 6 mg in a 35-day sleep laboratory trial in adults with chronic primary insomnia. Sleep 2011;34:1433–42.
26. Roth T, Rogowski R, Hull S, et al. Efficacy and safety of doxepin 1 mg, 3 mg, and 6 mg in adults with primary insomnia. Sleep 2007;30(11):1555–61.
27. Scharf M, Rogowski R, Hull S, et al. Efficacy and safety of doxepin 1 mg, 3 mg, and 6 mg in elderly patients with primary insomnia: a randomized, double-blind, placebo-controlled crossover study. J Clin Psychiatry 2008;69(10):1557.
28. Parmentier R, Ohtsu H, Djebbara-Hannas Z, et al. Anatomical, physiological, and pharmacological characteristics of histidine decarboxylase knock-out mice: evi-dence for the role of brain histamine in behavioral and sleep-wake control. J Neurosci 2002;22:7695e711.
29. Morin CM, Drake CL, Harvey AG, et al. Insomnia disorder. Nature Reviews, in press.
30. Herring WJ, Connor KM, Ivgy-May N, et al. Efficacy and safety of the Orexin receptor antagonist suvorexant in patients with insomnia: results form two 3-month randomized, double-blind, placebo-controlled, clinical trials. Biol Psychiatry 2014. [Epub ahead of print].
31. Michelson D, Snyder E, Paradis E, et al. Safety and efficacy of suvorexant during 1-year treatment of insomnia with subsequent abrupt treatment discontinuation: a phase 3 randomised, double-blind, placebo-controlled trial. Lancet Neurol 2014; 13:461–71.
32. Sakurai T. The role of orexin in motivated behaviours. Nat Rev Neurosci 2014;15: 719–31.
33. Krystal AD, Benca R, Kilduff T. Understanding the sleep-wake cycle: sleep, insomnia, and the orexin system. J Clin Psychiatry 2013;74(Suppl 1):3–20.
34. Scammell TE, Winrow CJ. Orexin receptors: pharmacology and therapeutic opportunities. Annu Rev Pharmacol Toxicol 2011;51:243–66.
35. Krystal AD, Davidson JR. The use of prazosin for the treatment of trauma night-mares and sleep disturbance in combat veterans with post-traumatic stress dis-order. Biol Psychiatry 2007;61:925–7.
36. Raskind MA, Peterson K, Williams T, et al. A trial of prazosin for combat trauma PTSD with nightmares in active-duty soldiers returned from Iraq and Afghanistan. Am J Psychiatry 2013;170(9):1003–10.
37. Taylor FB, Martin P, Thompson C, et al. Prazosin effects on objective sleep mea-sures and clinical symptoms in civilian trauma posttraumatic stress disorder: a placebo-controlled study. Biol Psychiatry 2008;63(6):629–32.
38. Raskind MA, Peskind ER, Hoff DJ, et al. A parallel group placebo controlled study of prazosin for trauma nightmares and sleep disturbance in combat veterans with post-traumatic stress disorder. Biol Psychiatry 2007;61(8):928–34.
39. Raskind MA, Peskind ER, Kanter ED, et al. Reduction of nightmares and other PTSD symptoms in combat veterans by prazosin: a placebo-controlled study. Am J Psychiatry 2003;160(2):371–3.

40. Goddard AW, Ball SG, Martinez J, et al. Current perspectives of the roles of the central norepinephrine system in anxiety and depression. Depress Anxiety 2010; 27(4):339–50.

41. Davey MJ. The pharmacology of prazosin, an alpha 1-adrenoceptor antagonist and the basis for its use in the treatment of essential hypertension. Clin Exp Hypertens A 1982;4(1–2):47–59.

42. Irwin M, Clark C, Kennedy B, et al. Nocturnal catecholamines and immune function in insomniacs, depressed patients, and control subjects. Brain Behav Immun 2003;17(5):365–72.

43. Vgontzas AN, Tsigos C, Bixler EO, et al. Chronic insomnia and activity of the stress system: a preliminary study. J Psychosom Res 1998;45(1):21–31.

44. Miyamoto M. Pharmacology of ramelteon, a selective MT1/MT2 receptor agonist: a novel therapeutic drug for sleep disorders. CNS Neurosci Ther 2009;15(1): 32–51.

45. Ferracioli-Oda E, Qawasmi A, Bloch MH. Meta-analysis: melatonin for the treatment of primary sleep disorders. PLoS One 2013;8:e63773.

46. Buscemi N, Vandermeer B, Hooton N, et al. The efficacy and safety of exogenous melatonin for primary sleep disorders. a meta-analysis. J Gen Intern Med 2005; 20:1151–8.

47. Kryger M, Wang-Weigand S, Roth T. Safety of ramelteon in individuals with mild to moderate obstructive sleep apnea. Sleep Breath 2007;11:159–64.

48. Kryger M, Roth T, Wang-Weigand S, et al. The effects of ramelteon on respiration during sleep in subjects with moderate to severe chronic obstructive pulmonary disease. Sleep Breath 2009;13:79–84.

49. Wirojanan J, Jacquemont S, Diaz R, et al. The efficacy of melatonin for sleep problems in children with autism, fragile X syndrome, or autism and fragile X syndrome. J Clin Sleep Med 2009;5(2):145–50.

50. Niederhofer H, Staffen W, Mair A, et al. Brief report: melatonin facilitates sleep in individuals with mental retardation and insomnia. J Autism Dev Disord 2003; 33(4):469–72.

Index

Note: Page numbers of article titles are in **boldface** type.

A

Psychiatr Clin N Am 38 (2015) 861–872
http://dx.doi.org/10.1016/S0193-953X(15)00110-0
0193-953X/15/$ – see front matter © 2015 Elsevier Inc. All rights reserved.

psych.theclinics.com

United States Postal Service
Statement of Ownership, Management, and Circulation
(All Periodicals Publications Except Requestor Publications)

1. Publication Title
Psychiatric Clinics of North America

2. Publication Number
0 0 0 0 - 7 0 0 3

3. Filing Date
9/18/15

4. Issue Frequency
Mar, Jun, Sep, Dec

5. Number of Issues Published Annually
4

6. Annual Subscription Price
$300.00

7. Complete Mailing Address of Known Office of Publication (Not printer) (Street, city, county, state, and ZIP+4®)
Elsevier Inc.
360 Park Avenue South
New York, NY 10010-1710

Contact Person
Stephen R. Bushing

Telephone (Include area code)
215-239-3688

8. Complete Mailing Address of Headquarters or General Business Office of Publisher (Not printer)
Elsevier Inc., 360 Park Avenue South, New York, NY 10010-1710

9. Full Names and Complete Mailing Addresses of Publisher, Editor, and Managing Editor (Do not leave blank)

Publisher (Name and complete mailing address)
Linda Belfus, Elsevier Inc., 1600 John F. Kennedy Blvd., Suite 1800, Philadelphia, PA 19103

Editor (Name and complete mailing address)
Lauren Boyle, Elsevier Inc., 1600 John F. Kennedy Blvd., Suite 1800, Philadelphia, PA 19103-2899

Managing Editor (Name and complete mailing address)
Adrianne Brigido, Elsevier Inc., 1600 John F. Kennedy Blvd., Suite 1800, Philadelphia, PA 19103-2899

10. Owner (Do not leave blank. If the publication is owned by a corporation, give the name and address of the corporation immediately followed by the names and addresses of all stockholders owning or holding 1 percent or more of the total amount of stock. If not owned by a corporation, give the names and addresses of the individual owners. If owned by a partnership or other unincorporated firm, give its name and address as well as those of each individual owner. If the publication is published by a nonprofit organization, give its name and address.)

Full Name	Complete Mailing Address
Wholly owned subsidiary of	1600 John F. Kennedy Blvd, Ste. 1800
Reed/Elsevier, US holdings	Philadelphia, PA 19103-2899

11. Known Bondholders, Mortgagees, and Other Security Holders Owning or Holding 1 Percent or More of Total Amount of Bonds, Mortgages, or Other Securities. If none, check box ☐ None

Full Name	Complete Mailing Address
N/A	

12. Tax Status (For completion by nonprofit organizations authorized to mail at nonprofit rates) (Check one)
The purpose, function, and nonprofit status of this organization and the exempt status for federal income tax purposes:
☐ Has Not Changed During Preceding 12 Months
☐ Has Changed During Preceding 12 Months (Publisher must submit explanation of change with this statement)

13. Publication Title
Psychiatric Clinics of North America

14. Issue Date for Circulation Data Below
September 2015

15. Extent and Nature of Circulation			Average No. Copies Each Issue During Preceding 12 Months	No. Copies of Single Issue Published Nearest to Filing Date
a. Total Number of Copies (Net press run)			691	625
b. Legitimate Paid and/Or Requested Distribution (By Mail and Outside the Mail)	(1)	Mailed Outside-County Paid/Requested Mail Subscriptions stated on PS Form 3541. (Include paid distribution above nominal rate, advertiser's proof copies and exchange copies)	283	191
	(2)	Mailed In-County Paid/Requested Mail Subscriptions stated on PS Form 3541. (Include paid distribution above nominal rate, advertiser's proof copies and exchange copies)		
	(3)	Paid Distribution Outside the Mails Including Sales Through Dealers And Carriers, Street Vendors, Counter Sales, and Other Paid Distribution Outside USPS®	163	176
	(4)	Paid Distribution by Other Classes of Mail Through the USPS (e.g. First-Class Mail®)		
c. Total Paid and/or Requested Circulation (Sum of 15b (1), (2), (3), and (4))		▲	446	367
d. Free or Nominal Rate Distribution (By Mail and Outside the Mail)	(1)	Free or Nominal Rate Outside-County Copies included on PS Form 3541	69	70
	(2)	Free or Nominal Rate In-County Copies included on PS Form 3541		
	(3)	Free or Nominal Rate Copies mailed at Other classes Through the USPS (e.g. First-Class Mail)		
	(4)	Free or Nominal Rate Distribution Outside the Mail (Carriers or Other means)		
e. Total Nonrequested Distribution (Sum of 15d (1), (2), (3) and (4))			69	70
f. Total Distribution (Sum of 15c and 15e)		▲	515	437
g. Copies not Distributed (See instructions to publishers #4 (page #3))		▲	176	188
h. Total (Sum of 15f and g)			691	625
i. Percent Paid and/or Requested Circulation (15c divided by 15f times 100)		▲	86.60%	83.98%

* If you are claiming electronic copies go to line 16 on page 3. If you are not claiming Electronic copies, skip to line 17 on page 3.

16. Electronic Copy Circulation	Average No. Copies Each Issue During Preceding 12 Months	No. Copies of Single Issue Published Nearest to Filing Date
a. Paid Electronic Copies		
b. Total paid Print Copies (Line 15c) + Paid Electronic copies (Line 16a)		
c. Total Print Distribution (Line 15f) + Paid Electronic Copies (Line 16a)		
d. Percent Paid (Both Print & Electronic copies) (16b divided by 16c X 100)		

☐ I certify that 50% of all my distributed copies (electronic and print) are paid above a nominal price

17. Publication of Statement of Ownership
If the publication is a general publication, publication of this statement is required. Will be printed in the *December 2015* issue of this publication.

18. Signature and Title of Editor, Publisher, Business Manager, or Owner

Stephen R. Bushing – Inventory Distribution Coordinator

Stephen R. Bushing – Inventory Distribution Coordinator

Date September 18, 2015

I certify that all information furnished on this form is true and complete. I understand that anyone who furnishes false or misleading information on this form or who omits material or information requested on the form may be subject to criminal sanctions (including fines and imprisonment) and/or civil sanctions (including civil penalties).

PS Form 3526, July 2014 (Page 1 of 3 (Instructions Page 3)) PSN 7530-01-000-9931 PRIVACY NOTICE: See our Privacy policy in www.usps.com

PS Form 3526, July 2014 (Page 3 of 3)